METHODS IN PHARMACOLOGY AND TOXICOLOGY

Series Editor
James Y. Kang
Sichuan University and University of Louisville
Prospect, Kentucky, USA

For further volumes:
http://www.springer.com/series/7653

Herbal Medicines

New Horizons

Edited by

Akio Inui

Department of Psychosomatic Internal Medicine,
Kagoshima University Graduate School of Medical & Dental Sciences,
Kagoshima, Japan

Humana Press

Editor
Akio Inui
Department of Psychosomatic Internal Medicine
Kagoshima University Graduate School of Medical
& Dental Sciences
Kagoshima, Japan

ISSN 1557-2153 ISSN 1940-6053 (electronic)
Methods in Pharmacology and Toxicology
ISBN 978-1-4939-4000-4 ISBN 978-1-4939-4002-8 (eBook)
DOI 10.1007/978-1-4939-4002-8

Library of Congress Control Number: 2016946606

Printed on acid-free paper

This Humana Press imprint is published by Springer Nature
The registered company is Springer Science+Business Media LLC New York

Preface

Complementary and alternative medicine continues to be used and may be included in cancer treatment with holistic spiritual practice, physical exercise, and herbal medicine for enhanced tumoricidal activity, reduction in treatment-related adverse events, and better quality of life. Herbal medicine has long been practiced in China, Korea, Japan, and other countries to achieve its key goal of restoring the balance of energy in the body.

Throughout the history of representative herbal medicine, traditional Chinese medicine, and other alternatives such as Japanese Kampo, the basic theories and the methods of diagnosis and treatment have differed considerably from those of Western medicine. Western medicine depends on disease-based diagnosis, while traditional Chinese medicine emphasizes patient-based diagnosis. Kampo is based on traditional Chinese medicine but is adapted to the Japanese culture. It can be considered as a simplified, positivistic, and pragmatic version of Chinese herbal medicine. Kampo practitioners treat patients based on the Kampo diagnosis (Sho: the patient's symptoms at a given moment) and choose the most suitable formula. The relationship between these steps is analogous to a lock and key; each pathological condition is related to its prescription. More than 200 Kampo recipes composed of mixtures of 2–15 components have been reported. Approximately 350 different components are used for these recipes. Most of them are medicinal herbs, but fungi, animal components, and minerals are also used. Approximately 120 of these crude drugs are listed in the Japanese Pharmacopoeia, and one-third of them are also listed in WHO monographs.

Herbal medicine continues to evolve in daily lifestyle and the treatment of cancer and many other illnesses. Herbal medicine has a significant effect on reducing fatigue and pain, improving respiratory tract infections and gastrointestinal problems including diarrhea, nausea, and vomiting, protecting liver function, and ameliorating the symptoms of cachexia. The stringent quality control of herbal medicine such as Kampo and reproducibility of preclinical findings, together with few adverse events, have made herbal medicine more and more attractive for the management of intractable diseases as well as common health problems. The multicomponent herbal medicine capable of targeting multiple sites could be useful for future drug discovery. Mechanistic studies and identification of active compounds could lead to new discoveries in biological and biomedical sciences.

This book summarizes the current state and translational aspect of herbal medicine in modern society. It provides a new horizon of herbal medicine to help establishing the rational therapy for the patients.

Kagoshima, Japan — *Akio Inui*

The original version of this book was revised. An erratum to the book can be found at 10.1007/978-1-4939-4002-8_16

Contents

Contributors

SHIH-LIANG CHANG • *Department of Medical Botanicals and Health Applications, Da-Yeh University, Dacun, Changhua, Taiwan; School of Chinese Medicine, China Medical University, Taichung, Taiwan*

JUEI-TANG CHENG • *Department of Medical Research, Chi-Mei Medical Center, Tainan City, Taiwan*

YUICHIRO DOKI • *Department of Gastroenterological Surgery, Osaka University Graduate School of Medicine, Osaka, Japan*

HIRONORI FUJIWARA • *Division of Medicinal Pharmacology, Department of Bioscience, Institute of Natural Medicine, University of Toyama, Toyama, Japan*

TOMOHISA HATTORI • *Tsumura Research Laboratories, Tsumura & Co., Ibaraki, Japan*

NORIO IIZUKA • *Department of Kampo Medicine, Hiroshima university, Ube, Yamaguchi, Japan*

AKIO INUI • *Department of Psychosomatic Internal Medicine, Kagoshima University Graduate School of Medical and Dental Sciences, Kagoshima, Japan*

MOSABURO KAINUMA • *Community Medicine Education Unit, Graduate School of Medical Science, Kyushu University, Higashi-ku, Fukuoka City, Japan*

YOSHIO KASE • *Tsumura Research Laboratories, Kampo Scientific Strategies Division, Tsumura & Co., Ibaraki, Japan*

JUNJI KOBAYASHI • *Department of General Medicine, Kanazawa Medical University, Ishikawa, Japan*

TORU KONO • *Center for Clinical and Biomedical Research, Sapporo Higashi Tokushukai Hospital, Sapporo, Hokkaido, Japan; Department of Pathophysiology and Therapeutics, Faculty of Pharmaceutical Sciences, Hokkaido University, Sapporo, Hokkaido, Japan; Department of Surgery, Institute of Health Biosciences, The University of Tokushima Graduate School of Medicine, Tokushima, Japan*

TOSHIRO KUBOTA • *Department of Obstetrics and Gynecology, Tokyo Medical and Dental University, Tokyo, Japan*

YUKINORI KUROKAWA • *Department of Gastroenterological Surgery, Osaka University Graduate School of Medicine, Osaka, Japan*

GEORGE BINH LENON • *School of Health and Biomedical Sciences, RMIT University, VIC, Australia*

TOMOKI MAKINO • *Department of Gastroenterological Surgery, Osaka University Graduate School of Medicine, Osaka, Japan*

KINZO MATSUMOTO • *Division of Medicinal Pharmacology, Department of Bioscience, Institute of Natural Medicine, University of Toyama, Toyama, Japan*

KANAKO MIYANO • *Division of Cancer Pathophysiology, National Cancer Center Research Institute, Tokyo, Japan*

YASUHIRO MIYAZAKI • *Department of Gastroenterological Surgery, Osaka University Graduate School of Medicine, Osaka, Japan*

MASAKI MORI • *Department of Gastroenterological Surgery, Osaka University Graduate School of Medicine, Osaka, Japan*

JUNJI MORIYA • *Department of General Medicine, Kanazawa Medical University, Ishikawa, Japan*

Miwa Nahata • *Tsumura Research Laboratories, Tsumura & Co., Ibaraki, Japan*
Koji Nakagawa • *Pathophysiology and Therapeutics, Hokkaido University, Faculty of Pharmaceutical Sciences, Sapporo, Hokkaido, Japan*
Kiyokazu Nakajima • *Department of Gastroenterological Surgery, Osaka University Graduate School of Medicine, Osaka, Japan*
Shunsuke Ohnishi • *Gastroenterology and Hepatology, Hokkaido University Graduate School of Medicine, Sapporo, Hokkaido, Japan*
Kosuke Okada • *Division of Medical Sciences, Institute of Clinical Medicine, University of Tsukuba, Tsukuba, Ibaraki, Japan*
Naoto Okubo • *Pathophysiology and Therapeutics, Hokkaido University, Faculty of Pharmaceutical Sciences, Sapporo, Hokkaido, Japan*
Chiharu Sadakane • *Tsumura Research Laboratories, Tsumura & Co., Ibaraki, Japan*
Yayoi Saegusa • *Tsumura Research Laboratories, Tsumura & Co., Ami, Ibaraki, Japan*
Mitsuo Shimada • *Department of Surgery, Institute of Health Biosciences, The University of Tokushima Graduate School of Medicine, Tokushima, Japan*
Junichi Shoda • *Division of Medical Sciences, Institute of Clinical Medicine, University of Tsukuba, Tsukuba, Ibaraki, Japan*
Tsuyoshi Sugiura • *Research Field in Dentistry, Medical and Dental Science Area, Research and Education Assembly, Kagoshima University Graduate School, Kagoshima, Japan*
Hajime Suzuki • *Department of Psychosomatic Internal Medicine, Kagoshima University Graduate School of Medical and Dental Sciences, Kagoshima, Japan*
Tsuyoshi Takahashi • *Department of Gastroenterological Surgery, Osaka University Graduate School of Medicine, Osaka, Japan*
Hiroshi Takeda • *Pathophysiology and Therapeutics, Hokkaido University, Faculty of Pharmaceutical Sciences, Sapporo, Hokkaido, Japan; Gastroenterology and Hepatology, Hokkaido University Graduate School of Medicine, Sapporo, Hokkaido, Japan*
Shuji Takiguchi • *Department of Gastroenterological Surgery, Osaka University Graduate School of Medicine, Osaka, Japan*
Hsiewe Ying Tan • *School of Health and Biomedical Sciences, RMIT University, VIC, Australia*
Masakazu Terauchi • *Department of Women's Health, Tokyo Medical and Dental University, Tokyo, Japan*
Yasuhito Uezono • *Division of Cancer Pathophysiology, National Cancer Center Research Institute, Tokyo, Japan; Division of Supportive Care Research, Exploratory Oncology Research and Clinical Trial Center, National Cancer Center, Tokyo, Japan; Innovation Center for Supportive, Palliative and Psychosocial Care, National Cancer Center Hospital, Tokyo, Japan*
Eiji Warabi • *Division of Biomedical Sciences, Faculty of Medicine, University of Tsukuba, Tsukuba, Ibaraki, Japan*
Chihiro Yamada • *Tsumura Research Laboratories, Tsumura & Co., Ibaraki, Japan*
Kojiro Yamaguchi • *Research Field in Dentistry, Medical and Dental Science Area, Research and Education Assembly, Kagoshima University Graduate School, Kagoshima, Japan*

JUN-ICHI YAMAKAWA • *Department of General Medicine, Kanazawa Medical University, Ishikawa, Japan*
MASAHIRO YAMAMOTO • *Tsumura Research Laboratories, Kampo Scientific Strategies Division, Tsumura & Co., Ibaraki, Japan*
MAKOTO YAMASAKI • *Department of Gastroenterological Surgery, Osaka University Graduate School of Medicine, Osaka, Japan*

Chapter 1

Chinese Herbal Medicine Including Historical Aspects

Shih-Liang Chang

Abstract

Chinese herbal medicine has been used in clinical applications for more than 2000 years in Chinese society. Many experiences supplying feedback from clinical applications have been described in the classic publications. Gradually, these experiences were summarized, forming an individual theory of the medical system, named Traditional Chinese Medicine (TCM), which directed the usages against clinical diseases that had been overviewed in the introduction. The development of TCM is in close relationship to historical development over time. Important concepts were proposed in each dynasty that helped in the development of TCM. This review attempts to summarize the important theories of historical aspects that were proposed in each dynasty of the Chinese people.

Taken together, without systemic knowledge about the applications of Chinese herbal medicine, that is, with just the experience of folk usage, even that cannot elevate the therapeutic effect for treating complex illnesses.

Key words Traditional Chinese medicine, Syndrome differentiation, Chinese herbal medicine, Four properties and five tastes, Channel tropism, The seven relations theory

1 Introduction

1.1 Traditional Chinese Medicine (TCM) and Chinese Herbal Medicine

The Traditional Chinese Medicine (TCM) has a long historical usage experience in China. People were struggling with diseases and tried to search for solutions from the feedback from treatments. The better experiences were written down in the classic publications, such as Nei-Jing 內經 (the Internal Canon of Medicine) [1] and Shanghan Lun 傷寒 (Treatise on Febrile Diseases) [2]. Gradually, this practice would form a systemic medical system with individual theories, diagnosis methods, and directions for the treatment of clinical diseases. From the original use to systemic application, there is a large gap because of the lack of large clinical experience feedback. Herbal medicine usually had a simple feedback from folk use of the medicinal plant, but the TCM had developed a systemic clinical medical system that summarized feedback from the ancient classics to current publications. Some basic theories of TCM had been formed over a long time of historical development, such as Yin-Yang and Five Elements (Wood, Fire,

Akio Inui (ed.), *Herbal Medicines: New Horizons*, Methods in Pharmacology and Toxicology, DOI 10.1007/978-1-4939-4002-8_1, © Springer Science+Business Media New York 2016

Earth, Golden, Water), Meridian, State of Internal Organs, and the Etiology and Pathogenesis theories of TCM. [3]. These basic theories direct the treatment very deeply and have a very close relationship with the clinical effect. Without the direction of the basic theories of TCM, Chinese herbal medicine is only folk herbal treatment by experience without systematic knowledge.

1.2 Diagnosis of TCM

How is the doctor of TCM to approach the patients? Usually through the four diagnosis (四診) methods "Observation," "Listening and Smelling," "Taking History," and "Pulse Feeling and Palpation" to collect the signs [4], and the TCM Eight Principal Syndromes (八綱) Yin, Yang, External, Internal, Cold, Hot, Deficiency, and Consolidation to analyze the syndromes for the character of the disease. Additionally, the meridian and state of internal organs are combined with the diagnosis of TCM for the location of disease. The characters and locations of disease are effective information for selection of Chinese herbal medicine or the formulas [5]. For example, the cold lung syndrome may use a heat herb such as *Ephedra*, and hot lung syndrome may use *Scutellaria* [6].

1.3 Treatment Based on Syndrome Differentiation

The core concept of TCM is "treatment based on syndrome differentiation." The thinking process follows four steps: Reason, Method, Formula, and Drug. Doctors use the four diagnosis methods "Observation," "Listening and Smelling," "Taking History," and "Pulse Feeling and Palpation" to collect signs from clinical patients. Comparison and analysis among the signs are used to summarize the syndromes, for example, Cold, Hot, Deficiency, and Consolidation syndromes, and these are the reasons that direct the treatment methods. For example, the cold syndrome is treated by a warm method, and the hot syndrome is treated by a cold method, etc. Therefore, according to these theories the doctor can use the drugs or the formulas to treat the disease.

According to the theory of TCM, there are some features such as the same disease having different treatments and different diseases having the same treatment. The same disease usually has different syndromes from the diagnosis of TCM that directs different methods of treatments. For example, a cough usually has various syndromes derived from the diagnosis of TCM: the cold syndrome of cough as treated by warm drugs or formulas such as Xiao-Qing-Long-Tang [5] (小青龍湯) from Shanghan Lun theory; and the hot syndrome of cough as treated by cold drugs or formula such as Yin-Qiao powder (銀翹散) and San-Gju-Yin decoction (桑菊飲) from therapeutic principles against febrile diseases. The different diseases had the same diagnosis of TCM that directs the same method of treatment; for example, an ancient formula from Shanghan Lun, Baihu (White tiger) Tang (白虎湯) that can treat different diseases such as bacterial infection and virus infection which cause different diseases [7, 8].

1.4 The Concept of Chinese Herbal Medicine

Chinese herbal medicine is known from the real clinical experiences of ancient Chinese people, such as the "Shen Nong" (神農), who tasted the herbs and wrote down their experience in Sheng Nong's herbal classic publication [9] (神農本草經). The principles of Chinese herbal medicine developed gradually. The four properties 四氣 (Cold, Cool, Heat, Warm) and five tastes 五味 (Sour, Bitter, Sweet, Spice, Salt) of herbs were derived from Yin-Yang and the five element theory. The channel tropism theory 歸經 is the action site of the human body after taking the Chinese herbal medicines that were recorded in the ancient classic publications directing the selection for clinical application [10]. For example: three yellow color drugs, *Radix Scutellariae*, *Rhizoma Coptidis*, and *Cortex Phellodendri*, are all cold property and bitter taste, but they are different channel tropisms and different action sites. The action site of *Radix Scutellariae* belongs to the chest respiration system with lung channel tropism, the action site of *Rhizoma Coptidis* belongs to the upper abdominal digestive system with stomach channel tropism, and the action site of *Cortex Phellodendri* belongs to the lower abdominal and pelvic urinary system with renal channel tropism. The function and the effect of Chinese herbal medicines were also recorded in the ancient classic publications in which were usually hidden many worthy experiences of clinical treatment from the ancient people of China [11].

1.5 The Formula of Chinese Herbal Medicine

Clinical diseases are usually very complicated. Thus, the application of a single Chinese herbal medicine cannot affect a complicated disease. Therefore, the concept of formula was developed. There were four parts: King君, Subjection臣, Assistant佐, and Guidance 使 separately. The main action of a herb is the King; the secondary action of herb is the subjection; a herb can help the action of the King and Subjection herbs as the Assistant herb; and a herb can guide the action of King and Subjection to the site of disease as the Guidance herb. The Si-Jun-Zi decoction (四君子湯) is a typical case. *Panax Ginseng* is the King herb, *Rhizoma Atractylodis* is the Subjection herb, and *Poria Cocos* and *Glycyrrhiza* are the Assistant and Guidance herbs [12].

Herbs' interaction were noticed very early in the classic publications of Chinese materia medica, and the seven relations theory (七情) was described as in the following list: (1) alone, (2) synergy, (3) the herb was decreased in disadvantage, (4) decreased the disadvantage of another herb, (5) elevating the effect of the king herb, (6) decreased the effect of the other herb, and (7) elevated the side effect of the other herb, to illustrate the concerted application among Chinese herbal medicines [13]. This concept or experience is very important for the formulation of Chinese herbal medicine.

1.6 Modern Research on Chinese Herbs and the Basic Theories of TCM

Although the application of Chinese herbal medicines had its principles and many experiences were accumulated in the Classic publications, such as six-meridian syndrome differentiation (六經辨證) from the Shanghan Lun Classic book, which directs the formula and herbs to treat the disease with excellent curative effect, the mechanisms of action were still subjected to few studies [14]. The basic theories of TCM were derived from philosophy, but modern research is based on science. How to integrate modern research into the application of TCM is the important issue. In clinical usage, the doctor generally obeys the principles of TCM in applying the herb or formula, and has support from modern research that is the better authority in the clinical application of Chinese herbal medicines [15].

2 Historical Aspects of Chinese Herbal Medicine

In this part, the important concepts in the application of Chinese herbal medicine are be summarized by the different dynasty periods. Also, the important classic publications and the important contributions of eminent physicians of TCM are described.

2.1 The Spring and Autumn Warring State Period

The medicinal plants or minerals or animals were usually applied in treatment for disease by ingestion, and many toxicities have been reported by experience and written down in classic publications such as Sheng Nong's herbal classic publication that classified the herbs into three classes: high, middle, and low [9]. There were 125 kinds of herbs in the low class, which were applied as assistant or guidance role in formulas; generally these had toxicities and cannot be consumed as a large dose or over a long period of time. The high class is safer than the middle class and the low class in clinical application. In this period, the basic principles of Chinese herbal medicine were just in the beginning of being founded. The Nei-Jing was the representative classic publication and even was called a bible of TCM [1].

2.2 The Han Dynasty

The utility of Chinese herbal medicines had more and more experience from a single herb into formula application in clinical treatment. The system of syndrome differentiation, the six-meridian syndrome differentiation, had been proposed in the Shanghan Lun classic publication that was derived from the Yin-Yang theory of Nei-Jing. Three Yang and three Yin were proposed to differentiate the stage of infectious diseases. Generally, the three Yang present the primary stage with different types of fever and the three Yin present the end stage of the disease with dysfunction of organs or meridian [16]. Also, the diseases cannot be classified into the six-meridian syndrome in which were described the miscellaneous diseases (雜病) such as edema, chest pain, and heart pain [17].

2.3 The Tang Dynasty

The theories and policies of TCM were more and more mature at this stage in history. Also, many specialists had developed, even with established diplomates. The large formulas that were used in clinical practice numbered many as 5000 to 6000. The "Immortal Sun's Precious Formulary" (千金方) is the representative classic publication [18]. The government publication "Xinxiu Bencao" (Newly Revised Materia Medica) (新修本草) appeared with strong impact on the development of Chinese herbal medicine [10]. This is the first Pharmacopeia published by the government in China. This pharmacopeia listed about 80 kinds of herbs usually used for diseases, which was very helpful in clinical application.

Many publications in a special division of herb application had been proposed at this stage. Especially, the special book "Lei Gong's Treatise" (雷公炮製) is the earliest book on preparation and boiling of materia medica that reflected the research and utilities of herbs more and more deeply and carefully [19].

2.4 The Period of Jin and Yuan Dynasty

A good basis for TCM was established in this stage. Many points of view about treatment of diseases had been proposed. Especially, the four eminent physicians in the Jin and Yuan period, Liu Wan-Su (劉完素), Chang Cong-Zheng (張從正), Li Dong-Heng (李東垣), and Zhu Zhen-Heng (朱震亨), presented their opinions. Dr. Liu was good at using the cold herbs for treating fever diseases; Dr. Chang summarized three methods—sweating, vomiting, and purging—for treating diseases; Dr. Li proposed to tonify the digestive system to elevate the person's nutritional state to regulate the ill state; and Dr. Zhu proposed the view "Yang usually over and Ying usually deficiency" is a dysfunction state that is a kind of unbalance in the Ying–Yang of a person. The fire (Yang) syndrome is usually caused by water (Ying) deficiency, so that the doctor regulated the ill or unbalanced state to a healthy balance by tonifying the useful water of the body using herbs such as *Radix Scrophulariae*, *Radix Ophiopogonis*, etc. [20].

2.5 The Period of Ming and Ching Dynasty

The treatment of febrile (warm) disease 溫病 was developed in this period [21]. Also, the individual differential diagnosis systems were proposed according to the infectious stages, such as the San-Jiao syndrome differentiation [22] (三焦辨證), and the defensive Qi and Nutrient Blood syndrome differentiation (衛氣營血辨證)., etc. [23]. In the primary stage of infection, the syndromes were focused on the respiratory system such as cough, throat, etc., that is, the upper-jiao syndrome; in the middle stage of infection, the syndromes were focused on the digestive system such as diarrhea or abdominal pain, that is, the middle-jiao syndrome; and in the end stage of infection, the syndromes were focused on fluid balance, such as dry mouth, edema, etc., that is, the lower-jiao syndrome. In the defensive Qi and Nutrient Blood syndrome differentiation, the syndrome from primary stage to middle stage of infection was regarded as defensive Qi, and the syndrome from middle stage to end stage was regarded as Nutrient Blood. Although they were different systems of syndrome differentiation in the infectious disease, the same stage of disease was treated by different experiences of application in Chinese herbal medicines and formulas from different specialists. There are some famous formulas that are still used at very high frequencies today by TCM doctors against infectious diseases from bacteria or viruses. Such will be a treasure in the development of new drugs as antibiotics or antivirus agents.

In this period, it is worthy to mention the huge Classic publication, "Compendium of Materia Medica," (本草綱目) by a Dr. Li Shi-Zhe (李時珍) who summarized the past 41 Classic publications of Chinese materia medica, including 1892 kinds of Chinese herbs. The book had advanced classification with detailed outlines that were different from the traditional three classes and corrected many mistakes found in traditional books of herbs. Also, 374 kinds of herbs usually used in clinical applications such as *Pseudo-Ginseng*, *Rhizoma Smilacis Glabrae*, etc., were added [9].

3 Summary

Chinese herbal medicines are still used in the present clinical setting for preventing or treating diseases in Chinese people, and even in Western people. This usage means that some diseases cannot be overcome by totally by modern or Western medicine. Reviewing the methods or theories from the historical experience of treating disease by TCM in using Chinese herbal medicine would be helpful in effective application, and even could help develop some new effective therapies or new drugs.

Also, TCM had its independent system of theory for directing the clinical application of Chinese herbal medicines. Many precious experiences were hidden in the traditional Classic publications that are worthy to be explored and integrated into modern research with evidence for application. This usage and integration could be helpful in promoting human health.

References

1. Wang QQ (2008) Methods for clinical study of Nei Jing. Zhong Xi Yi Jie He Xue Bao 6 (7):678–681. doi:10.3736/jcim20080704
2. Ma WH, Sun XH (2005) Discussion of time and space differentiation of three-yin and three-yang in Shanghan Lun. Zhong Xi Yi Jie He Xue Bao 3(4):257–259
3. Cheng JT (2000) Review: drug therapy in Chinese traditional medicine. J Clin Pharmacol 40 (5):445–450
4. Chen ZL (1984) Research on the "four methods of diagnosis" in traditional Chinese medicine and western medicine. Zhong Xi Yi Jie He Za Zhi 4(4):253–255
5. Chen C, Meng YM, Zhang P, Wang J, Zhao HH, Guo SZ, Wang W (2010) Diagnosis and treatment rule of traditional Chinese medicine for syndrome factors of chronic congestive heart failure: a study based on Shannon entropy method. Zhong Xi Yi Jie He Xue Bao 8(11):1080–1084

6. Brand E, Wiseman N (2008) Concise Chinese Materia Medica. Paradigm Publications, Taos, p 86
7. Zhang S, Wang D, Dong S, Yang F, Yan Z (2015) Differentially expressed genes of LPS febrile symptom in rabbits and that treated with Bai-Hu-tang, a classical anti-febrile Chinese herb formula. J Ethnopharmacol 169:130–137. doi:10.1016/j.jep.2015.04.021
8. Chen CC, Hsiang CY, Chiang AN, Lo HY, Li CI (2008) Peroxisome proliferator-activated receptor gamma transactivation-mediated potentiation of glucose uptake by Bai-Hu-Tang. J Ethnopharmacol 118(1):46–50. doi:10.1016/j.jep.2008.03.001
9. Unschuld PU (1986) Medicine in China: a history of pharmaceutics, vol 2. University of California Press, Oakland, CA
10. Zhu Y-P (1998) Chinese materia medica: chemistry, pharmacology and applications. CRC Press, Boca Raton, FL
11. Shang E, Duan JA, Fan X, Tang Y, and Su S (2008) Data Mining Technology for Studying the Compatibility of Nature, Flavor and Channel Tropism. World Science and Technology 1
12. Huang KC (1998) The pharmacology of Chinese herbs. CRC, Boca Raton, FL
13. Williamson EM (2001) Synergy and other interactions in phytomedicines. Phytomedicine 8(5):401–409
14. Chen FP, Chen FJ, Jong MS, Tsai HL, Wang JR, Hwang SJ (2009) Modern use of Chinese herbal formulae from Shang-Han Lun. Chin Med J (Engl Ed) 122(16):1889
15. Jian-guo J (2012) Discussion of the complex thinking of syndrome differentiation and treatment in 'Treatise on Febrile Diseases'. Shandong J Tradit Chin Med 2:001
16. Bao YJ, Sun TT, Lv WL, Hua BJ (2011) Essence and developmental history of classic formula: indications from the order of Three yin and Three yang in Shanghan Lun. China J Tradit Chin Med Pharm 9:007
17. Jingfeng C (1998) A historical overview of traditional Chinese medicine and ancient Chinese medical ethics. Ethik in Der Medizin 10(1)
18. Lin N, Wang L (2002) Collation and research on the different texts in Qian jin yao fang (Precious essential formulary, PEF). Zhonghua Yi Shi Za Zhi 32(2):87–91
19. Wu J-N (2005) An illustrated Chinese materia medica. Oxford University Press, Oxford, UK
20. Li CW, Si FC (2010) Study on basic theory innovation of TCM in Song, Jin, Yuan dynasties. China J Tradit Chin Med Pharm 7:010
21. Hanson M (2011) Speaking of epidemics in Chinese Medicine. Routledge, London
22. She Y, Wang J (2012) Preliminary exploration of WU Ju-tong to treat cold-dampness based on syndrome differentiation. China J Tradit Chin Med Pharm 8:009
23. Yan D, Yu X, Shi K, Song W, Zhang H, Wei J (2004) Discussion about treatment of severe acute respiratory syndrome based on syndrome differentiation. Zhong Xi Yi Jie He Xue Bao 2 (4):241–244

Chapter 2

Kampo Diagnosis Based on Sho

Mosaburo Kainuma

Abstract

In Japanese Kampo medicine, Sho is a diagnosis based on kampo principles and an indication of the prescription.

The patient's symptoms at any moment are recognized through the basic concepts of Yin-Yo; kyo-jitsu, ki, ketsu, and sui; six stages of disease; and the five parenchymatous viscera through Shi-shin. In addition, the doctor must identify any sign specific to the patient's clinical condition. Taken together, they establish the Sho: They select the Kampo formula corresponding to the Sho.

Key words Sho, Kamo diagnosis, Yin-Yo, Kyo-jitsu, Ki, ketsu, and sui, Six stages of disease, Shi-shin

1 Introduction

"Sho" is the traditional system used in East Asia, but the concept differs between Kampo and Traditional Chinese Medicine. In this chapter, I would like to explain some of the basic Kampo concepts on which Sho is founded and the way a Kampo diagnosis is made based on Kampo diagnosis, ShoSho. Sho is a method of diagnosis based upon the pathophysiological concepts of Kampo medicine. It is defined as the process of obtaining information about the physical and psychological condition of a patient by use of original parameters of Kampo medicine. It sums the particular pathological symptoms provided by the patient to describe the current status, which leads to the overall diagnosis and to the choice of the corresponding prescription.

2 Disease Condition (or Status) Categories: Yin-Yo, Jitsu-Kyo, Kan-Netsu, and Hyo-Ri

2.1 Yo Sho–Yin Sho

In medical terms, if the response to disease shown by the patient is feverish, active, or excitatory, the patient is said to be in Yo-Sho.

Akio Inui (ed.), *Herbal Medicines: New Horizons*, Methods in Pharmacology and Toxicology,
DOI 10.1007/978-1-4939-4002-8_2, © Springer Science+Business Media New York 2016

Conversely, if the response shown by the patient is chilly, inactive, or inhibitory, the patient is said to be in Yin-Sho.

2.2 Jitsu Sho–Kyo Sho

If the response to disease is strong, the patient is said to be in Jitsu-Sho. If the response is weak or lacking, the patient is said to be in Kyo-Sho.

2.3 Netsu Sho–Kan Sho

If the response to disease is febrile or the patient subjectively feels febrile, the patient is said to be in Netsu-Sho. Kan-Sho is the term used if the patient feels chilly. In clinical practice, the concepts of Yin-Yo and Kan-Netsu are almost identical, but the concept of Yin-Yo is superior to Kan-Netsu.

2.4 Hyo Sho–Ri Sho

If the site of a response to disease is exterior, the patient is said to be in Hyo-Sho. If the site is interior, the patient is said to be in Ri-Sho. Exterior refers to the body surface, including the skin, mucous membrane, throat, muscle, and joints. Interior refers to the digestive organs. In addition, the term HanpyoHanri means that the response site is between the exterior and interior, including the bronchi, lung, and liver. The locations expressed by exterior or interior are very rough descriptions that do not always represent specific viscera or tissue. Disease usually starts from Hyo and progresses to Ri.

3 The Three Constituent Categories: Ki, Ketsu, and Sui

Ki is regarded as the energy of a unified mind/body. In contrast to the Ki concept, Ketsu and Sui are considered to be blood and body fluids, respectively. In Kampo, Sho is mainly understood as disturbances of the three major constituents of life.

3.1 Ki-Kyo and Ketsu-Kyo (Kyo = Deficiency)

Ki is insufficient (strong) to sustain living functions. For example, fatigue, getting tired easily, feel lethargic or drowsy after meals, or appetite loss is often seen as Ki-kyo in Kampo terms. Likewise, a deficiency in Ketsu (blood), ketsu-kyo, is often seen as pallor, dry skin, leg cramps, or alopecia.

3.2 Ki-Utsu and Ki-Gyaku

Utsu literally means stagnation, while gyaku means counteraction. Thus, symptoms are sometimes seen as caused by the stagnation of Ki; for example, in depression, heavy-headedness, or nausea in Western terms. Likewise, a patient is considered to have a disease related to Ki-gyaku, counter-circulated Ki; for example, when they have palpitations, irritation, or paroxysmal headache.

3.3 O-Ketsu and Sui-Tai

O-ketsu refers to stagnation of the blood, which is sometimes seen in such conditions as lower limb varix, teleangiectasis, and pigmentation of the skin.

Table 1
Diagnostic criteria for oketsu syndrome

	Male	Female		Male	Female
Pigmentation of the orbicularis oculi	10	10	Tenderness/discomfort near the umbilicus/left side of lower abdomen	5	5
Dark facial complexion	2	2	Right side of lower abdomen	10	10
Rough and dry skin	2	5	Median lower abdomen	5	5
Dark red lips	2	2	Tenderness/discomfort in the ileocecal junction	5	2
Dark red gingiva	10	5	Tenderness/discomfort in the sigmoid colon	5	5
Dark red tongue	10	10	Tenderness/discomfort in the hypochondrium	5	5
Vasodilatation	5	5			
Hemorrhage under skin	2	10	Hemorrhoid	10	5
Palm erythema	2	5	Menstrual disorder		10

Determination: <20 points, no oketsu; 21–39 points, oketsu; >40 points, severe oketsu

Terasawa's diagnostic criteria are useful for identifying oketsu (Table 1) [1]. While there have been several sets of criteria proposed, Terasawa's are the most widely accepted. These criteria provide a common ground for the discussion of O-ketsu.

Sui-tai refers to the stagnation of body fluids and can be grouped into the three categories shown in Table 2 [2].

4 Six Stages of Disease Concept

The concept of Yin-Yo is used not only for the clinical condition in Kampo medicine but also for the staging of the disease.

"*ShangHanLun*" (傷寒論) classifies acute febrile diseases into six typical stages of disease transformation: TaiYo, ShoYo, YoMei, TaiYin, ShoYin, and KetsuY.

Most febrile disease transforms from Yo-sho to Yin-sho; however, occasionally it begins with the Sho Yin stage.

4.1 Tai Yo Stage

This is a stage of disease transformation identified by external hotness. The patient feels hot sensations accompanied, as a general rule, by chills from fever or the movement of air in the environment, headache, stiff neck and nape, and myalgia/arthralgia with floating pulse. These symptoms and signs are collectively termed the exterior pattern, meaning that the disorders are seen at an exterior location.

Table 2
Symptoms related to disorders of the body's fluid metabolism

Accumulation of water	Edema (teeth mark) Fluid and gas retention in the stomach Arthroedema, ascites, pleural effusion
Impaired water excretion	
Urination disorder	Decreased urination Frequent urination Delayed urination
Abnormal secretion	Ptyalism Excessive tearing Rhinorrhea Excessive sweating
Subjective symptoms	Heavy head, dizziness, dry mouth, stiffness, watery sputum, diarrhea, palpitation, tinnitus, borborygmus, heavy body

4.2 Sho Yo Stage

This is the stage of disease transformation with heat midway between exterior and interior. In the Sho Yo stage, the disease is converted into a heat type of alternating chills and fever: body temperature rises with chills and subsides with the appearance of the heat sensation. The chills and heat sensation appear alternately. Actually, body temperature does not rise in the morning, but rises gradually in the afternoon, reaches a peak in the evening, and subsides at night. Concurrently, with alternating chills and fever, Kyokyo Kũman appears as a specific feature in this stage. Patients have frequency sunken and string-like thin pulse, white tongue fur, bitterness or taste change in the mouth, or reduced appetite sometimes associated with nausea. Feelings of throat dryness, dizziness, or ear blockage also may occur.

4.3 YoMei Stage

This is a stage of disease transformation with heat at an interior location.

The YoMei stage has a tidal fever pattern. The patient does not have chills but suffers from heat-associated abdominal fullness and distention, constipation, and sunken excess pulse. In addition, the patient may talk in feverish delirium.

4.4 TaiYin Stage

This is a stage of disease transformation characterized by cold at an interior location.

The severity is mild, but it is likely to be associated with gastrointestinal symptoms such as abdominal fullness and pain, vomiting, anorexia, and diarrhea. Sunken pulse is also evident, which may often be accompanied by weak abdominal strength and occasionally by rectus abdominis muscle tension and epigastric discomfort and resistance.

4.5 Sho Yin Stage

This is a stage of disease transformation with cold at an interior location, sometimes accompanied by cold at an exterior location. The severity is moderate and it is featured by a pale face. The patient tires easily; wants to lie on his or her side; and complains of cold of the limbs, diarrhea, and systemic pain. The pulse is sunken and faint. Some febrile diseases begin with the Sho Yin stage, which is termed "direct Sho Yin stage."

4.6 Ketu Yin Stage

This is considered to be the end stage of disease, as in the preshock condition seen in acute febrile disease, with cold at an interior location, but it is likely to be associated with febrile symptoms. For example, the patient may present with mixed symptoms of cold and heat: true cold and false heat (kyonetsu). In this state medical condition is serious.

The patient suffers coldness from the distal to the proximal areas of the limbs, but feels heat in the trunk or cannot eat or may vomit even when hungry. They may have indigestion or diarrhea associated with a slow, sunken pulse despite the hot feeling on the body surface or upper body region.

5 The Five Solid Viscera Concept

Like the concept of Ki, Ketsu, Sui, there is a concept Stages of disease, Kampoof five solid viscera in which homeostasis is maintained in the liver, heart, spleen, lung, and kidney. The meaning of the five solid viscera is not defined by the anatomy of the individual organs but includes the functional unit to which each of them belongs. In older patients, there may be cases in which kidney and liver abnormality are indicated. This concept may be useful as background information to understand the classical literature, but abuse and overuse must be avoided in the clinical setting.

6 Shi-Shin

The disease conditions, seen as deviation or imbalance, are understood as such by the four physical approaches (Shi-Shin) as above defined.

6.1 Visual Observation (Boshin)

Observation is done with only the quickest glance to detect important signs of blood stagnation (Oketsu) and other important signs. These include the patient's complexion, facial expression, body shape, movement, gait when entering the room, pigmentation of the orbicularis oscli, rough and/or dry skin, dark red gingiva,

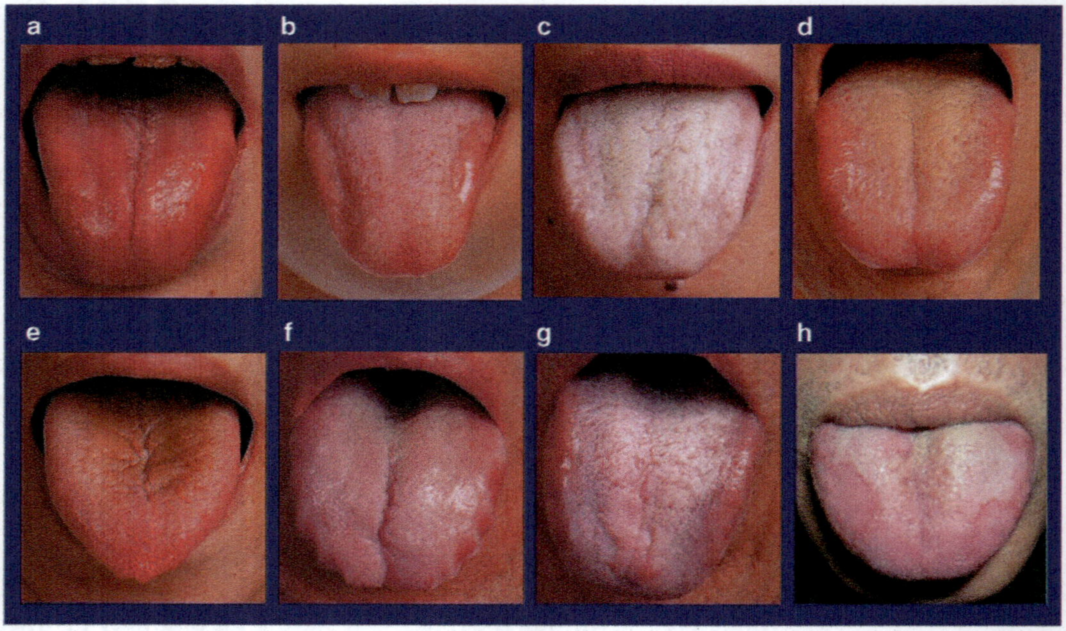

Fig. 1 The major features of tongue inspection.(**a**) No fur (**b**) Normal tongue (**c**) Thick, white fur (**d**) Yellow fur (**e**) Black fur (**f**) Dental indentations (**g**) Purple tongue (**h**) Geographical tongue

vasodilatation, hemorrhage under the skin, and palm erythema. Furthermore, one of the most important findings of *Boshin* is tongue inspection in which the tongue body, color, form, and motility are assessed. The major features of tongue inspection are as seen in Fig. 1.

1. No fur.
   The color of the tongue body is clearly visible without any fur. The absence of tongue fur may be attributed to atrophic or immature filiform papillae.
2. Normal tongue.
   A tongue of normal color is slightly red with little exfoliation of cells from keratinized filiform papillae. Small amounts of keratinized epithelial cells that are exfoliated but remain on the tips of filiform papillae develop into a thin white fur, which is commonly visible on the tongue of healthy persons.
3. Thick, white fur.
   A tongue covered with white fur has epithelial cells of filiform papillae that are degraded by keratinization but remain on the tips of the papillae. It indicates conditions such as the Sho Yo stage and stagnation or impairment of digestive function. In general, the thicker the fur the longer the duration of illness.

4. Yellow fur.
   Yellow fur indicates symptoms of stomach heat, such as heartburn, gastric acid reflux, stomachache, or constipation. Yellowing of the tongue fur is caused by further degradation of filiform papillae cells and bacterial proliferation.
5. Black fur.
   Black fur is seen at the peak of fever and in serious stages of disease. Black fur indicates an interior pattern and is commonly seen in patients receiving long-term antibiotic therapy and in terminally ill cancer patients.
6. Dental indentations.
   Dental indentations along the maxillary or mandibular dental arch are observed in patients with deficiency of the upper abdominal region, qi (Ki) deficiency, and fluid disturbance. If the tongue is thick, swollen, and large enough to force the mouth open and has margins that protrude beyond the lips and usually bearing dental indentation, we suspect fluid disturbance.
7. Purple tongue.
   A purple tongue indicates poor blood circulation and blood stasis. This accompanies changes in the venous system, such as venous dilation in the tongue.
8. Geographical tongue.
   A tongue with irregular peeling of the fur. This is a disorder that includes keratinization of the mucosal epithelium of the tongue, which is caused by partial atrophy, a keratinization disorder, and/or the disappearance of filiform papillae. Immature filiform papillae look red and depressed; mature filiform papillae look white and elevated. This type of tongue is commonly seen in patients with ki-deficiency.

*6.2 Listening and Smelling (*Bunshin*)*

Doctors directly listen to the sounds of the patient's voice, speech, breathing, cough, wheezing, belching, and stomach growling as part of their diagnosis process. Odors, such as from the body, breath, or stool may indicate an abnormality.

*6.3 Inquiry (*Monshin*)*

The importance of questioning the patient is the same for both Kampo and Western medicine. However, from the point of view of Kampo medicine the aim of the inquiry is to determine how the condition is imbalanced. Therefore, we ask the patients not only about their main complaints, medical history, past history, and family medical history, but also about coldness, appetite, urination, bowel movements, sleep, menstruation, and other factors that might aggravate the main complaint; for example, reaction to changes of the weather, especially atmospheric pressure, and dietary changes.

6.4 Palpation (Sessin)

1. Palpation of the skin, hands, and feet.
2. Pulse diagnosis.

   The kampo physician measures the pulse of the radial artery by placing his second, third, and fourth fingers on the internal area of the radius styloid process.

   (a) Depth (Floating ↔ Sunken).
   (b) Strength (Strong ↔ Weak).
   (c) Strain (Tight ↔ Relaxed).
   (d) Rate (Fast ↔ Slow).
   (e) Flow (Smooth ↔ Congested).

3. Palpation of the abdomen, abdominal diagnosis (Fig. 2).

   (a) Abdominal strength.
   Abdominal strength is usually rated on a five-point scale of excessive, slightly excessive, moderate, slightly deficient, and deficient. The abdominal strength is used in the determination of Kyo-Jitsu.

   (b) Contracture of the rectus abdominis.
   This indicates excessive strain of the rectus abdominis muscles. This change is usually bilateral but may also be unilateral or appear only on the upper abdomen. Furthermore, the rectus abdominis muscles can be very thick or thin like plywood.

   (c) Epigastric discomfort and resistance.
   Resistance in the epigastric region can usually be divided into two categories, only subjective symptoms or objective resistance.

1) Abdominal strength
2) Contracture of the rectus abdominis
3) Epigastric discomfort and resistance
4) Hypochondrium resistance and discomfort
5) Splashing sound
6) Palpable abdominal aortic pulsation
7) Tender points in the lower abdomen
   1.Tenderness in the peri-umbilical region
   2.Tenderness in the ilieocecal region
   3.Tenderness in the sigmoid colon region
8) Weakness and muscle tension of the lower abdominal region

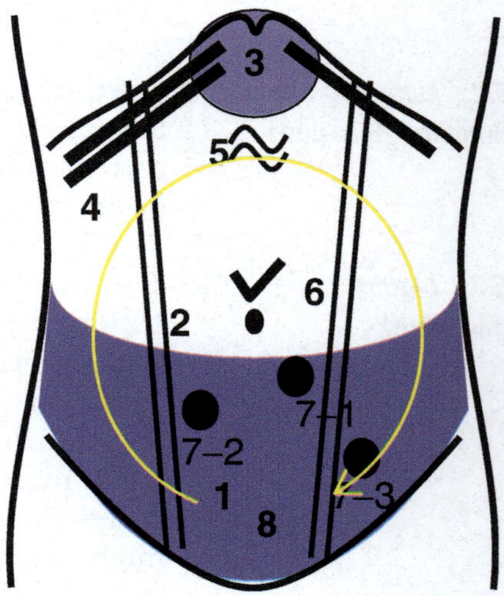

Fig. 2 Examination of abdominal findings

(d) Hypochondrium resistance and discomfort.
In the classical literature this is called "Kyokyo Kuman" and includes subjective discomfort and bilateral objective resistance or unilateral hypochondrium. Kyokyo Kuman is one of the characteristics of the Sho yo stage.

(e) Splashing sound.
This sound can be heard over the epigastric region or the third portion of the duodenum or jejunum when clapping with a flexible wrist. This finding indicates reduced abdominal tension in this area; air in the stomach; or fluid retention in stomach, duodenum, or jejunum.

(f) Palpable abdominal aortic pulsation.
When pulsation is palpable in the epigastric region, Kigyaku or Suitai are indicated.

(g) Tender points in the lower abdomen.
This is an important abdominal finding that indicates Oketsu. The prescription usually given differs by point of tenderness as follows.

- Tenderness in the periumbilical region.
- Tenderness in the ilieocecal region.
- Tenderness in the sigmoid colon region.

(h) Weakness of the lower abdominal region.

Abnormal sensation is felt in the infraumbilical region (numbness or supersensitivity), often accompanied by weakness (soft and feeble) in the infraumbilical region compared with the upper abdominal region. This is referred to in the clinical literature as Shofuku Fujin, and it is a sign of a deficiency of the kidney.

The patient's symptoms at any moment are recognized through the basic concepts of Yin-Yo, kyo-jitsu, ki,ketsu, and sui, the six stages of disease, the five parenchymatous viscera, and thorough Shi-shin. Of these concepts, we consider Yin-Yo to be the most important for determining Sho.

In addition, the doctor must identify any presenting sign specific to the patient's clinical condition. Taking the signs and symptoms together, the Sho is determined and a Kampo formula (herbal medicine) selected that corresponds to the Sho. The relation between Sho and the formula is similar to that between a lock and key. The accuracy of our Kampo diagnosis and prescription is only known by confirming if the various symptoms were relieved. If the patient's symptoms do not improve, our diagnosis is not correct so we again determine the Sho through Shi-shin (Fig. 3). Furthermore, because Sho is phenomenological it can change in hours; therefore, Kampo physicians should observe abdominal and pulse conditions that can discern the various Sho diagnoses at regular intervals.

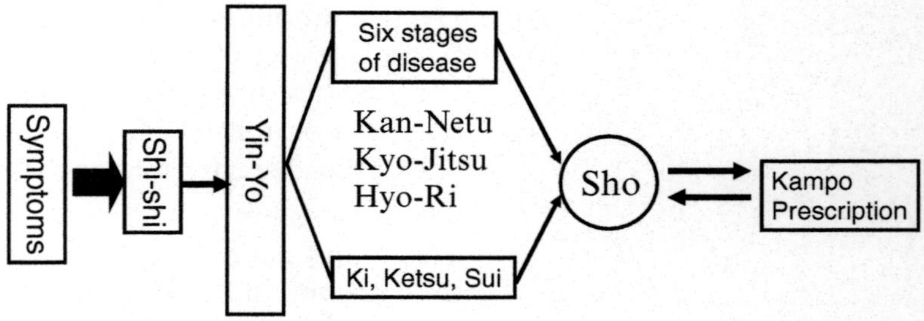

Fig. 3 Process of making a Kampo diagnosis

The particular characteristics of Sho are based on the results of several thousand years of experience; however, how and why particular signs and symptoms are related to Sho remain to be clarified. Future research will be required to objectively illustrate the mechanisms of Sho, which will make Kampo available to clinicians worldwide. In this regard, we have developed an objective tongue analysis system that clearly shows the relation between the gastroesophageal disease and Sho [3].

References

1. Katsutoshi Terasawa et al. (1983) Japanese Journal of Oriental Medicine 34: 1–17
2. Akira Imadaya (1993) Clinical Seminar o n the Traditional Oriental Medicine (the 43rd General Meeting). Japanese Journal of Oriental Medicine 43: 349–356
3. Kainuma M, et al (2015) The association between objective tongue color and endoscopic findings: results from the Kyushu and Okinawa population study (KOPS).BMC Complement Altern Med 15:372.

Chapter 3

Pain and Herbal Medicine: Effectiveness of Japanese Kampo Medicines on Pains Associated with Cancer Patients

Yasuhito Uezono and Kanako Miyano

Abstract

Pain derived from cancer therapy as well as cancer itself is one of the most incurable symptoms. Pain management is important in oncologic care and essential for maximizing patient outcomes. Accumulating evidence showed that unrelieved pain significantly comprised overall quality of life and effective pain control was associated with survival. In Asian countries, traditional herbal medicine is frequently combined with western medical approaches to treat cancer. Although an overview of systematic reviews about the complementary and alternative medicine (CAM) for cancer pain conducted, they showed that CAM may be beneficial for alleviating cancer pain, but the evidence levels were found to be low or moderate. In case of Japanese kampo medicine, recent progresses regarding cancer pain treatment have indicated that scientific evidence of both basic and clinical research has accumulated in many of the literatures. In this chapter, we discuss herbal medicines for pain relief of cancer patients, in particular, benefit of Japanese kampo medicines based on their accumulated evidence-based scientific reports. Further, we also introduced a novel screening assay, CellKey™ system, to find valuable ingredients or substances from kampo medicine possibly as well as other traditional herbal medicines in the world.

Key words Kampo medicine, Chemotherapy-induced peripheral neuropathy (CIPN), Cancer pain, Goshajinkigan, Hangeshashinto, CellKey™ system, Electrical impedance assay

1 Introduction

Pain evoked by stimulatory signal that is not released from significant tissue damage is regarded as beneficial sign. Persistent pain associated with hyperalgesia and tenderness, which differs in quality but is usually associated with the processes of inflammation, is also considered a normal protective response to a mild tissue injury [1]. This type of pain resolves once the injury has healed. A number of chronic pains occur in which the stimulus and pains are unrelated, and pain can no longer be regarded as a physiologically protective symptom. These types of pain syndromes such as migraine, lower-back pain, cancer pain, and neuropathic pain are not well understood and are difficult to treat. In particular, pain originally derived

Akio Inui (ed.), *Herbal Medicines: New Horizons*, Methods in Pharmacology and Toxicology,
DOI 10.1007/978-1-4939-4002-8_3, © Springer Science+Business Media New York 2016

from cancer itself and that from cancer therapy is complex and one of the most incurable symptoms [2].

A meta-analysis reported cancer pain in 64 % of patients with metastatic disease, 59 % of patients receiving antineoplastic therapy, and 33 % of patients who had received curative cancer treatment. Another report showed that 75–90 % cancer patients experienced pain during their illness and up to 50 % of cancer pain is undertreated [3, 4]. It was reported that one-quarter of the patients had newly diagnosed malignancies, one-third of the patients are undergoing treatment, and three-quarters of the patients with advanced disease experienced pain [5, 6]. Pain management is important in oncologic care and essential for maximizing patient outcomes [7, 8]. Accumulating evidence showed that unrelieved pain significantly comprised overall quality of life and effective pain control was associated with survival [7, 8]. For treatment of cancer pain in general, opioid therapies are mainly, and in some cases, adjuvant analgesics are used [2]. Although opioid therapy is very effective, it is with a lot of side effects, such as constipation, urinary retention, nausea, sedation, respiratory depression, myoclonus, delirium, sexual dysfunction, and hyperalgesia [9]. In these cases, several approaches are chosen and performed to reduce disease- or stage- or anticancer drug therapy-dependent pains (Table 1) [2]. Complementary and alternative medicine (CAM), which is noninvasive and generally considered to be relatively free of toxicity, has been used as an adjunct therapy together with standard pain management techniques (Table 1) [10]. A review showed that acupuncture, massage therapy, mind–body interventions, and music therapy could effectively reduce pain and enhance quality of life [10]. In Asian countries, traditional herbal medicine in each country is frequently combined with western medical approaches to treat cancer, usually in regimens that combine various traditional Asian herbs into one treatment strategy (Table 1) [11]. Alternative medicine has been used to meet patient needs in lieu of or as an adjunct to conventional medicine [11].

Although overviews of systematic reviews about CAM for cancer pain are conducted, they showed that CAM may be beneficial for alleviating cancer pain, but the evidence levels were found to be low or moderate. Future large and rigor randomized controlled studies are needed to confirm the benefits of CAM on adult cancer pain [6]. In case of Japanese kampo medicine, however, recent progresses regarding cancer pain treatment have indicated that scientific evidence of both basic and clinical research has accumulated in many of the literatures [12–14].

In this chapter, we discuss herbal medicines for pain relief of cancer patients, in particular, benefit of Japanese kampo medicines based on their accumulated evidence-based scientific reports.

Table 1
Several approaches of treatment for pain related to cancer

Approach	Type of treatment
1. Pharmacologic	Opioid analgesics Nonopioid analgesics (NSAIDs, etc.) Adjuvant analgesics
2. Interventional	Injection therapies (intrathecal therapy) Neural blockade Implant therapies
3. Rehabilitative	Modalities such as heat and cold Therapeutic exercise Occupational therapy Hydrotherapy Therapies for specific disorders (e.g., lymphedema)
4. Neurostimulation	Transcutaneous Transcranial Percutaneous peripheral nerve and spinal cord/root simulation
5. Psychologic	Psychoeducational interventions Cognitive-behavioral therapy Relaxation therapy, guided imagery, other types of stress management Other forms of psychotherapy
6. Integrative (complementary or alternative medicine (CAM))	Acupuncture Massage Yoga Movement therapies Traditional herbal medicines

Reference [2]

2 Japanese Kampo Medicine

Chinese herbal medicine, one of the oldest forms of traditional medicine, has been used in China and other countries for more than 3000 years. Traditional Japanese kampo medicine is originated from the Chinese herbal medicine after they were imported to Japan, and it subsequently modified and developed to suit Japanese culture and environmental factors [12, 15]. These kampo medicines, systemically developed in the sixteenth century into a more specifically Japanese form, have a wide range of indications for maintaining quality of life, rather than curing patients [12, 16].

Since Japan's Ministry of Health, Labour and Welfare approved more than 140 kampo medicines for use in clinical practice, they have been increasingly employed to help maintain the quality of life in patients with diseases such as gastrointestinal disorders, and lifestyle-related diseases and cancer [12, 13, 17]. However, there is scarce scientific evidence that supports reliable effects of kampo in the clinical study until twenty-first centuries. This is because kampo medicines are composed of several crude drug products mainly extracted from plants, so that it is difficult to maintain consistent quality and quantity of these ingredients. Recently, however, kampo medicines have been developed in Japan through clinical and laboratory studies based on western-adopted, scientific, experiment-based approaches [12, 13, 15, 18]. Accordingly, in order to support the use of kampo medicine, scientific evidence has been accumulated and is continuously increasing in the past decade.

3 Pain Classification and Pain Related to Cancer Pain

Pain is normally classified into two based on duration: acute and chronic. Generally, persisting chronic pain derives from the pathophysiologic changes in tissues. Cancer painCancer pain is a sort of heterologous combination of any types of pain described below so that it is difficult to relieve such kinds of complex pain [2, 19, 20].

3.1 Nociceptive Pain

This type of pain represents the normal response to injury of tissues or noxious insult of tissues. Its sensation is very important to warn alarm of body change status. It alerts us to external stimuli, such as pinprick or excessive heat, and internal stimuli, such as myocardial ischemia in patients with coronary artery disease. Certain diseases may generate recurrent or ongoing noxious stimuli to produce chronic nociceptive pain [19].

3.2 Inflammatory Pain

This type of pain is caused by tissue injury followed by its inflammatory response. To aid healing and repair of the injured body part, the sensory nervous system undergoes a profound change in its responsiveness; normally innocuous stimuli now produce pain and responses to noxious stimuli are both exaggerated and prolonged [19, 21]. Heightened sensitivity occurs within the inflamed area and in contiguous noninflamed areas as a result of plasticity in peripheral nociceptors and central nociceptive pathways [22–24]. Typically, inflammatory pain disappears after resolution of the initial tissue injury. However, in chronic disorders such as rheumatoid arthritis the pain persists for as long as inflammation is active [25].

3.3 Dysfunctional Pain

Dysfunctional pain occurs in situations in which there is no identifiable noxious stimulus nor any detectable inflammation or damage to the nervous system. It is unclear in most cases what causes the manifestation or persistence of dysfunctional pain [19]. In conditions such as fibromyalgia, irritable bowel syndrome, and interstitial cystitis, the pain appears to result from an autonomous amplification of nociceptive signals inside the CNS [26, 27] with a disturbed balance of excitation and inhibition in central circuits [28] and altered sensory processing that can be detected by functional imaging [29].

3.4 Neuropathic Pain

Pain and loss of function are intimately associated with the reaction of the nervous system to neural damage, and both provide important diagnostic clues that such damage has occurred [19]. Peripheral neuropathic pain results from lesions to the peripheral nervous system (PNS) caused by mechanical trauma, metabolic diseases, neurotoxic chemicals, infection, or tumor invasion and involves multiple pathophysiologic changes both within the PNS and in the central nervous system (CNS) [30, 31]. Although treatment targeted at the primary pathology is obviously essential, understanding the mechanisms responsible for the maladaptive plasticity offers specific therapeutic opportunities to prevent the development of neuropathic hypersensitivity and normalize function in established neuropathic pain. Once neuropathic pain is generated, the sensory hypersensitivity typically persists for prolonged periods, even though the original etiologic cause may have long since disappeared, as after nerve trauma. The syndrome can nevertheless progress if the primary disease, such as nerve compression continues to damage the nervous system. Neuropathic pain is not an inevitable consequence of neural lesions, though. On the contrary, the pain associated with acute neural damage usually transitions to chronic neuropathic pain in a minority of patients. This transition to chronicity is most obvious after surgical nerve lesions where the extent and timing of the lesion are defined [32].

4 Treatment of Cancer Pain with Western-Oriented Drugs

Target symptoms for several types of pain are many, and drugs are dependent on the types of pain. Inhibitors of pain evoking prostaglandin synthases (cyclooxygenase 1 (COX-1) and COX-2) are typical drugs, namely nonsteroidal anti-inflammatory drugs (NSAIDs). And drugs that activate opioid receptor systems are commonly used for treatment of cancer pain (Table 1) [2].

The approaches to analgesia may involve consideration of disease-modifying therapy or any of a variety of specific therapies (Table 1) [2]. Also, Auret and Schug [20] presented pain management for the cancer patient in current practice and also future development, showing methods of treatment of mild, moderate, and severe cancer pain with opioids, NSAIDs, and other pain-relieving drugs. In the homepage of "Cancer Research UK", a variety of western painkillers are shown to treat cancer pain [33].

5 Herbal Medicines for Pain Treatment

In Asian countries, traditional herbal medicine of their own has been frequently employed by themselves or in combination with Western medicines for the treatment of pain arising from a variety of disease symptoms [4, 6]. Herbal medicine combined with conventional therapy is reported to be efficacious as an adjunctive therapy for patients with cancer pain. However, they claim that more research, including well-designed, rigorous, and larger trials, is necessary [4]. In contrast, as far as Japanese kampo medicine, the effectiveness of kampo medicine has been recently recognized with scientific evidence-based experiments [12, 13, 34].

6 Pains in Cancer Patients and Kampo Medicine for the Treatment of Cancer Pain

For cancer pain, 75–90 % cancer patients experienced pain during their illness and up to 50 % of cancer pain is undertreated. It was reported that one-quarter of the patients had newly diagnosed malignancies, one-third of the patients are undergoing treatment, and three-quarters of the patients with advanced disease experienced pain [5]. For treatment of cancer pain, especially in Asian countries, traditional herbal medicine has been used and it has been used to meet patient needs in lieu of or as an adjunct to conventional medicine [11]. Although CAM may be beneficial for alleviating cancer pain, the evidence levels were found to be low or moderate and future large and rigor randomized controlled studies are needed to confirm the benefits of CAM on cancer pain [6]. Recent scientific evidence of both basic and clinical research has accumulated in many of the literatures in the case of Japanese kampo medicine [12, 13, 34]. Here, we show the examples of effectiveness of Japanese kampo medicine, for pain relief of cancer patients, as follows.

6.1 Chemotherapy-Induced Peripheral Neuropathy (CIPN)

Several chemotherapeutic drugs are known to be neurotoxic and can lead to CIPN. It is one of the main dose-limiting toxicities in oncologic treatments and a potential reason to terminate or suspend chemotherapy, in some cases leading to disease progression [35]. CIPNChemotherapy-induced peripheral neuropathy (CIPN) involves damage to the peripheral nervous system and can produce severe neuropathic pain [36, 37], sensory deficits, or gait impairment [38] and can severely decrease the patient's quality of life [39]. Sensory symptoms usually develop before motor symptoms, because motor neurons are more myelinated [36, 40]. Distal parts of the axons are the first affected, so sensory symptoms typically start symmetrically and bilaterally from the tips of the toes and fingers and progress proximally in a "stocking-glove"

Table 2
Ingredients of rokumigan (RMG), hachimijiogan (HJG), and goshajinkigan (GJG)

Herbal ingredients	Kampo medicine		
	Rokumigan (RMG)	Hachimijiogan (HJG)	Goshajinkigan (GJG)
Rehmanniae Radix			
Corni Fructus			
Dioscoreae Rhizoma			
Alismatis Rhizoma			
Poria			
Moutan Cortex			
Cinnamoni Cortex			
Processi Aconiti Radix (Bushi)			
Achyranthis Radix			
Plantaginis Semen			

distribution [41]. The incidence of CIPN can reach levels of up to 92 % [42, 43]. Some kampo medicines are reported to be useful for management of CIPN.

6.1.1 Goshajinkigan (GJG)

GJG, which is composed of ten herbal medicines (Table 2), has been widely used to treat disease-associated neuropathy (i.e. diabetic neuropathy) [44–46]. Animal investigations demonstrated that GJGGoshajinkigan (GJG) suppresses oxaliplatin-induced acutely occurred cold hyperalgesia [47] without affecting its antitumor effect [48]. Also, GJG prevented anticancer drug paclitaxel-induced mechanical allodynia without impairing the antitumor activity of paclitaxel [49].

More than half of patients treated with traditional Asian herbs are reported to have effective relief of pain symptoms [50]. In case of oxaliplatin therapy, it induces peripheral neuropathy that manifests itself as two distinct phases: acute cold hyperesthesia and chronic peripheral hypoesthesia/dysesthesia; and chronic status is a serious dose-limiting side effect that often leads to withdrawal of treatment [51]. Quite recently we developed a rat model expressing acute and chronic phases to investigate the action of GJG [51]. These rat models developed neuropathy for 8 weeks by injection of oxaliplatin twice a week. This model showed atrophy of axons of myelinated sciatic nerve fibers and co-administration of GJG ameliorated both abnormal sensations as well as histologic damage to the sciatic nerve. We further determined active ingredients in GJG and found that numerous neuroprotective components in GJG are rapidly absorbed into the blood. Also, GJG and some ingredients attenuated the generation of oxaliplatin-induced reactive oxygen species, which is a possible mechanism of oxaliplatin-induced neurotoxicity. From these results, we show that GJG is useful for oxaliplatin-induced neurotoxicity. These further promising prophylactic ingredients are included in GJG, expecting novel drugs for neuropathic pain [51].

6.1.2 Bushi

Bushi (*Processi Aconiti Radix*), which is derived from aconite, is contained in several kampo medicines such as GJG and hachimijogan (HJG). It is known to be effective for streptozotocin-induced diabetic autonomic neuropathy [52], paclitaxel-induced peripheral neuropathy, and some other types of pain [45, 53]. In addition and more importantly, Bushi has been effective for several types of chronic and persistent pain including neuropathic pain. By using rat nerve ligation (Seltzer) model mice, Shibata et al. showed that this neuropathy was associated with the activation of microglia and astrocytes in the spinal cord, and Bushi suppressed the activity of astrocytes, resulted in analgesia in the mice [54]. These results suggest that Bushi, even simple administration, could also be a useful therapeutic strategy for treating CIPN.

6.1.3 Rokumigan (RMG) and Hachimijiogan (HJG)

RMG, which is composed of six herbal ingredients, HJG of RMG + 2 other ingredients (8 components), and GJG of HJG + 2 other ingredients (10 components) are shown in Table 2. Andoh et al. compared the effects of reducing activity of mechanical allodynia induced by paclitaxel in mice [55], and found that the potency to reduce mechanical allodynia was GJG > HJG and RMGRokumigan (RMG) failed to induce anti-allodynia effects. Although underlying mechanisms for the effectiveness of reducing anticancer-induced mechanical allodynia were not well known, the herbal medicine *Achyranthis Radix* and *Plantaginis Semen*, the ingredients containing only in GJG, would contribute the inhibitory action of GJG on the exacerbation of paclitaxel-induced allodynia. Some reports suggested that *Plantaginis Semen* and *Achyranthis Radix* have an antioxidant activity [56, 57] and this action may be involved in the prevention of an exacerbation of paclitaxel-induced allodynia. Further, according to the results of the efficacy between GJG and HJGHachimijiogan (HJG) [55], it is possible that *Cinnamoni Cortex* and *Processi Aconiti Radix* (Bushi) also have some ability to produce anti-allodynia effects. As mentioned above, *Processi Aconiti Radix* (Bushi) by itself inhibited astrocytic activation to cause neuropathic pain [54].

6.1.4 Shakuyakukanzoto

Shakuyakukanzoto, a herbal medicine composed of two herbs *Paeoniae Radix* and *Glycyrrhizae Radix*, was reported to have anticholinergic and prostaglandin-production-inhibiting effects [58], and it has been reported to have ability to reduce muscle pain, muscle spasms, and numbness [59, 60]. In the status of CIPN induced by paclitaxel, shakuyakukanzoto is also effective. With the experimental rat model producing allodynial by single administration of paclitaxel, shakuyakukanzoto successfully relieved painful peripheral neuropathy [61].

6.1.5 Yokukansan

Yokukansan is a Japanese kampo medicine comprising seven herbal medicines (*Atractylodis Lanceae Rhizoma*, *Hoelen*, *Cnidii Rhizoma*, *Uncariae Uncis Cum Ramulus*, *Angelicae Radix*, *Bupleuri Radix*, and *Glycyrrhizae Radix*), and is used to control nighttime crying in children and to treat insomnia and neurosis. Recent studies indicate that yokukansan has been reported to improve behavioral and psychologic symptoms associated with dementia (BPSD), such as hallucinations, agitation, and aggressiveness in patients with Alzheimer's disease, dementia with Lewy bodies, and other forms of senile dementia [16, 62–64].

Recent reports also showed that yokukansan controls neuropathic pain as well as hallucinations and aggravation of dementia-associated symptoms [65]. In the CIPN rat model producing mechanical allochynia with nerve ligation, yokukansan improved mechanical allodynia through the regulation of the expression of interleukin-6, a well-known proinflammatory cytokine in the spinal cord [66].

6.2 Oral Mucositis

Chemotherapy-induced oral mucositis is a complication that is frequently encountered in cancer patients and may delay the treatment plan in the case of severe morbidity [67–69]. The oral mucosal injury involves chronic and/or intense pain, and affects nutritional intake and oral hygiene, as well as increases the risk for local and systemic infection, resulting in deterioration of the quality of life [67, 70].

A Japanese kampo medicine hangeshashinto (HST) consists of seven herbal crude drugs. From the sixteenth century to even now, HST has been prescribed in Japan as one of the main kampo medicine and targeted diseases and symptoms are as follows: acute or chronic gastrointestinal catarrh, fermentative diarrhea, dyspepsia, gastroptosis, nervous gastritis, gastrasthenia, hangover, belching, heartburn, neurosis as well as stomatitis [34, 71]. HST was demonstrated to inhibit pain and inflammation mediator prostaglandin E_2 (PGE_2) production in human gingival fibroblasts [72] and reduce the PGE_2 contents in the colons of several animal diarrhea models caused by anticancer drug, cholera toxin, or castor oil, resulting in amelioration of inflammatory damage [73–75]. HST was investigated for the preventive effects on inflammatory responses in lipopolysaccharide (LPS)-created human gingival fibroblasts as a model of oral mucositis [72]. They showed that HST decreased the typical mediator of inflammation and pain PGE_2 by suppression of cytoplasmic PGA_2, and LPS-induced cyclooxygenase-2 expression. Authors suggested that HST may be useful to improve gingival inflammation in periodontal disease [72].

We, with the experimental animal and cellular models, revealed that HST is a kind of multicomponent anti-PGE_2 agent with multi-targeting effects, at least having dual suppression of cyclooxygenase-2 expression and PGE_2 metabolic activity [69]. We demonstrated that inducible PGE_2, PGD_2, and $PGF_{2\alpha}$, metabolites of COX pathways were reduced by HST (10–300 μg/ml) without any cytotoxic effects [69]. The active ingredients of HST were quantified by LC-MS/MS, and [6]-shogaol, [6]-gingerol, wogonin, baicalien, baicalin, and berberine were shown to reduce PGE_2 production. We further demonstrated that a mixture of these six ingredients at concentrations equal to 300 μg/ml of HST strongly suppressed PGE_2 production to the same level as HST. [6]-Shogaol and [6]-gingerol did not decrease COX-2 mRNA expression and mostly inhibit PGE_2 metabolic activity in an assay using intact human oral keratinocyte cells, suggesting that they regulate PGE_2 synthesis at the posttranscriptional level. In the mean time, wogonin, baicalin, and berberine inhibited expression of COX-2 mRNA without affecting PGE_2 metabolic activity. These lines of evidence shows that HST includes several PGE_2-regulating ingredients that have different mechanisms and can function as a multicomponent and multitarget agent for treatment of chemotherapy-induced oral mucositis [69], indicating that HST may be beneficial in a new medial strategy for chemotherapy-induced oral mucositis treatment.

For the clinical study in 2010, Kono et al. [76] have shown that HST was effective for chemotherapy-induced oral mucositis in a pilot clinical study. In addition, double-blind, placebo-controlled, randomized phase II study was recently conducted, which have shown that the median duration of grade ≧2 oral mucositis of 5.5 versus 10.5 days ($p = 0.018$), indicating that HST had a significant effect in the treatment of grade ≧2 mucositis in patients with colorectal cancer [77]. These results strongly indicate that HST could be beneficial to the cancer patients who are suffering from oral mucositis.

7 New Assay Method for Detecting Cellular Protein Targets for Extracts of Kampo Medicines or Other Traditional Herbal Medicines

Electrical biosensors, also known as impedance-based biosensors, consist of a substrate, an electrode, and a cell layer in close contact with the electrode (Fig. 1) [12]. In the assay system, changes in cellular impedance (i.e., induced extracellular currents (iec) or induced transcellular currents (itc)) could be monitored in real-time, and the fluctuation of impedance depended on activation of cell surface target proteins followed by actin polymerization, thus linking this change to cellular motion [78]. Since then, electrical-based detections have been applied to study a wide variety of cellular events and it is now accepted that the impedance value corresponds to the sum of cellular events, including the relative density of cells over the electrode surface and the relative adherence

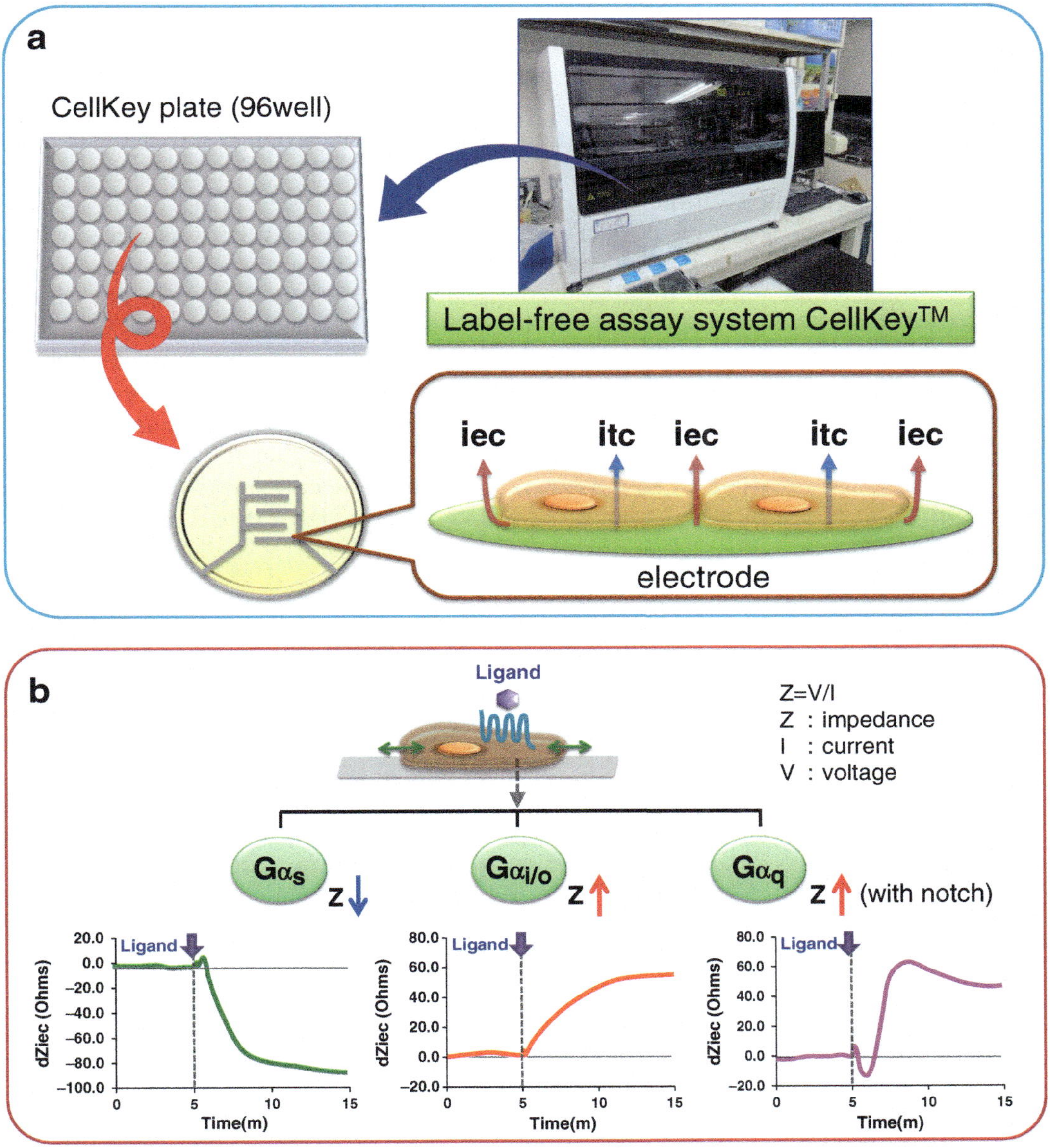

Fig. 1 (**a**) Photograph of the label-free assay system CellKey™ equipped with operation machine, and principles of CellKey™ impedance assay. *iec* induced extracellular currents, *itc* induced transcellular currents. (**b**) Schematic diagram of impedance assay with cells and representative waves mediated by typical different type of G protein-coupled, seven transmembrane receptors ($G\alpha_s$, $G\alpha_{i/o}$, and $G\alpha_q$)

of these cells [12]. We have been studying cellular responses caused by a variety of neurotransmitters or hormones that regulate cellular functions through their own target proteins such as G protein-coupled receptors (GPCRs), with a high-throughput system CellKey™, which is designed to detect acute cellular responses in 96- and 384-well formats (Fig. 1a). By using the CellKey™ system, others and we have observed distinct response profiles depending on activation of cell membrane excitability proteins such as several types of ion channels and GPCRs. By using this assay system, ligand-activated cellular responses thus were detected in a real-time (Fig. 1b) [12, 79, 80].

We observed that a kampo medicine rikkunshito actually modified and enhanced the orexigenic peptide ghrelin-induced receptor activation with the CellKey™ assay system [81]. This ghrelin-induced cellular enhancement by rikkunshito was already confirmed by measuring the rikkunshito-mediated enhancement of ghrelin-induced intracellular Ca^{2+} concentration with Ca^{2+} imaging assay [82]. By using the CellKey™ assay system, the actual ingredients in kampo medicines affecting cellular signaling would be identified as well [12, 79]. We previously described a review regarding the CellKey™ assay system as a State-of-the-Art biosensor assay [79]. In this review, we expected that the CellKey™ system will lead to innovative drug development, and that new attractive substances could be found from kampo extracts as well as from other traditional herbal medicines [79].

8 Conclusion

Pain derived from cancer therapy as well as cancer itself is one of the most incurable symptoms. Pain management is important in oncologic care and essential for maximizing patient outcomes. Recent progresses regarding cancer pain treatment indicated that Japanese kampo medicine could be useful for the treatment of cancer pain. We introduced effectiveness of kampo medicines for the treatment, in particular, CIPN and oral mucositis, in cancer patients treated with chemotherapy and/or radiation therapy. We also introduced a novel screening assay, CellKey™ system, to find valuable ingredients or substances from kampo medicine possibly as well as other traditional herbal medicines in all over the world.

Acknowledgments

This work was supported in part by a Grant-in-Aid for the Research Project for Improving Quality in Healthcare and Collecting Scientific Evidence on Integrative Medicine No. 15lk0310003h0001 from the Japan Agency for Medical Research and Development (AMED); Practical Research for Innovative Cancer Control No. 15Ack0106059h0002 from AMED; Foundation for Promotion of Cancer Research in Japan; Grants-in-Aid for Scientific Research (C) No. 15K08686, No. 15K10522, No. 15K008215, No. 15K09819, No. 25462442, Scientific Research (A) No. 15H02562 and Young Scientists (B) No. 25860199 from the Ministry of Education, Culture, Sports, Science and Technology of Japan; and a grant from Tsumura & Co. (Ibaraki, Japan).

References

1. Dray A, Urban L (1996) New pharmacological strategies for pain relief. Annu Rev Pharmacol Toxicol 36:253–280. doi:10.1146/annurev.pa.36.040196.001345
2. Portenoy RK, Ahmed E (2014) Principles of opioid use in cancer pain. J Clin Oncol 32 (16):1662–1670. doi:10.1200/jco.2013.52.5188
3. van den Beuken-van Everdingen MH, de Rijke JM, Kessels AG, Schouten HC, van Kleef M, Patijn J (2009) Quality of life and non-pain symptoms in patients with cancer. J Pain Symptom Manage 38(2):216–233. doi:10.1016/j.jpainsymman.2008.08.014
4. Lee JW, Lee WB, Kim W, Min BI, Lee H, Cho SH (2015) Traditional herbal medicine for cancer pain: a systematic review and meta-analysis. Complement Ther Med 23(2):265–274. doi:10.1016/j.ctim.2015.02.003
5. Running A, Seright T (2012) Integrative oncology: managing cancer pain with complementary and alternative therapies. Curr Pain Headache Rep 16(4):325–331. doi:10.1007/s11916-012-0275-x
6. Bao Y, Kong X, Yang L, Liu R, Shi Z, Li W, Hua B, Hou W (2014) Complementary and alternative medicine for cancer pain: an overview of systematic reviews. Evid Based Complement Alternat Med 2014:170396. doi:10.1155/2014/170396
7. Swarm RA, Abernethy AP, Anghelescu DL, Benedetti C, Buga S, Cleeland C, Deleon-Casasola OA, Eilers JG, Ferrell B, Green M, Janjan NA, Kamdar MM, Levy MH, Lynch M, McDowell RM, Moryl N, Nesbit SA, Paice JA, Rabow MW, Syrjala KL, Urba SG, Weinstein SM, Dwyer M, Kumar R (2013) Adult cancer pain. J Natl Compr Canc Netw 11(8):992–1022
8. Greer JA, Pirl WF, Jackson VA, Muzikansky A, Lennes IT, Heist RS, Gallagher ER, Temel JS (2012) Effect of early palliative care on chemotherapy use and end-of-life care in patients with metastatic non-small-cell lung cancer. J Clin Oncol 30(4):394–400. doi:10.1200/jco.2011.35.7996
9. Induru RR, Lagman RL (2011) Managing cancer pain: frequently asked questions. Cleve Clin J Med 78(7):449–464. doi:10.3949/ccjm.78a.10054
10. Cassileth B, Trevisan C, Gubili J (2007) Complementary therapies for cancer pain. Curr Pain Headache Rep 11(4):265–269
11. Eisenberg DM, Davis RB, Ettner SL, Appel S, Wilkey S, Van Rompay M, Kessler RC (1998) Trends in alternative medicine use in the United States, 1990–1997: results of a follow-up national survey. JAMA 280(18):1569–1575
12. Uezono Y, Miyano K, Sudo Y, Suzuki M, Shiraishi S, Terawaki K (2012) A review of traditional Japanese medicines and their potential mechanism of action. Curr Pharm Des 18 (31):4839–4853
13. Fujitsuka N, Uezono Y (2014) Rikkunshito, a ghrelin potentiator, ameliorates anorexia-cachexia syndrome. Front Pharmacol 5:271. doi:10.3389/fphar.2014.00271
14. Kono T, Shimada M, Yamamoto M, Kaneko A, Oomiya Y, Kubota K, Kase Y, Lee K, Uezono Y (2015) Complementary and synergistic therapeutic effects of compounds found in Kampo medicine: analysis of daikenchuto. Front Pharmacol 6:159. doi:10.3389/fphar.2015.00159
15. Yu F, Takahashi T, Moriya J, Kawaura K, Yamakawa J, Kusaka K, Itoh T, Morimoto S, Yamaguchi N, Kanda T (2006) Traditional Chinese medicine and Kampo: a review from the distant past for the future. J Int Med Res 34 (3):231–239
16. Mizukami K, Asada T, Kinoshita T, Tanaka K, Sonohara K, Nakai R, Yamaguchi K, Hanyu H, Kanaya K, Takao T, Okada M, Kudo S, Kotoku H, Iwakiri M, Kurita H, Miyamura T, Kawasaki Y, Omori K, Shiozaki K, Odawara T, Suzuki T, Yamada S, Nakamura Y, Toba K (2009) A randomized cross-over study of a traditional Japanese medicine (kampo), yokukansan, in the treatment of the behavioural and psychological symptoms of dementia. Int J Neuropsychopharmacol 12(2):191–199. doi:10.1017/s146114570800970x
17. Takeda H, Sadakane C, Hattori T, Katsurada T, Ohkawara T, Nagai K, Asaka M (2008) Rikkunshito, an herbal medicine, suppresses cisplatin-induced anorexia in rats via 5-HT2 receptor antagonism. Gastroenterology 134 (7):2004–2013. doi:10.1053/j.gastro.2008.02.078
18. Hattori T (2010) Rikkunshito and ghrelin. Int J Pept. doi:10.1155/2010/283549
19. Costigan M, Scholz J, Woolf CJ (2009) Neuropathic pain: a maladaptive response of the nervous system to damage. Annu Rev Neurosci 32:1–32. doi:10.1146/annurev.neuro.051508.135531
20. Auret K, Schug SA (2013) Pain management for the cancer patient—current practice and future developments. Best Pract Res Clin Anaesthesiol 27(4):545–561. doi:10.1016/j.bpa.2013.10.007

21. Juhl GI, Jensen TS, Norholt SE, Svensson P (2008) Central sensitization phenomena after third molar surgery: a quantitative sensory testing study. Eur J Pain 12(1):116–127. doi:10.1016/j.ejpain.2007.04.002
22. Huang J, Zhang X, McNaughton PA (2006) Inflammatory pain: the cellular basis of heat hyperalgesia. Curr Neuropharmacol 4 (3):197–206
23. Hucho T, Levine JD (2007) Signaling pathways in sensitization: toward a nociceptor cell biology. Neuron 55(3):365–376. doi:10.1016/j.neuron.2007.07.008
24. Woolf CJ, Salter MW (2000) Neuronal plasticity: increasing the gain in pain. Science 288 (5472):1765–1769
25. Michaud K, Bombardier C, Emery P (2007) Quality of life in patients with rheumatoid arthritis: does abatacept make a difference? Clin Exp Rheumatol 25(5 Suppl 46):S35–S45
26. Nielsen CS, Stubhaug A, Price DD, Vassend O, Czajkowski N, Harris JR (2008) Individual differences in pain sensitivity: genetic and environmental contributions. Pain 136 (1–2):21–29. doi:10.1016/j.pain.2007.06.008
27. Staud R, Rodriguez ME (2006) Mechanisms of disease: pain in fibromyalgia syndrome. Nat Clin Pract Rheumatol 2(2):90–98. doi:10.1038/ncprheum0091
28. Julien N, Goffaux P, Arsenault P, Marchand S (2005) Widespread pain in fibromyalgia is related to a deficit of endogenous pain inhibition. Pain 114(1–2):295–302. doi:10.1016/j.pain.2004.12.032
29. Staud R, Craggs JG, Perlstein WM, Robinson ME, Price DD (2008) Brain activity associated with slow temporal summation of C-fiber evoked pain in fibromyalgia patients and healthy controls. Eur J Pain 12 (8):1078–1089. doi:10.1016/j.ejpain.2008.02.002
30. Dworkin RH, Backonja M, Rowbotham MC, Allen RR, Argoff CR, Bennett GJ, Bushnell MC, Farrar JT, Galer BS, Haythornthwaite JA, Hewitt DJ, Loeser JD, Max MB, Saltarelli M, Schmader KE, Stein C, Thompson D, Turk DC, Wallace MS, Watkins LR, Weinstein SM (2003) Advances in neuropathic pain: diagnosis, mechanisms, and treatment recommendations. Arch Neurol 60(11):1524–1534. doi:10.1001/archneur.60.11.1524
31. Woolf CJ, Mannion RJ (1999) Neuropathic pain: aetiology, symptoms, mechanisms, and management. Lancet 353(9168):1959–1964. doi:10.1016/s0140-6736(99)01307-0
32. Kehlet H, Jensen TS, Woolf CJ (2006) Persistent postsurgical pain: risk factors and prevention. Lancet 367(9522):1618–1625. doi:10.1016/s0140-6736(06)68700-x
33. Cancer Research UK. http://www.cancerresearchuk.org/about-cancer/coping-with-cancer/coping-physically/pain/treatment/drugs/types-of-painkillers
34. Yamakawa J, Motoo Y, Moriya J, Ogawa M, Uenishi H, Akazawa S, Sasagawa T, Nishio M, Kobayashi J (2013) Significance of Kampo, traditional Japanese medicine, in supportive care of cancer patients. Evid Based Complement Alternat Med 2013:746486. doi:10.1155/2013/746486
35. Wilkes G (2007) Peripheral neuropathy related to chemotherapy. Semin Oncol Nurs 23 (3):162–173. doi:10.1016/j.soncn.2007.05.001
36. Lipton RB, Apfel SC, Dutcher JP, Rosenberg R, Kaplan J, Berger A, Einzig AI, Wiernik P, Schaumburg HH (1989) Taxol produces a predominantly sensory neuropathy. Neurology 39 (3):368–373
37. van Gerven JM, Moll JW, van den Bent MJ, Bontenbal M, van der Burg ME, Verweij J, Vecht CJ (1994) Paclitaxel (Taxol) induces cumulative mild neurotoxicity. Eur J Cancer 30A(8):1074–1077
38. Visovsky C, Collins M, Abbott L, Aschenbrenner J, Hart C (2007) Putting evidence into practice: evidence-based interventions for chemotherapy-induced peripheral neuropathy. Clin J Oncol Nurs 11(6):901–913. doi:10.1188/07.cjon.901-913
39. Hay JW (2002) Quality of life effects of chemotherapy-induced neuropathy in ovarian cancer. Am Soc Clin Oncol 21:222a
40. Hausheer FH, Schilsky RL, Bain S, Berghorn EJ, Lieberman F (2006) Diagnosis, management, and evaluation of chemotherapy-induced peripheral neuropathy. Semin Oncol 33(1):15–49. doi:10.1053/j.seminoncol.2005.12.010
41. Corse AM, Kuncl RW (1999) Peripheral neuropathy. In: Barker LR, Burton JR, Zieve PD (eds) Principles of ambulatory medicine, 5th edn. Williams & Wilkins, Baltimore
42. Oxaliplatin Prescribing Information (2013) Hospira Worldwide. http://www.drugs.com/pro/oxaliplatin.html.
43. Schroder S, Beckmann K, Franconi G, Meyer-Hamme G, Friedemann T, Greten HJ, Rostock M, Efferth T (2013) Can medical herbs stimulate regeneration or neuroprotection and treat neuropathic pain in chemotherapy-induced

peripheral neuropathy? Evid Based Complement Alternat Med 2013:423713. doi:10.1155/2013/423713

44. Uno T, Ohsawa I, Tokudome M, Sato Y (2005) Effects of goshajinkigan on insulin resistance in patients with type 2 diabetes. Diabetes Res Clin Pract 69(2):129–135. doi:10.1016/j.diabres.2004.11.017
45. Tawata M, Kurihara A, Nitta K, Iwase E, Gan N, Onaya T (1994) The effects of goshajinkigan, a herbal medicine, on subjective symptoms and vibratory threshold in patients with diabetic neuropathy. Diabetes Res Clin Pract 26(2):121–128
46. Usuki Y, Usuki S, Hommura S (1991) Successful treatment of a senile diabetic woman with cataract with goshajinkigan. Am J Chin Med 19 (3–4):259–263. doi:10.1142/s0192415x9100034x
47. Mizuno K, Kono T, Suzuki Y, Miyagi C, Omiya Y, Miyano K, Kase Y, Uezono Y (2014) Goshajinkigan, a traditional Japanese medicine, prevents oxaliplatin-induced acute peripheral neuropathy by suppressing functional alteration of TRP channels in rat. J Pharmacol Sci 125(1):91–98
48. Ushio S, Egashira N, Sada H, Kawashiri T, Shirahama M, Masuguchi K, Oishi R (2012) Goshajinkigan reduces oxaliplatin-induced peripheral neuropathy without affecting anti-tumour efficacy in rodents. Eur J Cancer 48(9):1407–1413. doi:10.1016/j.ejca.2011.08.009
49. Bahar MA, Andoh T, Ogura K, Hayakawa Y, Saiki I, Kuraishi Y (2013) Herbal medicine goshajinkigan prevents paclitaxel-induced mechanical allodynia without impairing antitumor activity of paclitaxel. Evid Based Complement Alternat Med 2013:849754. doi:10.1155/2013/849754
50. Rao JK, Mihaliak K, Kroenke K, Bradley J, Tierney WM, Weinberger M (1999) Use of complementary therapies for arthritis among patients of rheumatologists. Ann Intern Med 131(6):409–416
51. Kono T, Suzuki Y, Mizuno K, Miyagi C, Omiya Y, Sekine H, Mizuhara Y, Miyano K, Kase Y, Uezono Y (2015) Preventive effect of oral goshajinkigan on chronic oxaliplatin-induced hypoesthesia in rats. Sci Rep 5:16078. doi:10.1038/srep16078
52. Suzuki Y, Goto K, Ishige A, Komatsu Y, Kamei J (1999) Antinociceptive effect of Gosha-jinkigan, a Kampo medicine, in streptozotocin-induced diabetic mice. Jpn J Pharmacol 79 (2):169–175
53. Murayama M, Mori T, Bando H, Amiya T (1991) Studies on the constituents of Aconitum species. IX. The pharmacological properties of pyro-type aconitine alkaloids, components of processed aconite powder 'kako-bushi-matsu': analgesic, antiinflammatory and acute toxic activities. J Ethnopharmacol 35(2):159–164
54. Shibata K, Sugawara T, Fujishita K, Shinozaki Y, Matsukawa T, Suzuki T, Koizumi S (2011) The astrocyte-targeted therapy by Bushi for the neuropathic pain in mice. PLoS One 6(8): e23510. doi:10.1371/journal.pone.0023510
55. Andoh T, Kitamura R, Fushimi H, Komatsu K, Shibahara N, Kuraishi Y (2014) Effects of goshajinkigan, hachimijiogan, and rokumigan on mechanical allodynia induced by Paclitaxel in mice. J Tradit Complement Med 4 (4):293–297. doi:10.4103/2225-4110.128906
56. Li H, Wang Q (2004) Evaluation of free hydroxyl radical scavenging activities of some Chinese herbs by capillary zone electrophoresis with amperometric detection. Anal Bioanal Chem 378(7):1801–1805. doi:10.1007/s00216-004-2509-1
57. Zhu YZ, Huang SH, Tan BK, Sun J, Whiteman M, Zhu YC (2004) Antioxidants in Chinese herbal medicines: a biochemical perspective. Nat Prod Rep 21(4):478–489. doi:10.1039/b304821g
58. Imai A, Horibe S, Fuseya S, Iida K, Takagi H, Tamaya T (1995) Possible evidence that the herbal medicine shakuyaku-kanzo-to decreases prostaglandin levels through suppressing arachidonate turnover in endometrium. J Med 26(3–4):163–174
59. Yamamoto K, Hoshiai H, Noda K (2001) Effects of shakuyaku-kanzo-to on muscle pain from combination chemotherapy with paclitaxel and carboplatin. Gynecol Oncol 81 (2):333–334. doi:10.1006/gyno.2001.6168
60. Hyodo T, Taira T, Kumakura M, Yamamoto S, Yoshida K, Uchida T, Sakai T, Endo T, Baba S, Hidai H (2002) The immediate effect of Shakuyaku-kanzo-to, traditional Japanese herbal medicine, for muscular cramps during maintenance hemodialysis. Nephron 90(2):240
61. Hidaka T, Shima T, Nagira K, Ieki M, Nakamura T, Aono Y, Kuraishi Y, Arai T, Saito S (2009) Herbal medicine Shakuyaku-kanzo-to reduces paclitaxel-induced painful peripheral neuropathy in mice. Eur J Pain 13(1):22–27. doi:10.1016/j.ejpain.2008.03.003
62. Monji A, Takita M, Samejima T, Takaishi T, Hashimoto K, Matsunaga H, Oda M, Sumida Y, Mizoguchi Y, Kato T, Horikawa H, Kanba S (2009) Effect of yokukansan on the behavioral and psychological symptoms of dementia in

elderly patients with Alzheimer's disease. Prog Neuropsychopharmacol Biol Psychiatry 33 (2):308–311. doi:10.1016/j.pnpbp.2008.12.008

63. Matsumoto K, Zhao Q, Niu Y, Fujiwara H, Tanaka K, Sasaki-Hamada S, Oka J (2013) Kampo formulations, chotosan, and yokukansan, for dementia therapy: existing clinical and preclinical evidence. J Pharmacol Sci 122 (4):257–269
64. Okamoto H, Iyo M, Ueda K, Han C, Hirasaki Y, Namiki T (2014) Yokukan-san: a review of the evidence for use of this Kampo herbal formula in dementia and psychiatric conditions. Neuropsychiatr Dis Treat 10:1727–1742. doi:10.2147/ndt.s6525
65. Iwasaki K, Kosaka K, Mori H, Okitsu R, Furukawa K, Manabe Y, Yoshita M, Kanamori A, Ito N, Wada K, Kitayama M, Horiguchi J, Yamaguchi S, Shin Takayama S, Fukuhara R, Ouma S, Nakano S, Hashimoto M, Kinoshita T (2012) Improvement indelusions and hallucinations in patients with dementia with Lewy bodies upon administration of yokukansan, a traditional Japanese medicine. Psychogeriatrics 12(4):235–241
66. Ebisawa S, Andoh T, Shimada Y (2015) Yokukansan improves mechanical allodynia through the regulation of interleukin-6 expression in the spinal cord in mice with neuropathic pain. Evid Based Complement Alternat Med 2015:870687. doi:10.1155/2015/870687
67. Lalla RV, Peterson DE (2005) Oral mucositis. Dent Clin North Am 49(1):167–184. doi:10.1016/j.cden.2004.07.009, ix
68. Treister N, Sonis S (2007) Mucositis: biology and management. Curr Opin Otolaryngol Head Neck Surg 15(2):123–129. doi:10.1097/MOO.0b013e3280523ad6
69. Kono T, Kaneko A, Matsumoto C, Miyagi C, Ohbuchi K, Mizuhara Y, Miyano K, Uezono Y (2014) Multitargeted effects of hangeshashinto for treatment of chemotherapy-induced oral mucositis on inducible prostaglandin E2 production in human oral keratinocytes. Integr Cancer Ther 13(5):435–445. doi:10.1177/1534735413520035
70. Duncan GG, Epstein JB, Tu D, El Sayed S, Bezjak A, Ottaway J, Pater J (2005) Quality of life, mucositis, and xerostomia from radiotherapy for head and neck cancers: a report from the NCIC CTG HN2 randomized trial of an antimicrobial lozenge to prevent mucositis. Head Neck 27(5):421–428. doi:10.1002/hed.20162
71. Mori K, Kondo T, Kamiyama Y, Kano Y, Tominaga K (2003) Preventive effect of Kampo medicine (Hangeshashin-to) against irinotecan-induced diarrhea in advanced non-small-cell lung cancer. Cancer Chemother Pharmacol 51(5):403–406. doi:10.1007/s00280-003-0585-0
72. Nakazono Y, Ara T, Fujinami Y, Hattori T, Wang PL (2010) Preventive effects of a kampo medicine, hangeshashinto on inflammatory responses in lipopolysaccharide-treated human gingival fibroblasts. J Hard Tissue Biol 19(1):43–50
73. Kase Y, Hayakawa T, Aburada M, Komatsu Y, Kamataki T (1997) Preventive effects of Hange-shashin-to on irinotecan hydrochloride-caused diarrhea and its relevance to the colonic prostaglandin E2 and water absorption in the rat. Jpn J Pharmacol 75(4):407–413
74. Kase Y, Saitoh K, Yuzurihara M, Ishige A, Komatsu Y (1998) Effects of Hange-shashin-to on cholera toxin-induced fluid secretion in the small intestine of rats. Biol Pharm Bull 21 (2):117–120
75. Kase Y, Saitoh K, Makino B, Hashimoto K, Ishige A, Komatsu Y (1999) Relationship between the antidiarrhoeal effects of Hange-Shashin-To and its active components. Phytother Res 13(6):468–473
76. Kono T, Satomi M, Chisato N, Ebisawa Y, Suno M, Asama T, Karasaki H, Matsubara K, Furukawa H (2010) Topical application of hangeshashinto (TJ-14) in the treatment of chemotherapy-induced oral mucositis. World J Oncol 1(6):232–235. doi:10.4021/wjon263w
77. Matsuda C, Munemoto Y, Mishima H, Nagata N, Oshiro M, Kataoka M, Sakamoto J, Aoyama T, Morita S, Kono T (2015) Double-blind, placebo-controlled, randomized phase II study of TJ-14 (Hangeshashinto) for infusional fluorinated-pyrimidine-based colorectal cancer chemotherapy-induced oral mucositis. Cancer Chemother Pharmacol 76(1):97–103. doi:10.1007/s00280-015-2767-y
78. Giaever I, Keese CR (1991) Micromotion of mammalian cells measured electrically. Proc Natl Acad Sci U S A 88(17):7896–7900
79. Miyano K, Sudo Y, Yokoyama A, Hisaoka-Nakashima K, Morioka N, Takebayashi M, Nakata Y, Higami Y, Uezono Y (2014) History of the G protein-coupled receptor (GPCR) assays from traditional to a state-of-the-art biosensor assay. J Pharmacol Sci 126(4):302–309. doi:10.1254/jphs.14R13CP
80. Hisaoka-Nakashima K, Miyano K, Matsumoto C, Kajitani N, Abe H, Okada-Tsuchioka M, Yokoyama A, Uezono Y, Morioka N, Nakata

Y, Takebayashi M (2015) Tricyclic antidepressant amitriptyline-induced glial cell line-derived neurotrophic factor production involves pertussis toxin-sensitive galphai/o activation in astroglial cells. J Biol Chem 290 (22):13678–13691. doi:10.1074/jbc.M114.622415

81. Fujitsuka N, Asakawa A, Morinaga A, Amitani MS, Amitani H, Katsuura G, Sawada Y, Sudo Y, Uezono Y, Mochiki E, Sakata I, Sakai T, Hanazaki K, Yada T, Yakabi K, Sakuma E, Ueki T, Niijima A, Nakagawa K, Okubo N, Takeda H, Asaka M, Inui A (2016) Increased ghrelin signaling prolongs survival in mouse models of human aging through activation of sirtuin1. Mol Psychiatry. doi:10.1038/mp.2015.220

82. Fujitsuka N, Asakawa A, Uezono Y, Minami K, Yamaguchi T, Niijima A, Yada T, Maejima Y, Sedbazar U, Sakai T, Hattori T, Kase Y, Inui A (2011) Potentiation of ghrelin signaling attenuates cancer anorexia-cachexia and prolongs survival. Transl Psychiatry 1:e23. doi:10.1038/tp.2011.25

Chapter 4

Gastrointestinal Surgery and Herbal Medicine, Including Rikkunshito

Yasuhiro Miyazaki, Shuji Takiguchi, Tsuyoshi Takahashi, Yukinori Kurokawa, Tomoki Makino, Makoto Yamasaki, Kiyokazu Nakajima, Masaki Mori, and Yuichiro Doki

Abstract

Anatomical and functional changes occur inevitably after gastrointestinal surgeries for several diseases such as malignancies, functional disorders of the digestive tract, postoperative complications such as bowel obstruction, and inflammatory bowel diseases. Since such changes induce various digestive symptoms and complications, it is indispensable for gastrointestinal surgeons to pay attention to not only curability, but also patients' quality of life.

Recently, several reports including randomized controlled trial, which investigated the clinical effects of herbal medicine to postoperative digestive symptoms, have been published. In this chapter, focused on the gastrointestinal surgeries, current evidences with regard to herbal medicine therapy in this field are reviewed and summarized.

Key words Gastrointestinal surgery, Gastrectomy, Colectomy, Ileus, Kampo, Herbal medicine, Rikkunshito, Daikenchuto, Ghrelin, Quality of life

1 Consideration of Gastrointestinal Surgeries and Herbal Medicine Therapy

Several herbal medicines are well-known to act on digestive tract, and they are often prescribed for treatment of many gastrointestinal diseases, such as functional dyspepsia [1], chronic constipation, and irritable bowel syndrome [2]. In addition, many recent reports including randomized controlled trial, which investigated the pleural clinical effects of herbal medicine to postoperative digestive symptoms, adverse events of chemotherapy in the associated field with gastrointestinal (GI) surgeries and digestive tract malignancies, have been published.

Here, herbal medicine therapy for patients with gastrointestinal surgeries is summarized.

Akio Inui (ed.), *Herbal Medicines: New Horizons*, Methods in Pharmacology and Toxicology, DOI 10.1007/978-1-4939-4002-8_4, © Springer Science+Business Media New York 2016

2 Surgery-Related Disorders and Herbal Medicine

Gastrointestinal (GI) surgeries are performed aimed at cure for several diseases such as malignancies, benignancy (such as functional disorders of the digestive tract, adhesive short bowel obstruction), and inflammatory bowel diseases, although anatomical and functional changes inevitably occur due to these procedures. These changes can involve a number of different obstacles for patients, such as stenosis, ileus, deep vein thrombus, digestive symptoms (nausea, vomiting, anorexia, diarrhea, constipation, and so on), so-called postgastrectomy symptoms [3], and others. The type and degree of various postoperative complications caused by these changes depend on the primary diseases, surgical site, and procedure. Here, the authors divided GI surgeries to two categories: upper GI surgery and lower GI surgery. According to these categories, treatments using herbal medicine for postoperative complications and symptoms are stated.

2.1 Upper GI Surgery

Various types of operations relevant to the upper GI tract are performed, such as esophagectomy, gastrectomy, bypass, pancreatoduodenectomy, and others. No bariatric surgery is picked up in this chapter since those obese patients' backgrounds are disease-specific and particular compared to other diseases.

Gastric cancer (GC) remains a major health problem, especially in eastern countries, although the mortality rate has steadily decreased in recent years. The primary treatment for GC is surgery, which corresponds to gastrectomy. Although patients may be rendered free of gastric cancer by gastrectomy, they will suffer from "post-gastrectomy syndrome (PGS)", which includes weight loss, dumping syndrome, stasis syndrome, reflux esophagitis, alkaline gastritis, and, finally, malnutrition [4, 5].

Several causes of these postoperative complications are derived from hormonal and neurological changes. Gastrectomy affects the digestive hormones such as ghrelin, motilin, vasoactive intestinal polypeptide, leptin, somatostatin, and ghrelin, resulting in impaired digestive function [6].

It is, of course, important to ameliorate PGS to restore postoperative quality of life (QOLQuality of life (QOL)). Currently, a number of herbal medicines are manufactured on a modern industrial scale under strict quality controls and prescribed as complementary and alternative medicine amongst patients with gastrectomy and esophagectomy [7]. In this section, representative herbal medicine therapy is presented and recent evidences of clinical trials are summarized (Table 1).

2.1.1 Rikkunshito (RKT)

Rikkunshito (RKT)Rikkunshito (RKT)Rikkunshito (RKT) (Tsumura, Tokyo, Japan), a traditional herbal medicine, is prepared by

Table 1
Clinical trials of herbal medicine for patients undergoing upper gastrointestinal surgery (GI)

	Herbal medicine	Prescription	Procedures and diseases	Study design and scale	Results	Author (year)
Upper GI	RKT	7.5 g/day, 4 weeks	PPG	• Crossover study • 11 patients	1. Improvement of stasis-related symptoms in the questionnaire survey 2. Accelerated gastric emptying of solid meals, not liquid in the scintigraphy	[19]
		7.5 g/day, 4 weeks	LDG LTG	• Single-arm • 4-week administration and 4-week withdrawal of RKT • 25 patients	1. Significant increase of the mean ratio of acyl-/total ghrelin level 2. Improvement of total DAUGS score and several symptom scores	[21]
		7.5 g/day, 4 weeks	OPG	• Prospective, single-arm study • 18 patients	1. Significant bodyweight increase 2. Ghrelin level had no practical impact of clinical results 3. GSRS score improvement	[43]
	DKT	15 g/day, 2 weeks	OTG with JP	• Crossover study • 14 patients	1. Reduction of stasis-related symptoms by DKT 2. Accelerated emptying of both and liquid meals from pouch by DKT 3. Increase of pouch contraction by DKT	[20]
		7.5 g/day, 3 months	OTG	• Prospective RCT • DKT ($n = 41$) and control ($n = 40$)	1. Improvement of bowel movements, stool properties, and bowel gas 2. No significant differences in QOL compared to control	[26]

RKT rikkunshito, *DKT* daikentuto, *PPG* pyloruspreserving gastrectomy, *LDG* laparoscopic distal gastrectomy, *LTG* laparoscopic total gastrectomy, *OPG*; open proximal gastrectomy, *OTG* open total gastrectomy, *JP* jejunal pouch

compounding eight herbal medicines: *Ginseng radix* (component ratio = 4), *Atractyloidis lanceae rhizoma* (=4), *Hoelen* (=4), *Pinelliae tuber* (=4), *Aurantii nobilis percarpium* (=2), *Zizyphi fructus* (=2), *Glycyrrhizae radix* (=1), and *Zingiberis rhizome* (=0.5). RKT has been traditionally used for dyspeptic symptoms, gastroesophageal reflux disease (GERD), chemotherapy-induced dyspepsia and anorexia (see Chap. 3.5.1) [1, 8]. Moreover, recent evidences have shown the efficacy for PGS.

In animal experiments, RKT is reported to ameliorate gastric distension via a nitric oxide (NO)-mediated pathway and improves delayed gastric emptying [9]. Other reports documented the dual action on the stomach which corresponded to relaxation of the proximal stomach and increased contractions of the distal stomach [1, 10]. In addition, most recent findings revealed the notable ability of RKT for stimulated secretion of ghrelin [11–13] and enhanced ghrelin's activity due to several mechanisms such as the ability of inhibiting the ghrelin-degrading enzyme in rodents and humans [12, 14] (see Chap. 10). For the stated effect-efficacy above ("prokinetic effects" and "ghrelin enhancer"), RKT is considered to be a very useful herbal medicine for the treatment of PGS. Three human clinical trials for the treatment of PGS existed and reviewed here.

2.1.2 RKT Effect on Stasis in Patients after Pylorus-Preserving Gastrectomy

Pylorus-preserving gastrectomy (PPG) [15] has been applied to early gastric cancer to avoid the dumping syndrome and to reduce bile reflux and also maintain normal mucosal integrity of the remnant stomach [16, 17]. However, in some patients, undesirable signs and symptoms, including residual food in the remnant stomach, epigastric fullness, nausea, and vomiting due to delayed gastric emptying still exists [18]. Others may use medication, although there is no evidence.

Takahashi et al. considered that RKT having prokinetic effects may decrease postoperative symptoms due to delayed gastric emptying after PPGPylorus-preserving gastrectomy (PPG) and conducted the clinical trial [19]. Eleven patients who underwent PPG for early gastric cancer over 1 year after surgery enrolled to this study. Study design was a crossover study due to the limited number of patients. Patients in group A took RKT 7.5 g/day before each meal for 4 weeks (on-treatment), after which the RKT was discontinued for 4 weeks (off-treatment). In contrast, group B patients initially started from the off-treatment stage. After that, on-treatment stage was performed. The authors evaluated the patients' QOL using the gastrointestinal Quality-of-Life Index (GIQLI) [20] and the gastric emptying of liquids and solids with emptying study (dual-phase scintigraphy).

The GIQLI scores for the on-treatment period (median score 118, range 71–134) were not different from those for the off-treatment period (122 (85–135)). Stasis-related symptom scores graded by the modified Visick scoring system were significantly decreased from 3.9 ± 4.4 during the off-treatment period to 2.7 ± 3.1 during the on-treatment period. In contrast, the Sigstad dumping scores for the on-treatment period was not statistically different from those for off-treatment period ($p = 0.355$).

Dual-phase scintigraphy showed the significant difference of only solid clearance, not liquid clearance between on- and off-treatment. Quantitative evaluation in these data revealed that solid-phase radioactivity during the on-treatment period was more rapidly evacuated from the remnant stomach than during the off-treatment period ($p = 0.0003$), whereas liquid-phase radioactivity showed no significant difference between the two periods (Fig. 1).

The authors concluded that RKT improved gastric emptying especially for solid contents and ameliorated PGS after PPG. Though in small quantity, this study revealed the prokinetic effect of RKT not only in the subjective symptoms using the questionnaire but also in the objective assessment with scintigraphy. As for the gastric motility, at least, RKT is considered to play an important role to alleviate PGS.

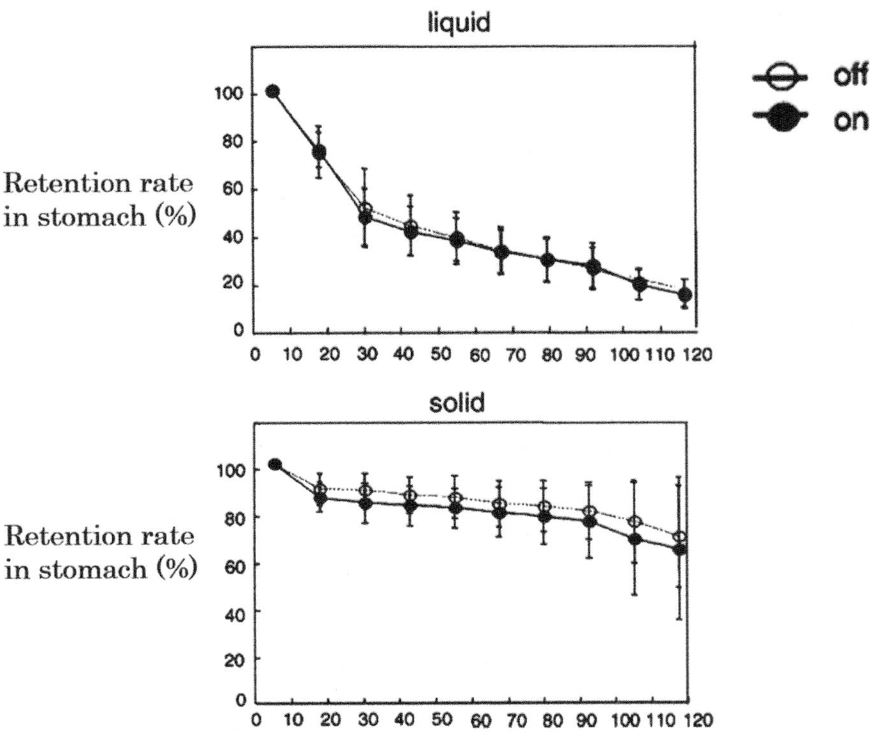

Fig. 1 Emptying of the remnant stomach after pylorus-preserving gastrectomy. Solid-phase radioactivity during the on-treatment period was more rapidly evacuated from the remnant stomach than during the off-treatment period ($p = 0.0003$), although liquid-phase radioactivity showed no significance

2.1.3 RKT Effect on Post-gastrectomy Syndromes as Ghrelin Enhancer

Takiguchi et al. reported the clinical trial to investigate the effect of RKT on PGS and ghrelin levels in early gastric cancer patients after gastrectomy [21]. Twenty-five patients (16 males and 9 females) who had undergone laparoscopic gastrectomy (17 distal gastrectomy, 8 total gastrectomy) 6 months to 5 years after surgery received RKT 7.5 g/day before each meal for 4 weeks, and a drug withdrawal period was established for the next 4 weeks.

Changes in gastrointestinal hormones, including ghrelin, and appetite visual analog scale scores were measured, and QOL was assessed by using the European Organization for Research and Treatment of Cancer core questionnaire QLQ-C30 [22]. The Dysfunction After Upper Gastrointestinal Surgery for Cancer (DAUGS) scoring system [23] was used to evaluate gastrointestinal symptoms after gastrectomy.

Hormonal studies showed that the mean ratio of the acyl-/total ghrelin concentration increased significantly after RKT administration (Pre: 7.8 ± 2.1, 4 weeks: 10.5 ± 1.7 %, $p = 0.0026$), although no statistical changes due to RKT administration with regard to nutritional status were observed. Serial changes in the ratio of the active/total ghrelin concentration were shown in Fig. 2. Administration and withdrawal of RKT increased and decreased the ratio of the acyl-/total ghrelin concentration significantly, although they had no significant influence on the concentrations themselves of acyl- and desacyl-ghrelin.

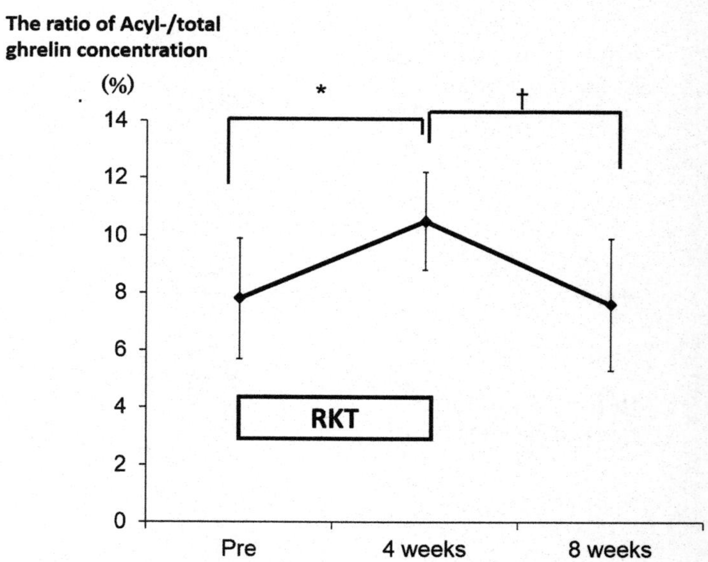

Fig. 2 Serial changes of the ratio of acyl-/total ghrelin concentration. Administration and withdrawal of RKT increased and decreased the ratio of the acyl-/total ghrelin concentration significantly (paired t test, Pre vs. 4 weeks $^{*}p = 0.0026$, 4 vs. 8 weeks, $^{\dagger}p = 0.0015$)

QOL assessments revealed total DAUGS score, as well as the scores reflecting limited activity due to decreased food consumption, reflux symptoms, dumping symptoms, and nausea and vomiting significantly improved after RKT administration. As to the results of QLQ-C30 score, almost all types of scores showed no statistical differences between administration and withdrawal of RKT. With regard to only the functional status, patients scored better after RKT administration and worse after withdrawal of RKT (pre: 86 ± 11, 4 weeks: 96 ± 7, $p < 0.01$; 8 weeks: 86 ± 9, $p < 0.01$).

In the present study, the administration of RKT did not increase the ghrelin concentration per se, which was different from previous study with healthy volunteers. Author's consideration with regard to influence to ghrelin due to RKT administration was described that it could be attributed to gastrectomy, because ghrelin is predominantly secreted by gastric endocrine cells. Previous study has already reported a persistent decline of serum ghrelin and bodyweight was commonly observed after total gastrectomy [24]. Therefore, authors documented that it is unlikely that RKT attenuates PGS through eliciting ghrelin secretion from the stomach. Conversely, even in this study, administration of RKT showed the elevation of ratio of acyl-/total ghrelin concentration as enhancement of ghrelin activity. The mechanism of this phenomenon was suggested to inhibition of ghrelin degrading enzyme due to the components of RKT, 10-gigerol [14].

2.1.4 RKT Effect on Post-gastrectomy Syndromes After Proximal Gastrectomy as Ghrelin Enhancer

Gunji et al. reported the effects of RKT on the PGS and plasma ghrelin levels in patients with gastric cancer who had undergone proximal gastrectomy (PG) [43]. In this study, 19 patients over 6 months after PG were enrolled and plasma ghrelin levels, bodyweight, appetite, and Gastrointestinal Symptom Rating Scale (GSRS) scores [25] were examined before and after 4-week administration of RKT.

The patients' bodyweight increased significantly after the administration of RKT (the average at baseline and after treatment; 56.8 and 57.2 kg, respectively ($p = 0.008$)). In the subgroup analysis, the mean total GSRS score improved significantly from 2.6 ± 0.6 before the administration of rikkunshito to 1.9 ± 0.7 after administration because of the significant improvement in the subscale scores for abdominal pain, acid reflux, diarrhea, and constipation. Similar to the Takiguchi et al. report, neither their appetite nor plasma acylated and deacylated ghrelin levels were significantly affected.

Their conclusions were that RKT significantly improved PGS, and its effect was possibly independent of the plasma ghrelin levels.

2.1.5 Daikenchuto (DKT)

Daikenchuto (DKTDaikenchuto (DKT)) extract powder is a mixture of dried extracts from ginger root, ginseng, and zanthoxylum fruit at a ratio of 5:3:2, by weight. DKTDaikenchuto (DKT) is one of the popular herbal medicines which are prescribed for abdominal pain and distension, for example postoperative ileus, after laparotomy. Although many experiments in vitro and vivo have already revealed the mechanisms of DKT, for example, enhancing gastrointestinal motility and suppressing postoperative inflammation (see Chap. 11), two human clinical trials of DKT for patients with gastrectomy are summarized, in this section.

2.1.6 Effects of DKT on Intestinal Motility After Total Gastrectomy

Small-scale prospective randomized trial for investigating the effects of DKT after total gastrectomy was reported by Akamaru et al. [26]. In this trial, patients with gastric cancer scheduled for a total gastrectomy were randomly assigned before surgery to receive either no treatment ($n = 40$; control group) or DKT (7.5 g/day, t.i.d.) for 3 months ($n = 41$) postoperatively. Stool attributes, the quantity of bowel gas, patients' QOL using GSRS, and the incidence of postoperative ileus were evaluated.

Significant differences were observed in the point of stool-related items and the quantity of bowel gas only during the hospital stay. The number of stools per day in the DKT group and controls was 1.1 ± 0.6 versus 0.8 ± 0.4, respectively ($p = 0.037$). Stool consistencies (Bristol scale ratings [27]) were 3.7 ± 0.8 vs. 3.1 ± 0.8, respectively ($p = 0.041$). The DKT group showed significant reductions in gas volume scores, calculated from abdominal radiographs, at 7 days, 1 month, and 3 months after surgery. The groups did not show significant differences in QOL or in the incidence of postoperative ileus.

The authors concluded that not any superiority in the DKT group was observed over untreated group in terms of clinical significance, although DKT improved bowel movements, stool properties, and bowel gas.

2.1.7 Effects of DKT on Stasis of Patients with Jejunal Pouch Interposition After Total Gastrectomy

Intestinal motility after gastric surgery frequently is disturbed and results in postoperative intestinal symptoms and poor QOL, especially for intestinal pouch reconstruction. Endo et al. reported the clinical trial to investigate the effects of DKT on intestinal motility of jejunal pouch and postoperative QOL of patients [20]. Seventeen patients who underwent total gastrectomy with jejunal pouch interposition for gastric cancer were enrolled. The patients were assigned randomly to the crossover study with or without 15 g/day of DKT.

Questionnaires, scintigraphy tests at the end of each treatment period, and a manometric study revealed the improvement of stasis-related symptoms by DKT ($p = 0.032$) and acceleration of emptying of both liquid ($p < 0.01$) and solid ($p = 0.015$) meals from the pouch due to DKT. In addition, the pouch showed bursts of contractions, which were increased significantly by oral intake of DKT ($p = 0.028$).

Combined with the reports of Akamaru et al. described above, effects of DKT on intestinal motility for patients with gastrectomy may be beneficial for elevated function of intestinal reconstruction, not PGS.

2.2 Lower GI Surgeries and Other Surgeries

In contrast to upper GI surgeries, bowel manipulation is mandatory in lower GI surgeries, which lead to intestinal adhesion. Therefore, most popular and dealt with surgery-related complications of lower GI surgeries is postoperative ileus (POI) including adhesive small bowel obstruction (ASBO), although POI occurs, of course, after other major abdominal surgeries including upper GI surgeries. A previous report showed that intestinal obstruction due to adhesion occurs in approximately 11 % of patients with total colectomy [28]. Despite the use of the enhanced recovery after surgery protocol that is supposed to stimulate and enhance gut motility [29], POI has been a major complication that remained to be solved.

In fact, in current reports, herbal medicine for patients who undergo lower GI surgeries and others including hepatectomy and pancreatoduodenectomy is DKT for prevention and treatment of POI and ASBO. In this section, recent evidences of clinical trials with regard to DKT in lower GI surgeries are presented (Table 2).

2.2.1 Daikenchuto (DKT)

Several animal studies reported that DKT administration into proximal small intestine dose dependently increased the motility of the duodenum and jejunum in dogs [30]. Prokinetic effect of DKT on intestinal dysmotility is derived from cholinergic and serotonergic mechanisms since DKT stimulated acetylcholine release in porcine ileal smooth muscle [31]. Prokinetic effects on ascending colon emptying were also reported in healthy adult human [32].

2.2.2 Clinical Effects of DKT on Gastrointestinal Function and Surgical Inflammatory Response Following Colon Surgery

Katsuno et al. reported a randomized, double-blind, multicenter, placebo-controlled study to determine whether DKT accelerates recovery of gastrointestinal function in patients who underwent "open" colectomy for colon cancer [33]. In this trial, patients received either placebo or Daikenchuto (15.0 g/day, t.i.d) between post-operative day (POD) 2 and POD 8. Primary endpoints included time to first bowel movement (BM), frequency of bowel movement, and stool form. Secondary endpoints were evaluation of QOL according to GSRS and Functional Assessment of Cancer Therapy-Colorectal FACT-C scale, serum C-reactive protein (CRP) levels, and the incidence of POI.

Finally, 336 patients (174 DKT group, 162 placebo group) were analyzed. Unfortunately, this study did not demonstrate the clinical benefits of DKT adequately. Concretely described, the time to first BM (Cox proportional hazards model, Log rank test: $p = 0.921$) was not different between the DKT and the control groups. As for frequency of BM, both groups demonstrated almost

Table 2
Clinical trials of herbal medicine for patients undergoing lower gastrointestinal (GI) surgery

	Herbal medicine	Prescription	Target procedures and diseases	Study design and scale	Results	Author (year)
Lower GI and others	DKT	15 g/day, 7 days	Colon surgery	• Prospective RCT, placebo-controlled, double-blind, multicenter • DKT ($n = 174$) and placebo ($n = 162$)	1. No significant differences in the time to first bowel movement, frequency of bowel movement, and other endpoints 2. Significantly greater number of hard stools in placebo than in the DKT group	[33]
		7.5 g/day, from 2 days prior to surgery until discharge	OC	• Prospective RCT • DKT ($n = 26$) and control ($n = 25$)	1. Significant faster time until first flatus, bowel movement, and colonic transit time in DKT group than control	[34]
		7.5 g/day, 7 days	LC	• Prospective comparative study • DKT ($n = 15$) and control ($n = 15$)	1. Significant lower CRP level on POD3 in DKT than control 2. Significant shorter the time until fast flatus in DKT than control	[35]
		7.5–15 g/day, at least 1 year	Bowel resection and Crohn's disease	• Retrospective observational study • Postoperative DKT(+) ($n = 100$), DKT(−) ($n = 158$)	Lower 3-year reoperation rate in the DKT group than in the non-DKT group	[36]

DKT daikentuto, *OC* open colectomy, *LC* laparoscopic colectomy

similar serial changes of number of BM after surgery. Rather, the frequency of BM in the DKT group at POD8 was significantly lower than that in the control group ($p = 0.024$). In addition, no significant differences with regard to all of secondary endpoints were observed.

The authors considered that, based on the negative results, open surgery (laparotomy), intestinal manipulation, and exposure to air may cause deterioration of gastrointestinal motility to a greater extent than expected. Additionally, further considerations with regard to the dose, method, and duration of DKT administration in open surgery, not laparoscopic surgery, are required for future clinical trials.

Yaegashi et al. reported the effect of DKT on preventing POI following open colectomy, a small-scale randomized trial [34]. DKT group (7.5 g/day, 2.5 g t.i.d, $n = 26$) had significantly faster time until fast flatus (67.5 ± 13.6 h) and bowel movement (82.9 ± 17.8 h) and colonic transit time (91.9 ± 19.8 h) which were measured using radiopaque markers and abdominal radiograph than control group ($n = 15$), (77.9 ± 11.8, 99.5 ± 18.9, 115.2 ± 12.8 h).

In the recent comparative study, Yoshikawa et al. showed the effect of DKT on the postoperative inflammation following laparoscopic colectomy [35]. Thirty patients who underwent laparoscopic colectomy for colorectal carcinoma were divided into two groups: a DKT group ($n = 15$) and a control group ($n = 15$). DKT group took 7.5 g/day of DKT from POD1 to POD7. Inflammation parameters, such as body temperature, WBC count, lymphocyte count, and CRP level were evaluated and compared between the two groups.

Although patients' mean age of DKT group and D3 lymph node dissection were significantly younger and more often than control group, the CRP level on the POD3 and the time until fast flatus in the DKT group were significantly lower and shorter than the control group (4.6 ± 0.6 vs. 8.3 ± 1.1 mg/dl, 1.8 ± 0.5 vs. 2.7 ± 0.5 days).

The conclusion of this study was that postoperative DKT administration significantly suppressed the CRP level and shortened the time until flatus. This is the first report that both of DKT effects, such as anti-inflammatory and enhancing gastrointestinal motility, were shown in human clinical trial. However, attention needs to be paid to interpretation of these results in this study since it was a non-randomized, small-scale study. Therefore, further large-scale, randomized comparative study will be warranted.

Kanazawa et al. reported that continuous administration of DKT over 1 year after surgery for Crohn's disease was a clinically useful and feasible maintenance therapy for the prevention of postoperative reoperation by the anti-inflammatory effect of DKT [36].

Since this study was a retrospective study and included several surgical procedures and a variety of patients' demographics, the results should be interpreted with caution.

2.2.3 Postoperative Ileus and Other GI Surgeries (Table 3)

One article of a placebo-controlled very small-scale randomized study which investigated the direct effect of DKT on POI after various abdominal surgeries existed [37]. Twenty-four patients with POI were randomly assigned to 15 g/day of oral DKT group ($n = 13$) or placebo group ($n = 11$). The results were that the frequency of surgical operation for POI was significantly lower in the DKT group ($n = 5$) than in the placebo group ($n = 10$). Another study as a propensity score analysis, which was a retrospective observational study using the diagnosis procedure combination (DPC) inpatient database in Japan, was performed to evaluate the effect of DKT on patients with POI following colorectal cancer surgery who received long-tube decompression (LTD) with or without DKT administration [38]. Although success rates of LTD were not significantly different between DKT users and non-users (84.7 vs. 78.5 %, $p = 0.224$), DKT users demonstrated shorter duration of LTD (8 vs. 10 days, $p = 0.018$) and shorter duration between long-tube insertion and discharge (23 vs. 25 days, $p = 0.018$).

No high-quality evidences, such as the results of prospective randomized study with sufficient sample sizes, can prove the clinical significance of DKT against POI. However, several published data suggest the usefulness of DKT on POI.

Since all of abdominal surgeries often induce disturbance of bowel movement and POI, several investigators have focused on the effect of DKT even in hepatobiliary and pancreatic surgeries other than GI surgeries.

Three articles reported the results with regard to the effects of DKT after hepatic resection [39–41]. Most current article among them was the multicenter, phase III trial in Japan with regard to DKT administration for patients with hepatectomy [41]. A total of 231 patients were randomly assigned to receive either oral doses 15 g/day of DKT or placebo control from preoperative day 3 to POD10. This large prospective study revealed that DKT could accelerate the first bowel movement, and in patients with grade B liver damage DKT tended to decrease serum CRP levels. Moreover, in addition to prospective cohort DKT study which demonstrated the reduction of the incidence of POI in pancreaticoduodenectomy (PD), phase III randomized control trials of 15 g/day DKT on postoperative bowel motility and paralytic ileus after PD have been already conducted in Japan [42].

Table 3
Clinical trials of herbal medicine for patients undergoing other surgery and for patients with postoperative ileus

	Herbal medicine	Prescription	Target procedures and diseases	Study design and scale	Results	Author (year)
Postoperative ileus and Other GI surgeries	DKT	15 g/day, 14 days	POI after several abdominal surgery	• Prospective RCT • DKT (n = 13) and placebo (n = 11)	Significantly lower frequency of operation for POI	Itoh et al. [37]
		NA	ASBO after abdominal surgery	• Retrospective study • Propensity score analysis • DKT users (n = 144) and non-users (n = 144)	Significant shorter duration of long-tube decompression for ASBO in DKT users than non-useres	Yasunaga et al. [38]
		7.5 g/day from POD1	Hepatic resection	• Prospective RCT • DKT (n = 16) and placebo (n = 16)	• Significant lower CRP and beta-D-glucan level on POD3 in DKT than control • Significant shorter the time until fast flatus, bowel movement, and the full recovery of oral intake in DKT than placebo	Nishi et al. [39]
		15 g/day, 7 days		• Proscpective RCT • DKT (n = 9) and DKT plus lactulose (n = 9)	Potential effectiveness of DKT for abdmoinal bloating after hepatectomy	Kanazawa et al. [36]
		15 g/day, 13 days		• Prospective RCT, placebo-controlled, multicenter • DKT (n = 108) and placebo (n = 101)	• Accelerated the time to first bowel movement by DKT • lower CRP levels in DKT than placebo for patients with liver damage B	Shimada et al. [41]
		15 g/day, 10 days	PD	• comparative cohort study • DKT (n = 30) and non-DKT (n = 15)	• Lower incidence of POI in DKT group • Significant shorter the time until fast flatus • Significant higher IL-9 and 10 level in the drainage in DKT group	Okada et al. [42]

GI gastrointestinal, *DKT* daikentuto, *NA* not assessed, *POD* postoperative days, *POI* postoperative ileus, *ASBO* adhesive small bowel obstruction, *PD* pancreaticoduodenectomy

3 Total Summary and Future Prospects of Herbal Medicine Gastrointestinal Surgeries

In this chapter, current evidences with regard to herbal medicine therapy in GI fields are reviewed and summarized. Rikkunshito in upper GI field and Daikenchuto in lower and other GI field play main roles not only in ameliorating postoperative symptoms and complications, but also improving patients' QOL.

Although many scientific and high-quality data even in this field are available in animal model, real human clinical data and evidences with regard to efficacy of herbal medicine in GI surgery remain insufficient due to the lack of large-scale randomized trials. Therefore, optimal dose and duration of herbal medicine in several GI surgical procedures have been uncertain yet and establishment of proper prescription, which is based on the high-quality evidences for treatment of patients with abdominal surgery, will be required in the near future.

References

1. Tatsuta M, Iishi H (1993) Effect of treatment with liu-jun-zi-tang (TJ-43) on gastric emptying and gastrointestinal symptoms in dyspeptic patients. Aliment Pharmacol Ther 7 (4):459–462
2. Iturrino J, Camilleri M, Wong BS et al (2013) Randomised clinical trial: the effects of daikenchuto, TU-100, on gastrointestinal and colonic transit, anorectal and bowel function in female patients with functional constipation. Aliment Pharmacol Ther 37(8):776–785. doi:10.1111/apt.12264
3. Nakada K, Ikeda M, Takahashi M et al (2015) Characteristics and clinical relevance of postgastrectomy syndrome assessment scale (PGSAS)-45: newly developed integrated questionnaires for assessment of living status and quality of life in postgastrectomy patients. Gastric Cancer 18(1):147–158. doi:10.1007/s10120-014-0344-4
4. Hioki K, Nakane Y, Yamamoto M (1990) Surgical strategy for early gastric cancer. Br J Surg 77(12):1330–1334
5. Sawai K, Takahashi T, Suzuki H (1994) New trends in surgery for gastric cancer in Japan. J Surg Oncol 56(4):221–226
6. Yamashita Y, Toge T, Adrian TE (1997) Gastrointestinal hormone in dumping syndrome and reflux esophagitis after gastric surgery. J Smooth Muscle Res 33(2):37–48
7. Lu P, Liang QD, Li R et al (2006) Effect of traditional Chinese medicine on survival and quality of life in patients with esophageal carcinoma after esophagectomy. Chin J Integr Med 12(3):175–179
8. Yagi M, Homma S, Kubota M et al (2004) The herbal medicine Rikkunshi-to stimulates and coordinates the gastric myoelectric activity in post-operative dyspeptic children after gastrointestinal surgery. Pediatr Surg Int 19 (12):760–765. doi:10.1007/s00383-003-1053-y
9. Kido T, Nakai Y, Kase Y et al (2005) Effects of rikkunshi-to, a traditional Japanese medicine, on the delay of gastric emptying induced by N (G)-nitro-L-arginine. J Pharmacol Sci 98 (2):161–167
10. Hayakawa T, Arakawa T, Kase Y et al (1999) Liu-Jun-Zi-Tang, a kampo medicine, promotes adaptive relaxation in isolated guinea pig stomachs. Drugs Exp Clin Res 25(5):211–218
11. Hattori T (2010) Rikkunshito and ghrelin. Int J Pep 2010:1–3. doi:10.1155/2010/283549
12. Matsumura T, Arai M, Yonemitsu Y et al (2010) The traditional Japanese medicine Rikkunshito increases the plasma level of ghrelin in humans and mice. J Gastroenterol 45 (3):300–307. doi:10.1007/s00535-009-0166-z
13. Takeda H, Sadakane C, Hattori T et al (2008) Rikkunshito, an herbal medicine, suppresses cisplatin-induced anorexia in rats via 5-HT2 receptor antagonism. Gastroenterology 134

(7):2004–2013. doi:10.1053/j.gastro.2008.02.078

14. Sadakane C, Muto S, Nakagawa K et al (2011) 10-Gingerol, a component of rikkunshito, improves cisplatin-induced anorexia by inhibiting acylated ghrelin degradation. Biochem Biophys Res Commun 412(3):506–511. doi:10.1016/j.bbrc.2011.08.002
15. Maki T, Shiratori T, Hatafuku T et al (1967) Pylorus-preserving gastrectomy as an improved operation for gastric ulcer. Surgery 61 (6):838–845
16. Kodama M, Koyama K (1991) Indications for pylorus preserving gastrectomy for early gastric cancer located in the middle third of the stomach. World J Surg 15(5):628–633, Discussion 633–624
17. Imada T, Rino Y, Takahashi M et al (1998) Postoperative functional evaluation of pylorus-preserving gastrectomy for early gastric cancer compared with conventional distal gastrectomy. Surgery 123(2):165–170
18. Nishikawa K, Kawahara H, Yumiba T et al (2002) Functional characteristics of the pylorus in patients undergoing pylorus—preserving gastrectomy for early gastric cancer. Surgery 131(6):613–624
19. Takahashi T, Endo S, Nakajima K et al (2009) Effect of rikkunshito, a Chinese herbal medicine, on stasis in patients after pylorus-preserving gastrectomy. World J Surg 33 (2):296–302. doi:10.1007/s00268-008-9854-8
20. Endo S, Nishida T, Nishikawa K et al (2006) Dai-kenchu-to, a Chinese herbal medicine, improves stasis of patients with total gastrectomy and jejunal pouch interposition. Am J Surg 192(1):9–13. doi:10.1016/j.amjsurg.2006.01.022
21. Takiguchi S, Hiura Y, Takahashi T et al (2013) Effect of rikkunshito, a Japanese herbal medicine, on gastrointestinal symptoms and ghrelin levels in gastric cancer patients after gastrectomy. Gastric Cancer 16(2):167–174. doi:10.1007/s10120-012-0164-3
22. Aaronson NK, Ahmedzai S, Bergman B et al (1993) The European Organization for Research and Treatment of Cancer QLQ-C30: a quality-of-life instrument for use in international clinical trials in oncology. J Natl Cancer Inst 85(5):365–376
23. Takiguchi S, Yamamoto K, Hirao M et al (2012) A comparison of postoperative quality of life and dysfunction after Billroth I and Roux-en-Y reconstruction following distal gastrectomy for gastric cancer: results from a multi-institutional RCT. Gastric Cancer 15 (2):198–205. doi:10.1007/s10120-011-0098-1
24. Takachi K, Doki Y, Ishikawa O et al (2006) Postoperative ghrelin levels and delayed recovery from body weight loss after distal or total gastrectomy. J Surg Res 130(1):1–7. doi:10.1016/j.jss.2005.08.003
25. Svedlund J, Sjodin I, Dotevall G (1988) GSRS—a clinical rating scale for gastrointestinal symptoms in patients with irritable bowel syndrome and peptic ulcer disease. Dig Dis Sci 33(2):129–134
26. Akamaru Y, Takahashi T, Nishida T et al (2015) Effects of daikenchuto, a Japanese herb, on intestinal motility after total gastrectomy: a prospective randomized trial. J Gastrointest Surg 19(3):467–472. doi:10.1007/s11605-014-2730-y
27. Lewis SJ, Heaton KW (1997) Stool form scale as a useful guide to intestinal transit time. Scand J Gastroenterol 32(9):920–924. doi:10.3109/00365529709011203
28. Dijkstra FR, Nieuwenhuijzen M, Reijnen MM et al (2000) Recent clinical developments in pathophysiology, epidemiology, diagnosis and treatment of intra-abdominal adhesions. Scand J Gastroenterol Suppl 232:52–59
29. Fearon KC, Ljungqvist O, Von Meyenfeldt M et al (2005) Enhanced recovery after surgery: a consensus review of clinical care for patients undergoing colonic resection. Clin Nutr 24 (3):466–477. doi:10.1016/j.clnu.2005.02.002
30. Jin XL, Shibata C, Naito H et al (2001) Intraduodenal and intrajejunal administration of the herbal medicine, dai-kenchu-tou, stimulates small intestinal motility via cholinergic receptors in conscious dogs. Dig Dis Sci 46 (6):1171–1176
31. Satoh K, Hayakawa T, Kase Y et al (2001) Mechanisms for contractile effect of Dai-kenchu-to in isolated guinea pig ileum. Dig Dis Sci 46(2):250–256
32. Manabe N, Camilleri M, Rao A et al (2010) Effect of daikenchuto (TU-100) on gastrointestinal and colonic transit in humans. Am J Physiol Gastrointest Liver Physiol 298(6): G970–G975. doi:10.1152/ajpgi.00043.2010
33. Katsuno H, Maeda K, Kaiho T et al (2015) Clinical efficacy of Daikenchuto for gastrointestinal dysfunction following colon surgery: a randomized, double-blind, multicenter, placebo-controlled study (JFMC39-0902). Jpn J Clin Oncol 45(7):650–656. doi:10.1093/jjco/hyv056
34. Yaegashi M, Otsuka K, Itabashi T et al (2014) Daikenchuto stimulates colonic motility after

laparoscopic-assisted colectomy. Hepato-Gastroenterology 61(129):85–89

35. Yoshikawa K, Shimada M, Nishioka M et al (2012) The effects of the Kampo medicine (Japanese herbal medicine) "Daikenchuto" on the surgical inflammatory response following laparoscopic colorectal resection. Surg Today 42(7):646–651. doi:10.1007/s00595-011-0094-4
36. Kanazawa A, Sako M, Takazoe M et al (2014) Daikenchuto, a traditional Japanese herbal medicine, for the maintenance of surgically induced remission in patients with Crohn's disease: a retrospective analysis of 258 patients. Surg Today 44(8):1506–1512. doi:10.1007/s00595-013-0747-6
37. Itoh T, Yamakawa J, Mai M et al (2002) The effect of the herbal medicine dai-kenchu-to on post-operative ileus. J Int Med Res 30 (4):428–432
38. Yasunaga H, Miyata H, Horiguchi H et al (2011) Effect of the Japanese herbal kampo medicine dai-kenchu-to on postoperative adhesive small bowel obstruction requiring long-tube decompression: a propensity score analysis. Evid Based Complement Alternat Med: eCAM 2011:264289. doi:10.1155/2011/264289
39. Nishi M, Shimada M, Uchiyama H et al (2012) The beneficial effects of Kampo medicine Dai-ken-chu-to after hepatic resection: a prospective randomized control study. Hepato-Gastroenterology 59(119): 2290–2294. doi:10.5754/hge10115
40. Hanazaki K, Ichikawa K, Munekage M et al (2013) Effect of Daikenchuto (TJ-100) on abdominal bloating in hepatectomized patients. World J Gastrointest Surg 5 (4):115–122. doi:10.4240/wjgs.v5.i4.115
41. Shimada M, Morine Y, Nagano H et al (2015) Effect of TU-100, a traditional Japanese medicine, administered after hepatic resection in patients with liver cancer: a multi-center, phase III trial (JFMC40-1001). Int J Clin Oncol 20(1):95–104. doi:10.1007/s10147-014-0678-2
42. Okada K, Kawai M, Hirono S et al (2015) Perioperative administration of Daikenchuto (TJ-100) reduces the postoperative paralytic ileus in patients with pancreaticoduodenectomy. Hepato-Gastroenterology 62(138):466–471
43. Gunji S, Ueda S, Yoshida M, et al. (2013) Effects of rikkunshito, a kampo medicine, on quality of life after proximal gastrectomy. J Surg Res 185(2):575–80. doi:10.1016/j.jss.2013.06.010

Chapter 5

Constipation and Herbal Medicine

Norio Iizuka

Abstract

Constipation is unsatisfactory defecation characterized by a variety of bowel symptoms such as difficulty passing stool, hard stool, and a feeling of incomplete evacuation. The multifactorial causes of constipation might limit the clinical efficacy of current conventional treatments that use a single drug that acts through only one pathway. Herbal medicines capable of targeting multiple organs and cellular sites are great fascinating from the standpoint of a holistic approach, making it possible to complement the shortcomings of the current Western medical system. In Japan, herbal medicines have been used throughout history as foods and medicines and currently Japanese physicians can use a standardized form of herbal combination with high quality.

This review provides an overview of the clinical application and pharmacological action of two types of Japanese herbal medicines (JHMs), Rhei rhizoma-based JHMs including Daiokanzoto and Mashiningan, and Kenchuto-based JHMs including Daikenchuto and Keishikashakuyakuto, in the treatment of constipated patient by combining the molecular basis of action drawn from many literatures and the unique theory of Japanese traditional medicine, known as Kampo medicine.

Key words Constipation, Herb, Herbal medicine, Kampo, Traditional medicine

1 Introduction

Constipation is a syndrome characterized by a variety of bowel symptoms such as difficulty passing stool, hard stool, and feelings of incomplete evacuation. It is reported that 12–19 % of people throughout the world suffer from constipation with symptoms varying by geographic location [1–3].

Constipation is usually caused by a wide variety of primary and secondary causes [4]. Primary constipation arises from intrinsic defects in colonic function or malfunction of the defecation process, whereas secondary constipation is related to organic disease, systemic disease, or medications [4]. Thus, the multifactorial causes of constipation would limit the clinical efficacy of current conventional Western treatments since these drugs act through a single pathway [5]. To complement these shortcomings and provide a complete holistic approach, herbal medicines capable of targeting

Akio Inui (ed.), *Herbal Medicines: New Horizons*, Methods in Pharmacology and Toxicology,
DOI 10.1007/978-1-4939-4002-8_5,

multiple organ sites may be used [6, 7]. Many traditional herbs and herbal combinations have been used throughout history as foods and medicines in the world [8–12] and are applied to current western medical practices as complementary or alternative therapies by using standardized herbal combinations with consistent quality and quantity of constituents in Japan [13]. These herbs contain a variety of components; however, it remains unclear how their components exert their biological effects and interact with other components in the herb. To better understand the biological activities of herbs as complex drugs derived from nature, many studies have elucidated the roles of each of major components in the biological activity of an herb [7]. Especially, consistent quality of herb and constituents are very important in the viewpoint of the evidence level on clinical trials; therefore, this review highlights basic and clinical studies with use of Japanese herbal medicines (JHMs)Japanese herbal medicines (JHMs).

This review provides a framework to better understand the clinical and pharmacological efficacy of JHMs on constipation by (1) explaining the unique history and theory of Japanese traditional medicine, Kampo medicine (KM); (2) summarizing classic JHMs used for constipation; (3) explaining the clinical application and pharmacological action of Rhei Rhizoma-based JHMs and Kenchuto-based JHMs including Daikenchuto.

2 The Unique History of Kampo Medicine (KM)

KM is another term for traditional Japanese medicine based on traditional Chinese medicine (TCM) [14] that was likely introduced to Japan directly or by way of Korea around the Fifth or Sixth Century. During the Edo period (Seventeenth to Eighteenth Century), KM evolved uniquely as holistic medicine and gained the first popularity; however, in the Meiji period (i.e., Nineteenth Century), it began to decline by rapid introduction of western medicine such as German medical system and was outside of the mainstream of the medical system and education in Japan. In the Showa period (i.e., 1960s), KM gained the second popularity in support with integration into Japan's health care system.

Currently, Japanese physicians can use fixed combinations of herbs, 148 government-regulated prescription JHMs, in standardized proportions on the basis of the classical literature of TCM [15]. Notably, it was reported that 70 % of the 200,000 physicians prescribed JHMs in their daily clinical practice in 1993 [13]. However, most of physicians who graduated from medical universities or colleges without KM education 15 years ago cannot understand the differences in the thinking process and approach of Western and KM medical systems, and cannot make good use of JHMs in the daily medical practice. This problem would be solved in the near future, because KM has been integrated to medical education program at all the 80 Japan's medical universities and colleges for the last decade. Exclusively, the current problem that we Japanese physicians face is to standardize the education for KM to uniform various modes of medical system caused by different schools such as the Kohoha and Goseiha.

3 The Unique Theory of KM

There is a marked difference between Western medicine and traditional Asian medicines such as TCM, KM, and traditional Korean medicine [7]. Western medicine specifically and efficiently attacks abnormal organs or cells by targeting the cause of the disease. More specifically, Western medicine focuses on pathogenesis rather than host reaction. In contrast, KM is concerned with the host's reaction to the pathogen, and thus focuses on the host's inherent ability to promote health by targeting multiple organs or cells concurrently. This is largely due to the fact that JHMs contain a combination of herbs, and thus a vast array of constituents. An evidence-based approach fails to assess efficacy when studying individualized medicines under the KM system because the end points are somewhat unclear. This is an issue that requires further investigation in future studies.

Similar to TCM, KM uses patterns (*Sho* in Japanese) to determine a suitable herbal combination for each patient. While TCM is based on the theory of the Ming Dynasty, KM was separated from this theory and then reestablished based on a different theory, Shang Han Lun, during the Edo period [13]. While organ systems are very important for determining medication patterns in TCM, they are not utilized in KM because Japanese KM specialists wish to avoid overlap with terms used in Western medicine. Thus, KM patterns are quite unique. One possible reason for this may be the fact that TCM prescriptions are individualized at the herbal level, while KM prescriptions are individualized at the formula level [13].

KM defines chronic health conditions as, for example, deficiency, intermediate (i.e., between deficiency and excess), and excess patterns in the whole body and Qi-blood-fluid. Qi, or life energy, is sourced from food and air. There are three types of abnormal Qi patterns: Qi deficiency, Qi stagnation, and Qi counterflow. Blood is a red fluid moved by Qi. There are two types of abnormal blood patterns: blood deficiency and blood stasis. Fluid, in contrast to blood, is a colorless and transparent liquid. In KM, illness is caused by an imbalance of these three elements. In determining KM patterns (i.e., *Sho*), physicians specializing in KM also use several parameters (i.e., yin–yang, deficiency–excess, cold–heat, interior–exterior, and six stages of acute febrile diseases) other than Qi blood fluid [7, 13, 16]. They can individualize constipation treatments by determining KM patterns with use of the following four traditional examination methods: inspection, listening and smelling, interviewing, and palpation [16]. Under KM theory, constipation is thought to be caused mainly by deficiency and cold patterns, specifically Qi deficiency, and other patterns (intermediate or excess) caused by Qi stagnation, blood deficiency, or blood stasis (Fig. 1).

4 JHMs Used for Constipation

JHMs are composed of various medicinal herbs. Figure 1 shows representative JHMs and their ingredients (i.e., herbs) used for constipation. There are two classes of JHMs, Rhei Rhizoma-based JHMs (class A) and Kenchuto-based JHMs (class B), both of which are frequently used for constipation [7, 17]. Information concerning herbs in KM were obtained from an online list of package inserts (http://plaza.umin.ac.jp/~kconsort/framepage.html).

Physicians specializing in KM usually use Rhei Rhizoma-based JHMs (class A) to treat constipated patients with excess or intermediate patterns, most of whom show atonic constipation [7, 17] (Fig. 1). One possible reason for this is that sennoside A, aloe-emodin, and rhein, which are the main components of Rhei

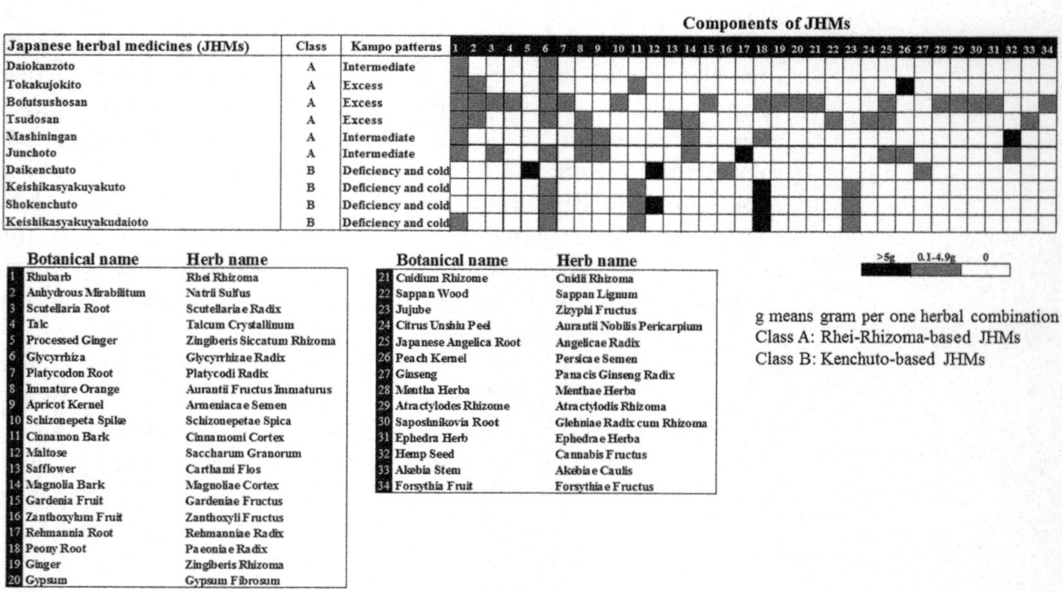

Fig. 1 Representative Japanese herbal medicines (JHMs) used for constipation. Note that there are two representative JHMs, Rhei-Rhizoma-based JHMs (class A) and Kenchuto-based JHMs (class B) that are classified by combination patterns of herbs that are obtained from the package insert of Tsumura Kampo Formulation for Prescription (http:/plaza.umin.ac.jp/~kconsort/framepage.html)

Rhizoma, have anti-inflammatory activities [18], and as a result, draw heat from the patient. Therefore, their pharmacological actions may cause harm in constipated patients with deficiency and cold patterns.

The word "Kenchuto" means an herbal combination that can improve the dysfunction of the alimentary tract [19]. Kenchuto is classified into two types, Daikenchuto and Keishikashakuyakuto, based on herb combinations. Interestingly, although these two types of JHMs have different herb combinations, they have similar functions in terms of promoting bowel movements (Fig. 1). KM physicians typically use Kenchuto-based JHMs (class B) to treat constipated patients with deficiency and cold patterns who also report general fatigue due to Qi deficiency (Fig. 1). In Japan, Kenchuto-based JHMs are frequently prescribed when patients with deficiency and cold patterns develop constipation-predominant irritable bowel syndrome (IBS) [16]. In particular, contraction of the rectus abdominis muscle (*Fukuhikokyu* in Japanese) is often found in patients with constipation-predominant IBS. KM physicians recognize empirically that Paeoniae Radix, a main component of Kenchuto-based JHMs, promotes relaxation of the rectus abdominis muscle [16] as well as smooth muscle of the intestinal tract. Therefore, for patients with IBS, contractions of the rectus abdominis muscle can be used as a selection criterion for Kenchuto-based JHMs.

5 Clinical Application and Pharmacology of Rhei-Rhizoma-Based JHMs

Rhei Rhizoma (Rhubarb in English and *Daio* in Japanese) is one of the most frequently used herbs for constipation throughout the world. Rhei Rhizoma contains dianthrone glycosides (sennosides A to F) and anthraquinones (e.g., rhein, aloe-emodin, emodin, physcion, chrysophanol) [20–22]. Among these components, sennosides (i.e., stimulative laxatives) have been well documented for their pharmacological action on constipation [23]. Sennosides A and B play a central role in the motility of the alimentary tract as prodrugs that are converted to an active principle, rheinanthrone, by intestinal microbiota [20, 21]. More recently, it was reported that sennoside A may exert a laxative effect by inhibiting water transfer from the intestinal tract to the vascular side via decreasing aquaporin-3 expression in the colon [24]. Thus, sennoside A would contribute to ameliorate both difficulty passing stool and hard stool in the constipated patient.

Daiokanzoto is a representative *Rhei rhizoma*-based JHM that is widely used to treat constipated patients with intermediate patterns (Fig. 1). Notably, it comprises only two herbs (*Rhei rhizoma* and *Glycyrrhizae radix*). Therefore, the pharmacological action of Daiokanzoto appears similar to that of sennoside, a main component of Rhei Rhizoma (Fig. 1). Inversely, a patient's response to sennoside may predict the clinical efficacy of Rhei Rhizoma-based JHMs. For example, KM physicians would not empirically prescribe Daiokanzoto for constipated patients deemed unresponsive to sennoside in the medical interview [17]. Alternatively, Daiokanzoto has beneficial effects on oral mucositis, a disease that results from increased cell death induced by chemotherapeutic agent 5-fluorouracil (5-FU) [25]. Taken together, Daiokanzoto may improve both constipation and quality of life in cancer patients treated with 5-FU-based chemotherapy, although further studies are required to gain deeper insight into its pharmacological actions.

Bofutsushosan, Tsudosan, and Tokakujokito also belong to "jokito" group that contains two main herbs: Rhei Rhizoma and Anhydrous Mirabilitum (*Bosho* in Japanese) (Fig. 1). Anhydrous Mirabilitum is a sodium sulfate similar to magnesium sulfate that acts as a salt-based laxative [7, 17]. Bofutsushosan, Tsudosan, and Tokakujokito are considered strong laxatives due to their stimulative and salt-based functions [17]. Among these three JHMs, Tsudosan and Tokakujokito are used for constipated patients with blood stasis (*Oketsu* in Japanese) [7]. Several herbs (Carthami Flos, Sappan Lignum, Angelica Radix, and Persicae Semen) used in Tsudosan and Tokakujokito improve blood stasis by inhibiting blood coagulation and causing vasodilation [7]. For example, Angelica Radix contains coumarin derivatives, which have inhibitory effects on platelet aggregation and blood coagulation [26]. Bofutsushosan is also used for constipated patients with Qi stagnation (*Kitai* in Japanese) [7]. Daiokanzoto and these three JHMs are frequently used in patients with atonic constipation without deficiency and cold patterns.

Junchoto and Mashiningan are unique Rhei Rhizoma-based JHMs that contain small amounts of Rhei Rhizoma and Cannabis Fructus (*Mashinin* in Japanese) (Fig. 1). In Japan, KM physicians prescribe Junchoto and Mashiningan exclusively for elderly patients who have spastic constipation (i.e., type 1 of Bristol Stool Chart) [7, 17]. Cannabis Fructus is an herb obtained from Hemp Seed that is a rich source of plant oil: therefore, this herb also contains large amounts of fatty oils, including olein, linolein, and linolenin, with actions similar to the bulk-forming laxative, polycarbophil calcium [27]. It was reported that intake of meals containing Cannabis Fructus reduced H_2O_2 toxicity markedly, indicating that Cannabis Fructus exerts a profound antioxidant effect [28]. For example, this antioxidant effect of Cannabis Fructus would confer another benefit in the management of bowel movement of elderly patients with Alzheimer's disease and cardiovascular disease.

In most patients with constipation, Junchoto or Mashiningan soften stool. Generally, constipated stool is dry, hard, and difficult to pass. Therefore, the combination of Rhei Rhizoma, which promotes movement of the alimentary tract, and Cannabis Fructus, which softens stool, may prove effective for any type of constipation, including atonic and spastic constipation [7, 17]. Mashiningan has been proven efficacious for functional constipation in a randomized double-blind, placebo-controlled study [29]. In that study, responder rates for the Mashiningan and placebo groups were 43.3 and 8.3 % during treatment and 30.0 and 15.0 % at 8-week follow-up, respectively ($P < 0.05$). The authors suggest that Mashiningan increases complete spontaneous bowel movement, relieves the severity of constipation and straining to evacuate, and effectively reduces the need for a laxative.

6 Clinical Application and Pharmacology of Daikenchuto, One of Kenchuto-Based JHMs

Daikenchuto, one Kenchuto-based JHMsmember of the Kenchuto-based JHM family, has a wide range of pharmacological actions and therefore is the most commonly prescribed JHM, which is composed of four herbs: processed ginger (*Kankyo* in Japanese), Ginseng Radix Rubra (*Ninjin* in Japanese), Zanthoxyli Fructus (Japanese pepper, *Sansho* in Japanese), and Saccharum Granorum (maltose powder derived from rice, *Koi* in Japanese) [30] (Fig. 1).

Among the four herbs, due to a lack of relevant studies, the precise pharmacological action of Saccharum Granorum, a disaccharide with high osmotic pressure, remains unclear. However, it is not difficult to suspect that it might affect stool consistency and the motility of the alimentary tract in a manner similar to that of lactulose, an osmotic laxative [7, 17].

Zanthoxyli Fructus contains hydroxy-sanshools (alpha and beta), which act as a serotonin receptor agonist via the cholinergic neuron system to enhance intestinal peristalsis [30]. Its pharmacological action is similar to that of the serotonin receptor agonist mosapride [17]. Indeed, this concept is supported by the findings that the intestinal motility increased by Daikenchuto is inhibited by several serotonin receptor antagonists [31–33]. Recently, Kono et al. demonstrated that hydroxy-sanshools activate intestinal epithelial transient receptor potential cation channel, subfamily A, member 1 (TRPA1) [34], which is highly expressed in enterochromaffin cells (serotonin-releasing cells) and may prove to be a novel target for constipation. In addition to the effects of these individual constituents, a recent study showed that Daikenchuto activates nicotinic acetylcholine receptors, which accounts for its effects on motility [35]. Kikuchi et al. reported that pretreatment with atropine, hexamethonium, ondansetron, (5-hydroxytryptamine-3 receptor antagonist), or capsazepine (antagonist for transient receptor potential cation channel, subfamily V, member 1

(TRPV1)) inhibited Daikenchuto-induced colonic contractions in a dog model [36]. This suggests that orally administered Daikenchuto stimulates colonic motility via TRPV1, muscarinic, nicotinic, and 5-hydroxytryptamine-3 receptors.

Processed ginger contains 6-gingerol and 6-shogaol, which have vanilloid structures, and possibly act as stimulators of TRPV1, formerly known as vanilloid receptor 1 [7, 17] as well as hydroxy-sanshools [37]. These constituents play an important role in promoting the movement of alimentary tract via sensory nerves. In addition, both gingerols and shogaols have anti-inflammatory and circulatory effects in the alimentary tract via modulation of mitogen-activated protein kinase (MAPK), protein kinase B (Akt), and NF-kB activities [38–41].

Ginseng radix plays an important role in increasing blood supply to the alimentary tract via vasodilation [42]. It was reported that Ginseng radix is mainly responsible for the increase in colonic vascular conductance (CVC)Colonic vascular conductance (CVC) induced by Daikenchuto at 15 min, whereas Zanthoxyli Fructus is mainly responsible for the increase in CVC induced by Daikenchuto at 45 min and later [42]. Ginseng Radix has also been shown to increase blood supply to other organs, including brain tissues [43].

In conjunction with the pharmacological actions of individual herbs, it is likely that Daikenchuto has two major pharmacological actions, amelioration of the motility of the alimentary tract and promotion of blood supply to the alimentary tract via vasodilation [30–33, 42, 44]. Many studies have shown that Daikenchuto ameliorates the motility of the alimentary tract via the cholinergic neuron system (serotonin and nicotinic acetylcholine receptors), substance P, motilin, and TRPV1 in several rodent and dog models with use of receptor antagonists or inhibitors [32, 33, 36, 45, 46]. Several studies have shown that oral administration of Daikenchuto by healthy individuals increases plasma levels of substance P and motilin, which promote, either directly or indirectly, the motility of the alimentary tract [45, 46]. Increased intestinal blood supply by Daikenchuto is very fascinating from the standpoint of long-term maintenance of digestive function. To the best of our knowledge, no other pharmaceutical laxatives produce the effect on blood supply to the alimentary tract. Both 6-shogaol extracted from processed ginger and hydroxyl-alpha-sanshool extracted from Zanthoxyli Fructus have been shown to increase intestinal circulation via calcitonin gene-related peptide (CGRP) and adrenomedullin (ADM) [42]. Ginseng Radix has also been shown to increase blood supply to other organs, including brain tissues [43]. These findings help explain why KM physicians frequently use Daikenchuto to treat constipated patients with deficiency and cold patterns from poor blood supply.

7 Clinical Application and Pharmacology of Other Kenchuto-Based JHMs

Secondary members of the Kenchuto-based JHM family include Keishikashakuyakuto, Keishikashakuyakudaioto, and Shokenchuto, which are more frequently used in patients with constipation-predominant IBS [47]. It is intriguing that Keishikashakuyakuto has shown antidiarrheal effects via the inhibition of excessively accelerated small intestinal movement [48]; it has also been effective for relieving abdominal pain in patients with diarrhea-predominant IBS [49]. Taken together, these reports suggest that Keishikashakuyakuto likely normalizes both accelerated and inhibited intestinal movements. This dual effect illustrates how certain herbal combinations, such as JHMs with multiple components, can help maintain host homeostasis.

Keishikashakuyakuto is composed of the following five herbs: Cinnamomi Cortex, Paeoniae Radix, Zingberis Rhizoma, Zizyphi Fructus, and Glycyrrhizae Radix (Fig. 1). Among these herbs, Paeoniae Radix and Glycyrrhizae Radix play a central role in ameliorating bowel dysfunction in patients with IBS. These two herbs has been shown to suppress the neurogenic contractions of the ileum induced by electrical stimulation and ganglionic-stimulating agents in guinea pigs via inhibition of acetylcholine (Ach) release from cholinergic nerves and inhibition of Ach action on ileum smooth muscle [50]. Likewise, their antispasmodic effect on the human colon has been confirmed [51].

In addition to its spasmolytic and smooth muscle-relaxing effects [52–54], Paeoniae Radix has been shown to have anti-inflammatory and analgesic effects, to inhibit gastric acid secretion and stress-induced ulceration [55], and to have sedative [52, 55] and antidepressant-like effects in rodent models [56]. Mao et al. (2012) suggested that Paeoniae Radix has antidepressant-like effects, which could be mediated in part by inhibiting monoamine oxidase activity, hypothalamic-pituitary-adrenal axis activation, oxidative stress, and upregulated brain-derived neurotrophic expression [56].

Glycyrrhizin, a main component of Glycyrrhizae Radix, and its metabolite, 18β-glycyrrhetinic acid, have been reported as likely responsible for ameliorating dysfunctional glutamate transport in astrocytes via the inhibition of protein kinase activity [57]. It has also been reported that after administration of 18β-glycyrrhetinic acid, about 13 % passes through the blood–brain barrier [56]. These findings suggest that 18β-glycyrrhetinic acid in the brain can scavenge excess glutamate via a transporter, which might be related to the pathophysiology of bipolar disorder, major depressive disorder [58], and schizophrenia [59]. Interestingly, brain–gut interactions have been suggested to play a central role in the pathogenesis of IBS [60]. Therefore, Keishikashakuyakuto orchestrates brain–gut interactions in IBS patients; Paeoniae Radix, in addition to its direct effect on the alimentary tract, has both sedative and antidepressant-like effects, and Glycyrrhizae Radix induces upregulation of astrocyte glutamate transport. Thus, JHMs prove useful because they are capable of targeting multiple and/or distant organs such as the brain or alimentary tract concomitantly.

Shokenchuto is composed of the five herbs used in Keishikashakuyakuto and Saccharum Granorum (Fig. 1). Keishikashakuyakudaioto is composed of the five herbs used in Keishikashakuyakuto, plus a small amount of Rhei Rhizoma (Fig. 1). Considering that Saccharum Granorum and Rhei Rhizoma both enhance intestinal movement, it seems that Shokenchuto and Keishikashakuyakudaioto are stronger laxatives than Keishikashakuyakuto. However, the manner in which these three JHMs play important roles in controlling intestinal movement remains unclear. Further studies are needed to elucidate their specific pharmacological action on constipation.

8 Conclusion

The authors have provided an overview of classic JHMs used to treat constipation by combining the molecular basis of action of herbs and the unique theory of KM. The actions of many herbs and herbal medicines are now being examined at the pharmacologic and molecular levels; however, there are limitations in the evaluation of the clinical efficacy of JHMs in a randomized clinical study setting because a placebo formulation that matches the texture, flavor, and other characteristics of the active drug is not always available. In addition, it is very difficult to accurately evaluate herbal efficacy on individual patients with the current study model. A new strategy for evaluating various herbal combinations, including JHMs, and exploring pharmacological data may be needed to provide individualized treatment to constipated patients and offer holistic JHMs capable of targeting multiple organ and cellular sites.

References

1. Eoff JC (2008) Optimal treatment of chronic constipation in managed care: review and roundtable discussion. J Manag Care Pharm 14:1–15
2. Cheng C, Chan AO, Hui WM et al (2003) Coping strategies, illness perception, anxiety and depression of patients with idiopathic constipation: a population-based study. Aliment Pharmacol Ther 18:319–326
3. Talley NJ, Weaver AL, Zinsmeister AR et al (1993) Functional constipation and outlet delay: a population-based study. Gastroenterology 105:781–790
4. Andrews CN, Storr M (2011) The pathophysiology of chronic constipation. Can J Gastroenterol 25(Suppl B):16B–21B
5. Gallagher P, O'Mahony D (2009) Constipation in old age. Best Pract Res Clin Gastroenterol 23:875–887
6. Suzuki H, Inadomi JM, Hibi T (2009) Japanese herbal medicine in functional

gastrointestinal disorders. Neurogastroenterol Motil 21:688–696
7. Iizuka N, Hamamoto Y (2015) Constipation and herbal medicine. Front Pharmacol 6:73. doi:10.3389/fphar.2015.00073
8. Iizuka N, Oka M, Yamamoto K et al (2003) Identification of common or distinct genes related to antitumor activities of a medicinal herb and its major component by oligonucleotide microarray. Int J Cancer 107:666–672
9. Eisenberg DM, Kessler RC, Foster C et al (1993) Unconventional medicine in the United States. Prevalence, costs, and patterns of use. N Engl J Med 328:246–252
10. Cassileth BR (1999) Alternative and complementary medicine. Cancer 86:1900–1902
11. McCann J (1997) Texas center studies research alternative treatments. J Natl Cancer Inst 89:1485–1486
12. DiPaola RS, Zhang H, Lambert GH et al (1998) Clinical and biologic activity of an estrogenic herbal combination (PC-SPES) in prostate cancer. N Engl J Med 339:785–791
13. Yakubo S, Ito M, Ueda Y et al (2014) Pattern classification in kampo medicine. Evid Based Complement Alternat Med 2014:535146
14. Tang JL, Liu BY, Ma KW (2008) Traditional Chinese medicine. Lancet 372:1938–1940
15. Watanabe K, Matsuura K, Gao P et al (2011) Traditional Japanese Kampo medicine: clinical research between modernity and traditional medicine—the state of research and methodological suggestions for the future. Evid Based Complement Alternat Med 2011:513842
16. Sato Y, Hanawa T, Arai M, The Japan Society for Oriental Medicine et al (2005) Introduction to Kampo—Japanese traditional medicine. Elsevier, Tokyo, Japan
17. Iizuka N (2011) Benpi daiokanzoto and daikenchuto. Shindan-to-Chiryo 99:759–764, In Japanese
18. He XY, Liu QC, Peng W et al (2013) Bioactivities and serum pharmacochemistry of Qi-Wei-Xiao-Yan-Tang. Pharm Biol 51:629–634
19. Satoh K, Kase Y, Yuzurihara M et al (2003) Effect of Dai-kenchu-to (Da-Jian-Zhong-Tang) on the delayed intestinal propulsion induced by chlorpromazine in mice. J Ethnopharmacol 86:37–44
20. Hardcastle JD, Wilkins JL (1970) The action of sennosides and related compounds on human colon and rectum. Gut 11:1038–1042
21. Dreessen M, Eyssen H, Lemli J (1981) The metabolism of sennosides A and B by the intestinal microflora: in vitro and in vivo studies on the rat and the mouse. J Pharm Pharmacol 33:679–681
22. Ngoc TM, Minh PT, Hung TM et al (2008) Lipoxygenase inhibitory constituents from rhubarb. Arch Pharm Res 31:598–605
23. de Witte P (1993) Metabolism and pharmacokinetics of anthranoids. Pharmacology 47:86–97
24. Kon R, Ikarashi N, Nagoya C et al (2014) Rheinanthrone, a metabolite of sennoside A, triggers macrophage activation to decrease aquaporin-3 expression in the colon, causing the laxative effect of rhubarb extract. J Ethnopharmacol 152:190–200
25. Yoshida K, Yoshioka M, Okamura H et al (2014) Preventive effect of Daiokanzoto (TJ-84) on 5-fluorouracil-induced human gingival cell death through the inhibition of reactive oxygen species production. PLoS One 9(11): e112689
26. Lee YY, Lee S, Jin JL, Yun-Choi HS (2003) Platelet anti-aggregatory effects of coumarins from the roots of Angelica genuflexa and A. gigas. Arch Pharm Res 26:723–726
27. Montserrat-de la Paz S, Marín-Aguilar F, García-Giménez MD, Fernández-Arche MA (2014) Hemp (Cannabis sativa L.) seed oil: analytical and phytochemical characterization of the unsaponifiable fraction. J Agric Food Chem 62:1105–1110
28. Cheng CW, Bian ZX, Zhu LX et al (2011) Efficacy of a Chinese herbal proprietary medicine (hemp seed pill) for functional constipation. Am J Gastroenterol 106:120–129
29. Lee MJ, Park MS, Hwang S et al (2010) Dietary hempseed meal intake increases body growth and shortens the larval stage via the upregulation of cell growth and sterol levels in Drosophila melanogaster. Mol Cell 30 (1):29–36. doi:10.1007/s10059-010-0085-0
30. Kono T, Kanematsu T, Kitajima M (2009) Exodus of Kampo, traditional Japanese medicine, from complimentary and alternative medicines: is it time yet? Surgery 146:837–840
31. Shibata C, Sasaki I, Naito H et al (1999) The herbal medicine Dai-Kenchu-Tou stimulates upper gut motility through cholinergic and 5-hydroxytryptamine 3 receptors in conscious dogs. Surgery 126:918–924
32. Satoh K, Hashimoto K, Hayakawa T et al (2001) Mechanism of atropine-resistant contraction induced by Dai-kenchu-to in guinea pig ileum. Jpn J Pharmacol 86(1):32–37
33. Satoh K, Hayakawa T, Kase Y et al (2001) Mechanisms for contractile effect of Dai-kenchu-to in isolated guinea pig ileum. Dig Dis Sci 46:250–256

34. Kono T, Kaneko A, Omiya Y et al (2013) Epithelial transient receptor potential ankyrin 1 (TRPA1) dependent adrenomedullin upregulates blood flow in rat small intestine. Am J Physiol Gastrointest Liver Physiol 304: G428–G436
35. Endo M, Hori M, Ozaki H et al (2014) Daikenchuto, a traditional Japanese herbal medicine, ameliorates postoperative ileus by antiinflammatory action through nicotinic acetylcholine receptors. J Gastroenterol 49:1026–1039
36. Kikuchi D, Shibata C, Imoto H et al (2013) Intragastric Dai-Kenchu-To, a Japanese herbal medicine, stimulates colonic motility via transient receptor potential cation channel subfamily V member 1 in dogs. Tohoku J Exp Med 230:197–204
37. Koo JY, Jang Y, Cho H et al (2007) Hydroxy-alpha-sanshool activates TRPV1 and TRPA1 in sensory neurons. Eur J Neurosci 26:1139–1147
38. Hung JY, Hsu YL, Li CT et al (2009) 6-shogaol, an active constituent of dietary ginger, induces autophagy by inhibiting the AKT/mTOR pathway in human non-small lung cancer A549 cells. J Agric Food Chem 57:9809–9816
39. Wu H, Hsieh MC, Lo CY et al (2010) 6-shogaol is more effective than 6-gingerol and curumin in inhibiting 12-O-tetradecanoylphorbol 13-acetate-induced tumor promotion in mice. Mol Nutr Food Res 54:1296–1306
40. Huang HC, Chiu SH, Chang TM (2011) Inhibitory effect of [6]-gingerol on melanogenesis in B16F10 melanoma cells and a possible mechanism of action. Biosci Biotechnol Biochem 75:1067–1072
41. Li XH, McGrath KC, Tran VH et al (2013) Attenuation of proinflammatory responses by S-[6]-gingerol via inhibition of ROS/NFKappaB/ COX-2 activation in HuH7 cells. Evid Based Complement Alternat Med 2013:951758. doi:10.1155/2013/951758
42. Kono T, Koseki T, Chiba S et al (2008) Colonic vascular conductance increased by Daikenchuto via calcitonin gene-related peptide and receptor-activity modifying protein 1. J Surg Res 150:78–84
43. Kim CS, Park JB, Kim KJ et al (2002) Effect of Korea red ginseng on cerebral blood flow and superoxide production. Acta Pharmacol Sin 23:1152–1156
44. Manabe N, Camilleri M, Rao A et al (2010) Effect of daikenchuto (TU-100) on gastrointestinal and colonic transit in humans. Am J Physiol Gastrointest Liver Physiol 298: G970–G975
45. Sato Y, Katagiri F, Inoue S et al (2004) Daikenchu-to raises levels of calcitonin gene-related peptide and substance P in human plasma. Biol Pharm Bull 27:1875–1877
46. Nagano T, Itoh H, Takeyama M (1999) Effect of Dai-kenchu-to on levels of 3 brain-gut peptides (motilin, gastrin and somatostatin) in human plasma. Biol Pharm Bull 22:1131–1133
47. Oka T, Okumi H, Nishida S et al (2014) Effects of Kampo on functional gastrointestinal disorders. Biopsychosoc Med 8:5
48. Saitoh K, Kase Y, Ishige A et al (1999) Effects of Keishi-ka-shakuyaku-to (Gui-Zhi-Jia-Shao-Yao-Tang) on diarrhea and small intestinal movement. Biol Pharm Bull 22:87–89
49. Sasaki D, Uehara A, Hiwatashi Y et al (1998) Kabinsei Cho Shoukougun ni taisuru, keishika-shakuyakuto no rinsho kouka – tashisetsu kyodo musakui waritsuke gunkan hikaku rinsho shiken – (witten in Japanese). Jpn J Clin Exp Med 75:1136–1152
50. Maeda T, Shinozuka K, Baba K, Hayashi M, Hayashi E (1983) Effect of shakuyakukanzoh-toh, a prescription composed of shakuyaku (Paeoniae Radix) and kanzoh (Glycyrrhizae Radix) on guinea pig ileum. J Pharmacobiodyn 6:153–160
51. Ai M, Yamaguchi T, Odaka T et al (2006) Objective assessment of the antispasmodic effect of shakuyaku-kanzo-to (TJ-68), a Chinese herbal medicine, on the colonic wall by direct spraying during colonoscopy. World J Gastroenterol 12:760–764
52. Takagi K, Harada M (1969) Pharmacological studies on herb paeony root III. Effects of paeoniflorin on circulatory and respiratory systems and isolated organs. Yakugaku Zasshi 89:893–898
53. Hayashi M, Baba K, Maeda T (1990) Effect of shakuyaku-extract on electrical stimulation induced contraction of guinea pig ileum. Yakugaku Zasshi 110:139–143
54. Tsuji S, Yasuda K, Sumi G et al (2012) Shakuyakukanzo-to inhibits smooth muscle contractions of human pregnant uterine tissue in vitro. J Obstet Gynaecol Res 38:1004–1010
55. Takagi K, Harada M (1969) Pharmacological studies on herb paeony root II. Anti-inflammatory effect, inhibitory effect on gastric juice secretion, preventive effect on stress ulcer, antidiuretic effect of paeoniflorin and combined effects with licorice component FM100. Yakugaku Zasshi 89:887–892

56. Mao QQ, Ip SP, Xian YF et al (2012) Antidepressant-like effect of peony: a mini-review. Pharm Biol 50:72–77
57. Kawakami Z, Ikarashi Y, Kase Y (2010) Glycyrrhizin and its metabolite 18 beta-glycyrrhetinic acid in glycyrrhiza, a constituent herb of yokukansan, ameliorate thiamine deficiency-induced dysfunction of glutamate transport in cultured rat cortical astrocytes. Eur J Pharmacol 626:154–158
58. Hashimoto K, Sawa A, Iyo M (2007) Increased levels of glutamate in brains from patients with mood disorders. Biol Psychiatry 62:1310–1316
59. Schobel SA, Chaudhury NH, Khan UA et al (2013) Imaging patients with psychosis and a mouse model establishes a spreading pattern of hippocampal dysfunction and implicates glutamate as a driver. Neuron 78:81–93, See comment in PubMed Commons below
60. Fichna J, Storr MA (2012) Brain-gut interactions in IBS. Front Pharmacol 3:127

Chapter 6

Odontopathy and Herbal Medicine

Kojiro Yamaguchi and Tsuyoshi Sugiura

Abstract

This chapter highlights several refractory odontopathies, such as (1) stomatitis, (2) chronic pain [burning mouth syndrome (BMS), glossalgia, atypical facial pain (AFP)], (3) dryness of mouth, (4) taste abnormality, and (5) temporomandibular joint disorder, in which use of Kampo medicines, on the basis of Kampo theory, could exert the maximum effects on human body.

1. In stomatitis, heat may affect the head, chest, and middle abdominal region. Stomatitis is also related to the generation of reactive oxygen species. There are many antioxidants in the crude extracts of Kampo medicines. It is possible to control environmental factors (cold, heat, dampness, dryness) and vital energy, blood, and fluid of the organ systemically using Kampo medicines to treat stomatitis and eliminate local reactive oxygen species accumulation.
2. BMS, glossalgia, and AFP are multifactorial syndromes involving the interaction of biological and psychological factors. Local temperature decrease and edema often occur in chronic pain. These are local circulatory disturbances that can be resolved by improving the flow of blood and fluid. Tokishakuyakusan (TSS) and Kamishoyosan (KSS) are effective for enhancing peripheral circulation. Those medicines such as Saikokaryukotuboreito (SRB), Yokukansan (YKS), KSS, and Saibokutou (SBT) can reduce stress. The clinical efficacy of KM for BMS and AFP may depend on the regulation of the mesolimbic dopaminergic and descending glutamatergic pain modulation systems.
3. Heat- and cold-dryness stages exist in dry mouth. Byakkokaninjinto is useful for heat-dryness, whereas ninjinyoeito, bakumondoto, and hochuekkito (HET) have moisturizing effects in the cold-dryness stage.
4. Taste abnormality: Bitterness is an indicated Syoyobyo stage in the Kampo theory. Saiko-containing formulae are useful for this symptom. Intense sweetness is a sign indicative of digestive canal dampness and heat. Rikkunsito (RKT), Hangeshashinto, etc. are effective for this symptom. The intense astringency can be regarded as a pathological condition of Shoyobyo stage or glossalgia. It is effective to treat with Saiko-containing formulae. Taste loss is a sign of spleen and stomach deficiency. Hozai such as HET, Juzentaihoto, RKT et al. are effective for this symptom.
5. Temporomandibular joint disorder: It is usually treated with Shakuyakukanzoto or Kakkonto in the case with myotonia and/or muscle pain. KSS, TSS, and keishibukuryogan are used for blood circulation improvement. KSS, YKS, SRB, SBT, etc. are usually used in the case of psychogenesis.

Key words Kampo therapy, Stomatitis, Chronic pain, Taste abnormality, Dry mouth, Temporomandibular joint disorder

Akio Inui (ed.), *Herbal Medicines: New Horizons*, Methods in Pharmacology and Toxicology, DOI 10.1007/978-1-4939-4002-8_6, © Springer Science+Business Media New York 2016

1 Introduction

The human oral cavity is the initial digestive organ and is likely to be affected by various localized stimuli and microorganisms.

The oral cavity is an anatomically complex structure that has evolved to perform a multitude of functions, including mastication, swallowing, tasting, and articulation.

The cranial nerve system is set up in a complicated fashion around the oral and maxillofacial region. The oral cavity is also the initial digestive organ, and is thus critical for nutrition and gastrointestinal function. These functions require an extensive and highly integrated system of sensorimotor control pathways.

Furthermore, the oral environment is susceptible to salivation and the peripheral circulation.

Those changes are closely related to the work of the autonomic nervous system.

The systems of traditional Japanese herbal medicine treat oral discomfort and odontopathy by considering anatomic and intraoral environmental factors (i.e., cold, heat, dampness, and dryness), as well as a holistic perspective considering general physical and psychological health [1].

The object of this section is to introduce and summarize clinical applications of Japanese herbal medicines in various refractory oral diseases such as stomatitis, chronic pain [burning mouth syndrome (BMS), glossalgia (glossodynia), atypical facial pain (AFP)], dryness of the mouth, taste abnormality, and temporomandibular joint disorder.

1.1 Kampo Theory

Kampo theory, a branch of traditional Japanese medicine emphasizing the treatment of vital energy (Ki), blood (Ketsu), and fluid (Sui) abnormalities using herbal preparations, has proven to be useful and highly effective for the treatment of oral discomfort and odontopathy resulting from various diseases [1, 2].

Kampo theory encompasses Yin/Yo theory, Ki, Ketsu, and Sui theory, and the five parenchymatous viscera theory.

The five parenchymatous viscera generate Ki, Ketsu, and Sui, and function to circulate them. Ki, Ketsu, and Sui maintain the state of the body while having a mutual association. The five parenchymatous viscera, Ki, Ketsu, and Sui are controlled by the cerebrum (Fig. 1).

1.1.1 "Yin/Yo" Theory

The Yin/Yo theory is based on the philosophical concept of well-balanced pairs of complementary aspects, such as heaven and earth or day and night. Medical excess, heat, and "Ki" belong to the "Yo" category, whereas deficiency, cold blood, and fluid (visible circulating elements) belong to the "Yin" category [2, 3] (Fig. 1).

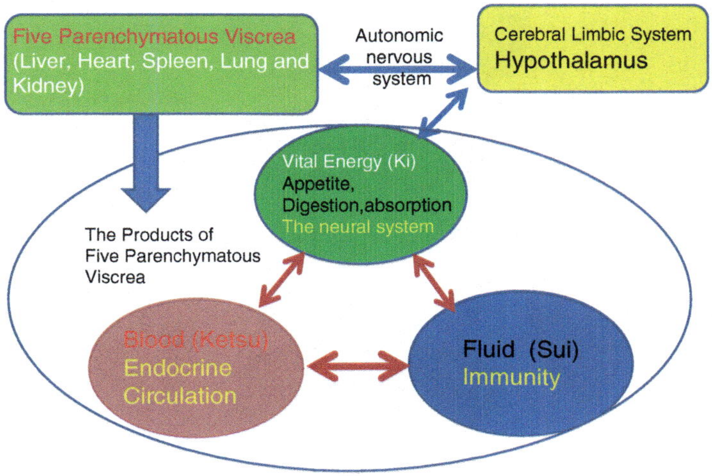

Fig. 1 Schematic view of the Kampo theory

1.1.2 "Ki, Ketsu, and Sui" Theory

"Ki" is invisible circulating vital energy and belongs to the "Yo" category. "Ki" disturbance is manifested by regurgitation of "Ki" and depression of "Ki." "Ketsu" indicates blood (one of the visible circulating elements) and belongs to the "Yin" category. "Ketsu" disturbance is manifested by blood stasis (Oketsu) and "Ketsu" deficiency. "Sui" is fluid (one of the visible circulating elements) that belongs to the "Yin" category. "Sui" disturbance is manifested by accumulation of "Sui" and impaired water excretion [2, 3] (Fig. 1).

1.1.3 Five Parenchymatous Viscera Theory

The five parenchymatous viscera (liver, heart, spleen, lung, and kidney) are used as functional units in Kampo theory. The concept of five parenchymatous viscera encompasses not only the viscera of Western medicine but also several differential functional units. Every viscera produces Yin and Yo products. In the abnormal stage, deficiency or excess in Yin and/or Yo, or a dual deficiency, is observed in the body [2, 3] (Fig. 1).

2 Stomatitis

Stomatitis develops with inflammatory manifestations including reddening, erosion, and ulceration in the oral mucosa. Occasionally, stomatitis may be multiple or recurrent.

In Kampo medicine, stomatitis treatment differs depending on whether the symptoms are intense, acute, or chronic. Stomatitis extends to four categories such as "heat and dampness pattern," "heat and dryness pattern," "cold and dampness pattern," and "cold and dryness pattern" (Fig. 2; Table 2).

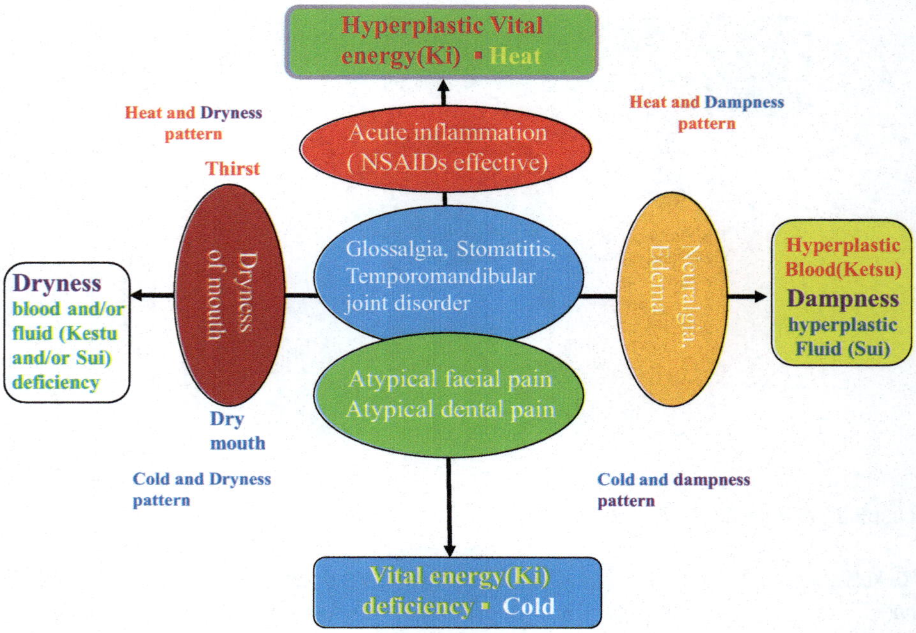

Fig. 2 The relationship between odontopathy and cold, heat, dampness, and dryness categories

2.1 Acute Type

In the acute type, heat from agitated vital energy may affect the head, chest, and middle abdominal region. Therefore, treatment is required to cool the heat in the heart, stomach, and liver with hangeshashinto (HST), orento (ORT), orengedokuto (OGT), Inchinkoto, byakkokaninjinto (BNT), kamishoyosan (KSS), etc.. Kanzoto and kikyoto (KKT), possessing antiinflammatory and heat pattern-treating effects, are also useful as an oral rinse [3].

2.2 Chronic Type

In the chronic type, prolonged head, chest, and middle abdominal heat causes fluid deficiency. Therefore, formulae are required not only to alleviate the heat but also to treat vital energy and blood and to increase wetness by increasing fluid retention.

The following formulations can be selected: middle-region deficiency-treating formulae including kenchuto group, rokumigan (RKG) and hachimijiogan (HJG); Ki deficiency-treating formulae including hochuekkito (HET) and rikkunshito (RKT); dual deficiency-treating formulae including juzentaihoto (JTT) and ninjinyoeito (NYT); and other formulations such as jiinkokato, unseiin, and tokishakuyakusan (TSS).

Kampo formulae may also suppress the underlying causes of stomatitis, particularly infection, inflammation, and concomitant oxidative stress and the drug-induced type.

The crude drugs, such as Scutellariae Radix and Cinnamomi Cortex, inhibit several bacterial infections and have an antifungal effect. Glycyrrhizae Radix and Scutellariae Radix inhibit viral

Table 1
The effects of crude drugs in stomatitis treatment

Effect	Crude drugs
Inhibited bacterial infection	Scutellariae Radix, Coptidis Rhizoma, Cinnamomi Cortex, Glycyrrhizae Radix, Astragali Radix, Phellodendri Cortex
Antifungal effect	Scutellariae Radix, Cinnamomi Cortex, Anemarrhenae Rhizome, Menthae Herba
Inhibited viral infection	Glycyrrhizae Radix, Scutellariae Radix, Cinnamomi cortex
Antiinflammatory effects	Astragali Radix, Scutellariae Radix, Phellodendri Cortex, Coptidis Rhizoma, Glycyrrhizae Radix, Platycodi Radix, Bupleuri Radix, Paeoniae Radix, Atractylodis, Lanceae Rhizoma, Cimicifugae Rhizoma, Cnidii Rhizoma, Angelicae Radix, Poria, Processi Aconiti Radix Ephedrae Herba
Anodyne effects	Paeoniae Radix, Cimicifugae Rhizoma, Cnidii Rhizoma, Angelicae Radix, Processi Aconiti Radix

infection. Several crude drugs have antiinflammatory effects, anodyne effects, and antioxidant effects [3, 4] (Table 1).

HST has a preventive effect on stomatitis associated with chemotherapy and radiation therapy [5]. OGT significantly improves mucositis caused by anticancer agents [6].

The expression of stomatitis is related to generation of reactive oxygen species and that antioxidants contained in medicinal herbs can effectively mitigate this damage [3, 5, 7–12].

3 Chronic Pain (Burning Mouth Syndrome, Glossalgia, Atypical Facial Pain, and Atypical Dental Pain)

Recently, Hagelberg et al. reported the relationship in putamenal/striatal dopamine receptor expression in patients with BMS or atypical facial pain using positron emission tomography (PET) imaging [13–15]. Functional decline of the mesolimbic dopamine system (MDS) came to attract attention in chronic pain.

On the other hand, Yilmaz et al. investigated lingual biopsy specimens of the BMS patients and found that transient receptor potential vanilloid receptor-1 (TRPV1)-positive nerve fibers were significantly increased in those specimens [16].

Effective blocking of the TRPV1 receptor will be able to use one of the treatments for orofacial chronic pain including BMS and AFP in the future.

3.1 Burning Mouth Syndrome and Glossalgia

Burning mouth syndrome (BMS) is characterized by chronic pain in the tongue or other oral mucous membranes in the absence of any visible abnormality or organic disease [17–20]. Burning mouth patients typically exhibit pain symptoms bilaterally in the mouth, the most commonly affected sites being the tongue and lips.

The etiology of BMS is currently unknown; however, most studies support a multifactorial syndrome involving the interaction of biological and psychological factors (particularly paresthesia, altered taste sensation, blood stasis, and mouth dryness from lack of fluid, and depression) [1, 3, 17–20] (Table 2).

Glossalgia is a disease that is regarded as a partial symptom of BMS. The clinical condition is characterized by tongue-confined pain that occurs without organically abnormal findings in the tongue.

Its clinical characteristic features are as follows.

1. It is common in women at a cancer-prone age (middle age and older). Climacteric or postmenopausal hormone changes, stress, anxiety, and nervousness are involved in the aggravation and continuation of symptoms.
2. It occurs more frequently in the tip and lateral margin of the tongue and infrequently in the back of the tongue.
3. The pain mitigates or resolves on talking or eating [1].

BMS and glossalgia extend to four categories such as "heat and dampness pattern," "heat and dryness pattern," "cold and dampness pattern," and "cold and dryness pattern" (Fig. 2).

3.1.1 Treatment with Kampo Medicines in BMS and Glossalgia (Table 2)

Given the relationship between the frequent onset sites for glossalgia and the anatomic compartments of the tongue, it seems that the tip of the tongue corresponds to the heart and lungs, the margin of the tongue to the liver and gallbladder, and the back of the tongue to the spleen and stomach. The causes include blood stasis, vital energy depression, and dryness resulting from lack of fluid.

3.2 Deficiency Pattern (Table 2)

1. Hochuekkito (HET): Effective for BMS and glossalgia in patients with deficiency pattern associated with vital energy depression.
2. Kamishoyosan (KSS): Used with most confidence for nonspecific women's complaints and upper heat-lower cold in deficiency-pattern patients. Redness in the tip of the tongue indicates upper-body heat and is a good indication for this formula.
3. Tokishakuyakusan (TSS): Used for BMS and glossalgia associated with general malaise, fatigue proneness, menstrual disorder, palpitation, or autonomic nerve imbalance, particularly in patients who have white fur tongue and dark-red punctate color change on the lingual tip and margin.

Table 2
Symptoms of abnormality for Ki, blood, and fluid in the whole body and oral cavity and those supporting Kampo medicines

	The concomitant symptom	Oral and maxillofacial disease	Kampo medicines
Ki counterflow	Upper heat and lower cold, palpitation, mood becomes unstable, red flushed face, fretfulness, dizziness, surprise, perspiration of the foot and hand, etc.	Glossalgia, temporomandibular joint disorder (TMD), oral discomfort, atypical facial pain, atypical dental pain, taste abnormality (TAB)	SBT, HKT, YKS, KSS, SRB, ORT, HST, etc.
Ki stagnation and depression	Depressive condition, abnormal sensation in the laryngopharynx, asthma, dull headache, abdominal distension from gas retention, etc.	BMS, glossalgia, TMD, neuralgia, atypical facial pain, atypical dental pain, TAB	SBT, HKT, YKS, HST, KSS, SRB, kousosan, orengedokuto, etc.
Ki deficiency	Entail digestive dysfunction, geographical tongue, feeling tired and lazy, inactive or low spirit condition, weak abdominal strength, etc.	Stomatitis, atypical facial pain, TAB, BMS, atypical dental pain, wound healing disorder, taste loss	HET, NYT, JTT, KKT, RKT, Ougikenchuto etc.
Blood stasis	Dry mouth, subjective feeling of abdominal fullness, feeling of heat, capillary and venous distension, purpura of skin and oral mucosa, irritable, angry, dark red or blue tongue, purple spots on the lingual margin (static spots, static macules), red flush face, et al.	Bruise, occlusal trauma, postoperative swelling and/or pain, peripheral circulation disorder	KBG, TSS, KSS, Jidabokuippou, etc.
Blood deficiency	Anemia, feeling tired and lazy, dry skin, skin and/or mucosal atrophy, abnormal condition of hair, represents poor nutritional and circulatory conditions, decreased activity, cold, etc.	Stomatitis, atypical facial pain, atypical dental pain, neuralgia, wound healing disorder, TAB	JTT, NYT, KKT, TSS, KJT, Unseiin etc.

(continued)

Table 2 (continued)

	The concomitant symptom	Oral and maxillofacial disease	Kampo medicines
Modulation of fluid metabolism, Dryness	Marginal edema, splashing sound in the epigastric region, vomiting, excess of saliva, urine volume disorder, thirst, dry mouth, headache, vertigo, dizziness upon standing, dental identation, shortage of fluid, yellow fur heat body (including false heat), etc.	Edematous pain, chronic pain, neuralgia, paralysis of the nerve, TMD, TAB, dry mouth, salivation disorder	BMT, GRS, TSS, KJT, BNT, NYT, Bukuryoin, Ryoukeijutukanto, Kakkonkajutubuto, Saireito Jiinkokato, etc.

Yamaguchi et al. reported that HET, TSS, and/or KSS reduced visual analogue scale (VAS) pain score by 92.4 % after 19.4 weeks in BMS patients [21].

3.3 Heat Pattern (Table 2)

1. Byakkokaninjinto (BNT): Appropriate for patients with interior heat pattern associated with oral dryness. Effective especially for glossalgia associated with nocturnal thirst.
2. Kikyoto (KKT): Antiinflammatory and heat pattern-treating (Seinetsu) effects can be expected.

Yamaguchi et al. reported a case of BMS treated with BNT, which reduced the VAS score from 44 mm to almost 0 after 18 weeks [22]. Thus, BNT is appropriate for patients with an interior heat pattern associated with oral dryness; therefore, it is effective, particularly for glossalgia associated with nocturnal thirst. KKT is also effective as an antiinflammatory and heat pattern-treating formulation. Yamaguchi et al. reported a case of glossodynia with erythrokeratoderma treated with both internal and gargled Kikyoto [23].

3.4 Pain Control (Table 2)

1. Rikkosan (RKS): Effects can be expected through the analgesic action of saishin and bofu and the antiinflammatory action of ryutan and shoma. Horie et al. demonstrated that RKS reduced PGE_2 by selectively inhibiting cyclooxygenase-2 activity [3, 7]. The crude drugs of Asiasari Radix include methyleugenol and Pellitorine. Those structures resemble capsaicin. Therefore, the Kampo medicine that includes Asiasari Radix, such as RKS, may affect the TRPV1 receptor; the Kampo medicines that include Asiasari Radix, such as RKS, may affect the TRPV1 receptor [3].

2. Keishikajutsubuto (KJT): Used for fluid retention in patients with dampness, cold, or deficiency pattern [24]. It is effective for water retention and exerts an analgesic effect under warming to contain Processi Aconiti Radix.

3.5 Psychosomatic Pattern (Table 2)

1. Saibokuto (SBT): SBT is effective for glossalgia (including laryngopharyngeal discomfort) associated with fluid retention (fluid disturbance) in Shoyobyo stage (the stage of disease transformation with heat halfway between exterior and interior, characterized by bitter taste). It is offered to patients who complain of pain in the median part of the back of the tongue [3].

   SBT reduced pain and burning sensation in glossodynia patients more effectively than diazepam plus vitamin B complex therapy. The majority of SBT-treated patients (92 %) reported good or excellent responses after 3 months compared to only 69 % in the diazepam group [3, 25].
2. Saikokaryukotsuboreito (SRB) and Keishikaryukotuboreito (KRB): SRB suppressed the increase in amygdalar, hypothalamic, and thalamic dopamine, and 3,4-dihydroxy-phenyl acetic acid (DOPAC) in mice exposed to psychological stress and conditioned fear. SRB ameliorated the stress-induced depressive state and reversed the decrease in both extracellular serotonin and dopamine in the prefrontal cortex (PFC) [3, 26, 27].
3. Yokukansan (YKS) and Yokukansankachinpihange (YKSCH): YKS reversed the age-related decreases in extracellular dopamine and serotonin.

   Suzuki et al. reported suppression of mechanical and thermal allodynia by YKS in the chronic constriction injury model of chronic pain. In addition, YKS significantly reduced the increase in cerebrospinal fluid glutamate induced by mechanical or cold stimuli, whereas glutamate transporter inhibitors suppressed these antiallodynic effects [28]. Herbal medicines can reduce stress and associated pain by altering glutamatergic and monoaminergic transmission in hypothalamus and amygdala [29]. The clinical efficacy of Kampo medicines for BMS and atypical facial pain may depend on regulation of the mesolimbic dopaminergic and descending glutamatergic pain modulation systems [3].
4. Other formulae: KSS, Kososan, and kambakutaisoto are used for psychogenic conditions.

3.6 Atypical Facial Pain and Atypical Dental Pain

Both atypical facial pain (AFP) and atypical dental pain (ADP) are generic terms for chronic persistent pain in the oral cavity, jaw, face, and/or teeth without identifiable organic causes. However, those symptoms are related to somatoform disorder and psychological factors. The pain is inconsistent with nerve tracts [1].

AFP and ADP extend to two categories such as "cold and dampness pattern" and "cold and dryness pattern" (Fig. 2).

3.7 Treatment with Kampo Medicines in AFP and ADP (Table 2)

In Kampo medicine, it is important to determine whether the pain is caused by cold or heat, or lack or stagnation of vital energy, blood, or fluid.

Internal warming formulations, fluid disturbance-treating formulae, and blood stasis-treating formulae are used in treatment.

Dual deficiency of vital energy and blood is categorized in the cold and dryness pattern (Fig. 2). Tongue inspection includes enlarged tongue, tongue fur dryness, and geographical tongue. For dual deficiency of vital energy and blood with prolonged pain, mainly HET and TSS, renjuin, JTT, NYT, daibofuto, kamikihito (KKT), and other deficiency pattern-treating formulae are used. Bushi-containing formulae such as KJT are effective in vital energy deficiency with cold pattern (Fig. 2).

Keishikaryukotsuboreito, SRB, YKS, and YKSCH are offered in the vital energy depression pattern (Fig. 2). Static blood with dampness pattern shows dark-red punctate color change and sublingual vein distension on tongue inspection (Fig. 2). TSS, KSS, and KBG are appropriate in this pattern. Fluid retention with dampness patterns shows enlarged tongue and teeth-marked tongue on tongue inspection (Fig. 2). Goreisan (GRS), ryokeijutsukanto, etc. are used in this pattern [3, 24].

4 Dryness of the Mouth

Kampo medicine divides dryness of the mouth into thirst and dry mouth.

Dryness of the mouth may occur as a result of reduced saliva secretion or as a sensation of dryness (thirst) in the presence of normal saliva secretion. Prescriptions are selected according to the condition of dryness (thirst or true dry mouth).

Dryness of mouth extends to two categories such as "heat and dryness pattern" and "cold and dryness pattern" [3] (Fig. 2).

4.1 Thirst (Heat and Dryness Pattern) (Table 2)

Patients with this condition are constantly thirsty and tend to drink copious amounts of water. Frequently they have thirst at night, and want to cool the mouth with ice, as is explained by the presence of heat pattern [interior heat (Rinetsu)] and fluid retention.

BNT, Shosaikotokakikyosekko, Makyokansekito, and Kikyoto (KKT) have heat pattern-treating and saliva-secreting effects, whereas RKG and HJG are effective for thirst in aged individuals who have kidney deficiency [3, 24].

Yanagi et al. reported that BNT ameliorated thirst in several rat thirst models established by muscarinic receptor antagonists This effect was associated with increased expression of aquaporin 5, suggesting that BNT enhanced salivary secretion by muscarinic (M3) receptor-mediated upregulation of aquaporin 5 [30].

4.2 Dry Mouth (Cold and Dryness Pattern) (Table 2)

Patients have dryness in the mouth, but need moistening of the oral cavity rather than to drink much water. This condition is associated with dampness heat, splashing sound, vital energy depression, dual deficiency of spleen and stomach, dual deficiency of vital energy and blood, and dryness and heat because of lack of fluid, etc.

To treating vital energy and fluid deficiency, dry mouth can be effectively treated with NYT and Bakumondoto (BMT), which possess heat pattern-treating effects [3, 24].

Miyazaki et al. reported that NYT improved oxybutynin hydrochloride-induced xerostomia in 12 of 16 patients diagnosed with psychogenic frequency or unstable bladder (chronic cystitis, neurogenic bladder) [31]. Yamaguchi et al. reported a case of xerostomia after oral cancer treatment. A 73-year-old woman complained of lack of appetite and dry mouth following radiation therapy (40 Gy), TS-1 applied at 2240 mg, and surgery for tongue cancer. NYT 6 g/day was administered for treatment of tongue pain, dry mouth, and anorexia. Two weeks later, appetite had improved. Both dry mouth and appetite improved after 2 months of treatment [32].

Nishizawa et al. found BMT was effective and safe for the relief of subjective symptoms and salivary hyposecretion associated with primary Sjögren's syndrome in four separate randomized controlled trials. In fact, it was more effective and safer than the mucolytic bromhexine hydrochloride [33–36].

Ohno reported that 27 of 30 Sjögren's syndrome patients in a quasi-randomized controlled trial showed increased salivary secretion following Kampo treatment (12.0 ± 1.4 ml versus 8.2 ± 1.2 ml at baseline; $p < 0.005$) [37].

Dry mouth can be favorably treated with jiinkokato, unseiin, JTT, and seishoekkito, which all possess heat pattern-treating effects.

Otherwise, GRS can be used to regulate moisture content in the body. KSS and KKT are recommended for psychogenic or stress-induced dry mouth.

5 Taste Abnormality ([24]; Table 2)

The etiology of taste abnormality varies widely from dominant nerve disorder and taste abnormality related to systemic disease (zinc-deficiency disorder, drug-induced illness, endocrine abnormality, etc.) to oral mucosa abnormality (inflammation, oral dryness, tongue papilla atrophy, etc.) and psychogenic causes. Kampo medicines must be selected according to the patient's condition. Electrogustometry, qualitative taste testing, and serum zinc and copper testing should be carried out.

5.1 Intense Bitterness

Oral candidiasis (thrush) manifests with oral bitterness. Therefore, it should be ruled out beforehand. If the symptom remains even in those have been treated for candidiasis, they are candidates for Kampo therapy. The symptom of bitterness is indicated Syoyobyo stage in the Kampo theory. Saiko-containing formulae, such as Shosaikoto, Saikokeishito, and SBT, may be considered for intense bitterness in Shoyobyo stage patients [3].

5.2 Intense Sweetness

The symptom of intense sweetness is a sign indicative of digestive canal dampness and heat (Shitsunetsu). HST, Inchinkoto (ICK), and Rikkunshito (RKT) are effective to improve digestive function, dampness, and heat [24].

5.3 Intense Astringency

It has been considered that astringent substances interact with proteins in the tongue and oral mucosa, and via denaturation (astringent effect) the intense astringency is produced. There is one hypothesis that such taste abnormality is close to pain and tactile sensation, and another proposes it is only a taste. Physiologically, astringency is also categorized as a kind of bitterness. Therefore, intense astringency can be regarded as a pathological condition of Shoyobyo stage or glossalgia. It is effectively treated with Saiko-containing formulae, such as KSS or HET [24].

5.4 Taste Loss (Table 2)

Except for taste cell atrophy cause by zinc deficiency, a loss of taste may be a sign of spleen and stomach deficiency, for which RKT and HET are effective. JTT, NYT, and other deficiency pattern-treating formula(e) (Hozai) are helpful for lack of fluid and blood [24].

5.5 Miscellaneous

ORG or BNT is effective to control taste abnormality with heat. HKT and SBT are appropriate for taste abnormality in patients with severe fluid retention [24].

6 Temporomandibular Disorder ([38]; Fig. 2; Table 2)

Temporomandibular disorder (TMD) is a comprehensive diagnosis of which the pain of temporomandibular joint and masticatory muscles disorder, clicking, crepitus, and trismus in jaw movement abnormality are main symptoms. Masticatory muscle ache disorder, temporomandibular joint arthralgia disorder, temporomandibular joint disk disorder, and arthrosis deformans of temporomandibular joint are included in the TMD condition. The Kampo medicine is used for the case which cannot be given a muscle relaxant or NSAIDs and by combination with the Western medicine.

In temporomandibular disorders, the Kampo medicine is used for the treatment of the pain, numbness, and movement disorder of the muscle, ligament, and articular.

Also, temporomandibular disorder can easily cause a muscle contraction headache.

In cases with myotonia and muscle pain, these are usually treated with Shakuyakukanzoto or Kakkonto. KSS, TSS, and KBG are used for blood circulation improvement, and Keishikajutsubuto is used if cold and dampness are strong. In the case of psychogenesis, KSS, SRB, Shigyaku-san, YKS, SBT, and HKT are usually used. In addition, JTT is also effective in the weakness type [38].

References

1. Yamaguchi K (2013) Atypical maxillofacial pain, glossalgia, atypical dental pain. Pain Kampo Med 23:43–47 (in Japanese with English abstract)
2. The Japan Society for Oriental Medicine (2005) Chapter, diagnosis and treatment 22-52: Introduction to Kampo Japanese traditional medicine. Elsevier, Tokyo
3. Yamaguchi K (2015) Traditional Japanese herbal medicines for treatment of odontopathy. Front Pharmacol Ethnopharmacol 6:1–14
4. Toriizuka K (2003) Monographs of pharmacological research on traditional herbal medicines (Shoyaku no Yakuso·Yakuri). Ishiyaku, Tokyo (in Japanese)
5. Kono T, Satomi M, Chisato N et al (2010) Topical application of Hangeshashinto (TJ-14) in the treatment of chemotherapy-induced oral mucositis. World J Oncol 1(6):232–235
6. Okumi H, Koyama A (2014) Kampo medicine for palliative care in Japan. Biopsychosoc Med 8:1–6
7. Horie N, Hashimoto K, Kato T et al (2008) COX-2 as possible target for the inhibition of PGE_2 production by Rikko-san in activated macrophage. In Vivo 22:333–336
8. Zheng LW, Hua H, Cheung LK (2011) Traditional Chinese medicine and oral diseases: today and tomorrow. Oral Dis 17:7–12
9. Aoyama T, Nishikawa K, Takiguchi N et al (2014) Double-blind, placebo-controlled, randomized phase II study of TJ-14 (hangeshashinto) for gastric cancer chemotherapy-induced oral mucositis. Cancer Chemother Pharmacol 73:1047–1054
10. Li S, Kodama NE, Inoue Y et al (2010) Procyanidin B1 purified from Cinnamomi cortex suppresses hepatitis C virus replication. Antivir Chem Chemother 20:239–248
11. Dragland S, Senoo H, Wake K et al (2003) Several culinary and medicinal herbs are important sources of dietary antioxidants. J Nutr 133:1286–1290
12. Oka S (1995) The effects of Oren-to on stomatitis. Nihon Toyo Igaku Zasshi 46:439–445 (in Japanese with English abstract)
13. Hagelberg N, Forssell H, Aalto S et al (2003) Altered dopamine D2 receptor binding in atypical facial pain. Pain 106:43–48
14. Hagelberg N, Forssell H, Rinne JO et al (2003) Striatal dopamine D1 and D2 receptors in burning mouth syndrome. Pain 101:149–154
15. Hagelberg N, J□□skel□inen SK, Martikainen IK et al (2004) Striatal dopamine D2 receptors in modulation of pain in humans: a review. Eur J Pharmacol 500:187–192
16. Yilmaz Z, Renton T, Yiangou Y et al (2007) Burning mouth syndrome as a trigeminal small fiber neuropathy: increased heat and capsaicin receptor TRPV1 in nerve fibers correlates with pain score. J Clin Neurosci 14:864–871
17. Baker KE, Savage NW (2005) Burning mouth syndrome: an update on recent findings. Aust Dent J 50:220–223
18. Ferensztajn E, Lojko D, Rybakowski J (2013) Burning mouth syndrome: pathogenic and therapeutic concept. Psychiatr Pol 47:973–988
19. Klasser GD, Epstein JB, Villines D (2011) Management of burning mouth syndrome. J Can Dent Assoc 77:b151
20. Klasser GD, Fischer DJ, Epstein JB (2008) Burning mouth syndrome: recognition, understanding, and management. Oral Maxillofac Surg Clin N Am 20:255–271
21. Yamaguchi K, Mukai H, Kawashima K et al (2007) Effect of Kampo medicine on the burning mouth syndrome. Pain Kampo Med 17:43–47 (in Japanese with English abstract)
22. Yamaguchi K, Imamura H, Kasuga Y et al (2005) A case report of the burning mouth effectively treated with Byakkokaninjinto (TJ-34). Pain Kampo Med 15:73–76, In Japanese
23. Yamaguchi K, Mukai H, Kawashima K et al (2009) Kikyou-to (TJ138) effective for a case

of glossodynia with erythrokeratoderma. Pain Kampo Med 19:66–70

24. Yamaguchi K (2012) Therapy details, oral discomfort. In: Textbook of traditional Japanese medicine. Part 1: Kampo, pp 113–117. Health and Labour Sciences Research Grant: Research on the standardization of traditional Japanese medicine promoting integrated medicine
25. Bessho K, Okubo Y, Hori S et al (1998) Effective of Kampo medicine (Sai-boku-to) in treatment of patients with glossodynia. Oral Surg Oral Med Oral Pathol Oral Radiol Endod 86:682–686
26. Sasaki K, Suzuki K, Ueno M, Takao K, Yoshizaki F (1998) Increase in monoamine levels caused by emotional stress in mice brain regions is attenuated by Saiko-ka-ryukotsu-borei-to. Methods Find Exp Clin Pharmacol 20:27–30
27. Mizoguchi K, Yuzurihara M, Ishige A et al (2003) Saiko-ka-ryukotsu-borei-to, a herbal medicine, ameliorates chronic stress-induced depressive state in rotarod performance. Pharmacol Biochem Behav 75:419–425
28. Suzuki Y, Mitsuhata H, Yuzurihara M, Kase Y (2012) Antiallodynic effect of herbal medicine Yokukansan on peripheral neuropathy in rats with chronic constriction injury. Evid Based Complement Alternat Med 2012:1–8
29. Mizoguchi K, Tanaka Y, Tabira T (2010) Anxiolytic effect of a herbal medicine, yokukansan, in aged rats: involvement of serotonergic and dopaminergic transmissions in the prefrontal cortex. J Ethnopharmacol 127:70–75
30. Yanagi Y, Yasuda M, Hashida .K et al (2008) Mechanism of salivary secretion enhancement by Byakkokaninjinto. Biol Pharm Bull 31:431–435
31. Miyazaki Y, Yamada A, Saitou M (1994) Effect of Ninjin-Youei-tou on xerostomia induced by oxybutynin hydrochloride. Shinyaku to Rinsho 43:2613–2617 (in Japanese)
32. Yamaguchi K, Mukai H, Hamada T, Sugihara K (2012) Three cases report of intraoral discomforts with after cancer treatment successfully treated with Ninjinyoeito (TJ108). Pain Kampo Med 22:56–62 (in Japanese)
33. Nishizawa Y, Nishizawa K, Yoshioka F et al (2002) Long-term effects of traditional Chinese herbal medicine, mai-men-dong-tang (Japanese name: bakumondo-to) compared with bromhexine, hydrochloride on sicca syndrome, especially, salivary secretion in patients with primary Sjögren's syndrome: a multicenter, randomized well controlled group parallel comparative trial study with bromhexine. Nihon Daekisen Gakkaishi 43:62–66 (in Japanese)
34. Nishizawa Y, Nishizawa K, Yoshioka F et al (2003) Improving effect of Chinese herb medicine mai-men-dong- tang (Japanese name: bakumondo-to) comparative with sicca syndrome in especial salivary patients with secondary Sjögren's syndrome in multicenter, well controlled, long-term comparative study. Nihon Daekisen Gakkaishi 44:65–70 (in Japanese)
35. Nishizawa Y, Nishizawa K, Yoshioka F et al (2004) Long-term effect of traditional Chinese herbal medicine, mai-men-don-tang on sicca syndrome, especially, salivary secretion in patients with primary Sjögren's syndrome: a multicenter, randomized well controlled group-parallel double-blinded study. Nihon Daekisen Gakkaishi 45:66–74 (in Japanese)
36. Nishizawa Y, Nishizawa K, Goto GH et al (2004) The multicenter randomized comparative study of kampo herbal medicine, mai-men-dong-tang (Japanese name Bakumondo-to) compared with bromhexine on salivary secretion in secondary Sjögren's syndrome. Pain Kampo Med 14:10–17 (in Japanese)
37. Ohno S (2006) The effect of Kampo medicine on salivary secretion in Sjögren's syndrome. Kampo to Saishin-Chiryo 15:134–140 (in Japanese)
38. Wang PL, Sunagawa M, Yamaguchi K et al (2015) EBM of Kampo medicine in oral surgery. Oral Ther Pharmacol 34(1):23–30 (in Japanese)

Chapter 7

Menopausal Symptoms and the Kampo Medicine: Tokishakuyakusan, Kamishoyosan, and Keishibukuryogan

Masakazu Terauchi and Toshiro Kubota

Abstract

Women in the menopausal transition and the postmenopausal period are affected with variety of physical and psychological symptoms. In a recent series of studies, we investigated the effects of three major Kampo formulae (Tokishakuyakusan, Kamishoyosan, and Keishibukuryogan) on Japanese peri- and postmenopausal women, and reached the following conclusions: (1) Each of the three formulae alleviates sleep disturbances, with Kamishoyosan the most effective in improving difficulty in initiating sleep and non-restorative sleep; (2) Keishibukuryogan lowered the systolic and diastolic blood pressures, the pulse rate, and the resting energy expenditure of women with hypertension or high-normal blood pressure; and (3) Tokishakuyakusan could be an effective treatment for the women with both headaches and depression.

Key words Menopause, Postmenopause, Sleep disorder, Insomnia, Blood pressure, Hypertension, Headache, Depression

1 Introduction

Women in the menopausal transition and the postmenopausal period are affected with vasomotor symptoms, urogenital atrophy, sexual dysfunction, somatic symptoms, cognitive difficulty, sleep disturbance, and psychological problems. Some of these effects, particularly vasomotor symptoms and urogenital atrophy, are closely associated with estrogen deficiency, whereas the exact mechanism underlying the other symptoms is not fully understood.

In addition to conventional medicine, complementary and alternative medicines (CAM) are widely used across the world, especially by women and middle-aged individuals, people with higher levels of education and higher incomes, and people with chronic diseases or poor overall health [1]. It was reported that in the early 2000s, CAM was used by almost 50 % of the middle-aged women in Western countries to alleviate menopausal symptoms-Kampo medicine [1, 2]. The percentage might be even higher at

Akio Inui (ed.), *Herbal Medicines: New Horizons*, Methods in Pharmacology and Toxicology,
DOI 10.1007/978-1-4939-4002-8_7, © Springer Science+Business Media New York 2016

present because of the Women's Health Initiative (WHI) reports on the negative aspects of hormone replacement therapy [3, 4].

Kampo, a Japanese subdivision of traditional East Asian medicines, was founded in the sixth century as a local adaptation of the Chinese herbal medicine. Kampo is a more pragmatic approach to complementary and alternative medicine than the Chinese herbal medicine. In the Chinese herbal medicine, a medical practitioner confirms the treatment principle according to "Zheng" (the clinical diagnosis determined on the basis of an analysis of the patient's history, symptoms, and signs) and then mixes 10–15 herbs to create a specific formula for each patient. In Kampo, a practitioner chooses the best formula for a patient from approximately 150 ready-to-use formulae—each of which is typically composed of 5–9 herbs—on the basis of the patient's "Sho" (pattern of symptoms) [5, 6].

The use of Kampo medicine has been revived in Japan since its approval by the Ministry of Health and Welfare in 1976, and now it is one of the main treatment options for menopausal symptoms together with hormone therapy. Among the ~150 formulae that are currently available, three of them: Tokishakuyakusan (Tangkuei and peony powder), Kamishoyosan (Augmented rambling powder), and Keishibukuryogan (Cinnamon twig and poria pill), have been considered to be the best fits for women with menopausal symptoms. Tokishakuyakusan is mainly used for those who are easily fatigued and have generally weak muscles with their waist and lower limbs susceptible to cold, showing suidoku (fluid retention) and deficiency patterns (chills, heavy head, edema, vertigo, etc.). Kamishoyosan is indicated for those who have delicate constitution and are easily fatigued and apt to have autonomic disorders as well as vasomotor symptoms (hot flushes), shoulder stiffness, various psychoneurotic symptoms including anxiety and mood disturbance. Keishibukuryogan is indicated for those who show an oketsu (blood stagnation) pattern (hot flushes with cold legs, neck aches, and stiffness) with a solid constitution, ruddy face, and pain at either side of the navel on palpation. The composition of the three formulae is detailed in Table 1.

In a recent series of studies, we investigated the effects of these three Kampo formulae on Japanese peri- and postmenopausal women who were enrolled in the Systematic Health and Nutrition Education Program (SHNEP), conducted at the Menopause Clinic of the Tokyo Medical and Dental University Hospital, during 1995–2010 [7–9].

2 Effects of Three Kampo Formulae on Sleep Disturbances [7]

Insomnia is defined as difficulty in the initiation and/or maintenance of sleep and/or inadequate or poor quality of sleep that results in the impairment of daytime functioning, despite adequate

Table 1
Composition of the three Kampo Formulae: Tokishakuyakusan, Kamishoyosan, and Keishibukuryogan

	Tokishakuyakusan [Tangkuei and peony powder] (TJ-23) (%)	Kamishoyosan [Augmented rambling powder] (TJ-24) (%)	Keishibukuryogan [Cinnamon twig and poria pill] (TJ-25) (%)
Cinnamon bark			4.7
Bupleurum root		7.1	
Mentha herb		2.4	
Ginger		2.4	
Glycyrrhiza		3.6	
Peach kernel			4.7
Moutan bark		4.7	4.7
Peony root	9.7	7.1	4.7
Japanese angelica root	7.3	7.1	
Cnidium rhizome	7.3		
Gardenia fruit		4.7	
Poria sclerotium	9.7	7.1	4.7
Atractylodes lancea rhizome	9.7	7.1	
Alisma rhizome	9.7		

opportunities and circumstances for sleep. The symptom, known to affect 6–30 % of the general population [10], is not merely an issue of sleep disruption but is known to cause general health problems, such as obesity, diabetes and impaired glucose tolerance, hypertension, metabolic syndrome, eventually leading to increased mortality [11–15]. Difficulty in sleeping is also fairly common in middle-aged women, and the prevalence of the symptom is known to increase from pre- to peri-, and postmenopause [16–18]. Although the exact mechanisms underlying the increase in the prevalence of troubled sleeping with the advanced stage of menopause are not fully understood, the association of sleep disturbance with vasomotor symptoms and depressed mood, at this stage in a woman's life, has been well documented [19–22]. We recently reported that sleep disturbance is highly prevalent in Japanese peri- and postmenopausal women [23]. Sleep disturbance, more often coexist with mood disturbance, was shown to deteriorate their health-related quality of life (HR-QOL) significantly.

In our first study of Kampo medicine for the treatment of menopausal symptoms, we compared the effects of the formulae Tokishakuyakusan, Kamishoyosan, and Keishibukuryogan on the subjective sleep disturbance score and sleep quality measures in women with sleep disturbances [7]. We retrospectively analyzed the records of 1523 Japanese peri- and postmenopausal women who were enrolled in SHNEP between 1995 and 2009. The mean (SD) age of the participants was 53.0 (7.2) years. Among the patients, 28.3 % were classified to be in menopausal transition and 71.7 % as postmenopausal based on the pattern of their menstrual cycles. At each interview session of SHNEP, the women rated the severity of their menopausal symptoms using a 4-point scale that measured how often each symptom affected their daily life: none (never, 0 point), mild (rarely, 1 point), moderate (sometimes, 2 points), and severe (very often, 3 points). The severity of difficulty in sleeping scored in this system is referred to as "the subjective sleep disturbance score". Sleep quality was also assessed by the participants themselves and recorded in terms of sleep duration (h), sleep onset (easy, difficult, and neither easy nor difficult), sleep disruption (the number of awakenings per night), and sleep satisfaction (restorative, nonrestorative, and neither restorative nor nonrestorative) of the previous night. Of the 1474 participants who rated the severity of difficulty in sleeping at their first visit, 747 (50.7 %) reported that their daily life was either moderately (sometimes) or severely (very often) affected by difficulty in sleeping; these women were regarded as having sleep disturbances. Of these, 151 were selected for the first study, because they received only health/nutrition education, without any medical treatment (control; $n = 77$) or treatment with one of the three Kampo formulae: Tsumura Tokishakuyakusan Extract Granules (TJ-23; 7.5 g/day; $n = 42$), Tsumura Kamishoyosan Extract Granules (TJ-24; 7.5 g/day; $n = 16$), or Tsumura Keishibukuryogan Extract Granules (TJ-25; 7.5 g/day; $n = 16$), during the follow-up period of 144 ± 58 days (mean ± SD). At baseline, the TJ-25 group showed significantly higher body weight, body mass index, body fat, lean body mass, and resting energy expenditure than any other group. Further, the systolic pressure, diastolic pressure, and pulse rate were relatively high in the TJ-25 group although the differences were not statistically significant.

We compared the four treatment groups for the changes in the subjective sleep disturbance score and self-reported sleep quality measures after an interval of 5 months (Table 2; Fig. 1). Improvement in the sleep disturbance scores after intervention was

Table 2
The change in the subjective sleep disturbance score, sleep duration, and disrupted sleep in Japanese peri- and postmenopausal women with difficulty in sleeping after intervention ($n = 151$)

	Control ($n = 77$)	TJ-23 ($n = 42$)	TJ-24 ($n = 16$)	TJ-25 ($n = 16$)
Subjective sleep disturbance score				
Before	2.4 (2.27–2.50)	2.6 (2.39–2.71)	2.3 (2.01–2.49)	2.8 (2.51–2.99)
After	1.7 (1.47–1.94)***	2.0 (1.69–2.21)***	1.1 (0.80–1.46)**†	1.1 (0.80–1.46)***†
Sleep duration (h)				
Before	6.1 (1.1)	4.8 (1.0)	5.9 (0.6)	5.8 (1.3)
After	6.2 (1.0)	5.0 (1.0)	6.2 (0.7)	6.5 (1.0)
Disrupted sleep (per night)				
Before	0.9 (0.8)	0.9 (0.8)	1.4 (1.0)	0.9 (1.3)
After	0.6 (0.7)**	0.5 (0.6)**	0.5 (0.6)**	0.3 (0.4)

Data are expressed as mean (95 % confidence interval) for subjective sleep disturbance score and as mean (standard deviation) for sleep duration and disrupted sleep
**$p < 0.01$; ***$p < 0.001$ versus before intervention (Wilcoxon's matched pairs test)
†$p < 0.05$ versus control (Mann–Whitney test)

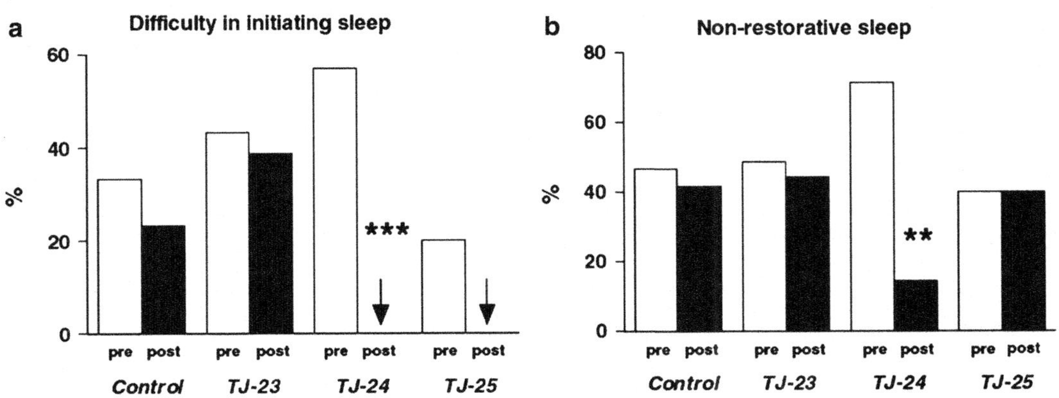

Fig. 1 Percentage of women reporting (**a**) difficulty in initiating sleep (DIS) and (**b**) nonrestorative sleep (NRS) in Japanese peri- and postmenopausal women with sleeping disorder, before and after intervention with either Tokishakuyakusan (TJ-23), Kamishoyosan (TJ-24), or Keishibukuryogan (TJ-25): *open bars*, before intervention; *filled bars*, after intervention. **$p < 0.01$; ***$p < 0.001$ versus pre-treatment, Fisher's exact test

observed in every group, of which the groups TJ-24 and TJ-25 showed a significantly greater decrease ($p < 0.05$, Mann–Whitney test) than the control group. The self-reported sleep duration did not change with treatment in any of the four groups. The percentage of women reporting difficulty in initiating sleep (DIS) and nonrestorative sleep (NRS) reduced substantially after intervention in the TJ-24 group (DIS, from 57 to 0 %, $p < 0.001$; NRS, from 71 to 14 %, $p < 0.01$, Fisher's exact test), while there was a significant decrease in the frequency of disrupted sleep per night in the TJ-23 and TJ-24 groups. These findings indicate that Kampo medicine, especially Kamishoyosan, considerably improved the sleep quality in Japanese peri- and postmenopausal women with sleep disturbances, although they did not extend the sleep duration.

As described above, the women who were prescribed TJ-25 showed higher, if not significantly different, systolic and diastolic pressures and pulse rate at baseline before intervention. The TJ-25 group showed a significant reduction in all the parameters (systolic pressure, 133.0–125.8 mmHg; diastolic pressure, 83.2–80.2 mmHg; pulse rate, 80.7–76.6 mmHg).

Although the exact mechanism by which these Kampo medicines alleviate sleep disturbances is unknown, Mizowaki et al. revealed that the anxiolytic effect of Tokishakuyakusan is mediated by gamma-amino-butyric acid (GABA)-A receptors in a study assessing the social interaction of male mice [24]. One of the common ingredients of Tokishakuyakusan and Kamishoyosan, Japanese Angelica Root, might be the key herb that acts through GABA-A receptors to facilitate sleep [25]. On the other hand, Shinno et al. speculated that the improvement in subjective and objective sleep parameters induced in patients with dementia by another Kampo formula, Yokukansan, is likely to be explained by its serotonergic effect [26]. As Yokukansan shares five of its seven ingredients with Kamishoyosan, their effects on sleep disturbance could have some mechanisms in common.

3 Effects of Keishibukuryogan on Blood Pressure [8]

Women in their youth are less vulnerable to cardiovascular disease (CVD) than men, although this advantage is rapidly reversed after the menopause [27]. This is regarded as proof of the protective effect of estrogen on the cardiovascular system. The prevalence of hypertension—one of the main risk factors for CVD—is known to increase with age [28], so proper management of blood pressure in peri- and postmenopausal women is essential for the prevention of CVD in later life.

The finding of the previous study that Keishibukuryogan did not only improve sleep disturbances but also decreased the blood pressure and pulse rate of insomniac women prompted further analysis of the effects of this formula on the blood pressure of peri- and postmenopausal women with hypertension or high-normal blood pressure.

Our second study of Kampo medicine for the treatment of menopausal symptoms was likewise a retrospective analysis of the records of 1448 Japanese peri- and postmenopausal women enrolled in SHNEP between 1995 and 2009 whose systolic and diastolic blood pressures were measured and recorded. Of these, 374 (25.8 %) women had hypertension (systolic pressure [SP] $\geqq$140 and/or diastolic pressure [DP] $\geqq$90) and 260 (18.0 %) had high-normal blood pressure (SP 130–139 and/or DP 85–89) according to the European Society of Hypertension and European Society of Cardiology criteria.

Of the women with hypertension or high-normal blood pressure, 77 were selected for the second study because they received health/nutrition education with or without Tsumura Keishibukuryogan Extract Granules (TJ-25) and no other medical treatments. The control group (education only) comprised 47 women; the treatment group (education and treatment with TJ-25) comprised 30 women.

After a follow-up period of 182 ± 76 days, there were no significant changes in body weight, body mass index, body fat, or lean body mass in either group. However, the systolic and diastolic blood pressures, the pulse rate, and the REE were significantly reduced in the TJ-25 group. The systolic pressure decreased from 148.4 ± 2.6 mmHg (mean ± standard error of the mean) to 134.8 ± 2.8 mmHg; the diastolic pressure decreased from 89.7 ± 2.1 mmHg to 83.7 ± 1.9 mmHg; the pulse rate decreased from 79.5 ± 1.7 beats/min to 73.5 ± 1.5 beats/min; and the REE decreased from 1552 ± 73 kcal/day to 1373 ± 56 kcal/day (Fig. 2).

Furthermore, the improvements in menopausal symptom scores for perspiration, difficulty sleeping, and headaches/dizziness were statistically significant in the TJ-25 group. The percentages of women who reported difficulty in initiating sleep and nonrestorative sleep were also significantly reduced in the TJ-25 group (from 26.9 to 3.8 %, from 38.5 to 7.7 %, respectively). In terms of the effects of health/nutrition education and TJ-25 on the HR-QOL, both groups showed significant improvements in the mental health and social involvement domains. In addition, women in the TJ-25 group had significant score increases in the physical health and life satisfaction domains.

The exact mechanism underlying the changes induced by Keishibukuryogan is elusive, but several ingredients of the formula are known to affect the vasculature. In a study analyzing the effect of peony root (Paeonia lactifolia) on the rat thoracic aorta [29], the active component gallotannin induced endothelium-dependent vasorelaxation. Similarly, the active components of moutan bark (Paeonia suffruticosa)—pinane glycosides and galloyl glucose—induced endothelium-dependent and nitric-oxide-mediated vasorelaxation [30]. Cinnamaldehyde, the active component of cinnamon, also exerts endothelium-dependent (nitric-oxide-mediated) and endothelium-independent vasorelaxant effects on the rat

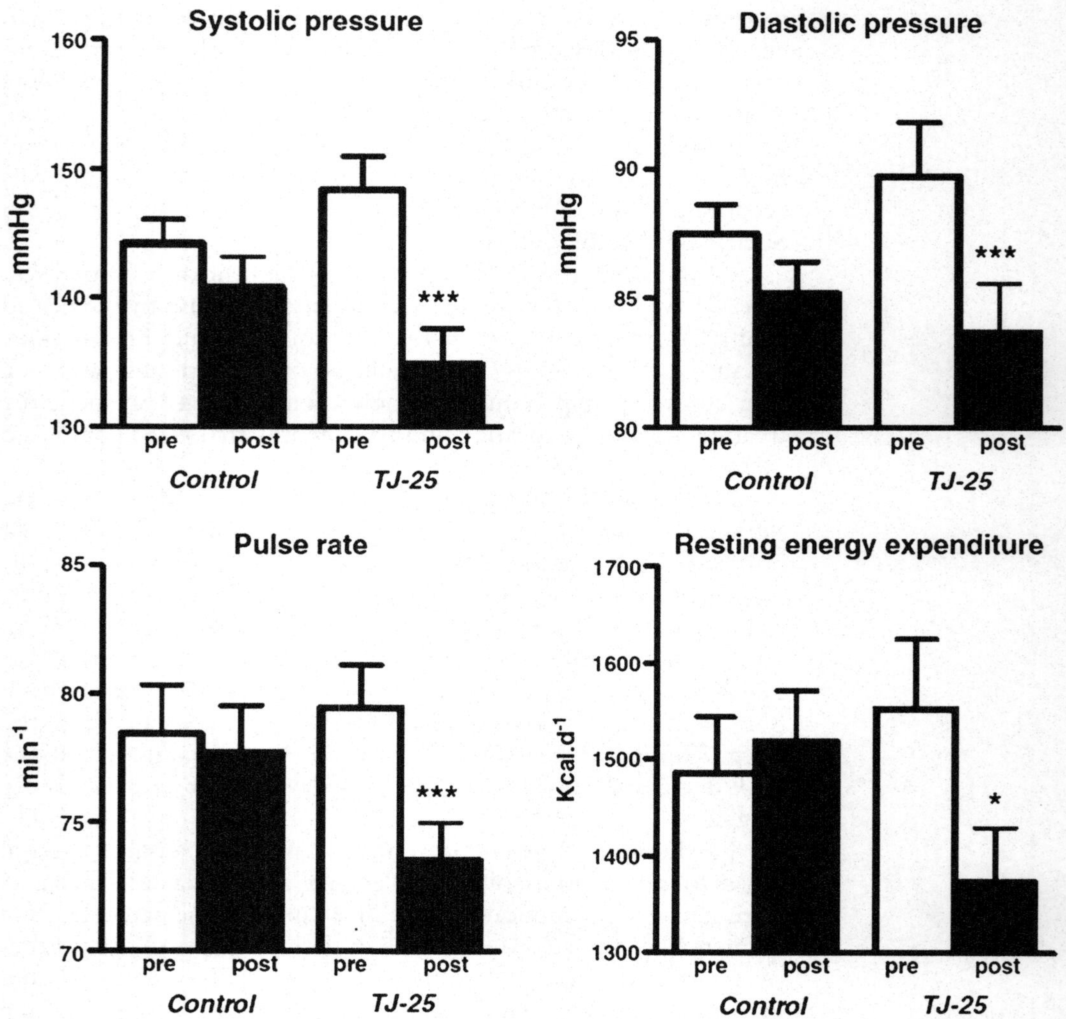

Fig. 2 Cardiovascular parameters before and after the intervention with or without Keishibukuryogan (TJ-25). *Open bars* denote baseline; *filled bars* denote postintervention. The data are presented as mean and standard error. *$P < 0.05$ versus baseline, paired *t* test. ***$P < 0.001$ versus baseline, paired *t* test

thoracic aorta [31]. In addition, the herb reduced the blood pressure of spontaneously hypertensive rats in a dose-dependent manner when mixed in their diet [32]. Moreover, Keishibukuryogan itself induced endothelium-dependent vascular relaxation by inhibiting the release of superoxide from neutrophils [33].

The Keishibukuryogan formula has additional vascular and hemorheological effects. It reduced the number of atheromatous plaques in the aorta of cholesterol-fed rabbits by inhibiting lipid peroxide formation [34], and it promoted the viscoelasticity of red-blood-cell membranes by increasing the intracellular ATP content, thus enhancing red-blood cell deformability [35]. The combination of these mechanisms, which were demonstrated in rodents, could explain the blood-pressure lowering effect of Keishibukuryogan in humans.

In the study, Keishibukuryogan was also effective in the treatment of menopausal symptoms and, as expected, it alleviated perspiration and headaches/dizziness. The observation that Keishibukuryogan improved sleep disturbances in peri- and postmenopausal women with hypertension or high-normal blood pressure supports our previous study. The significant improvements in the physical health and life satisfaction domains induced by Keishibukuryogan could be explained by improvements in menopausal symptoms such as sleep disturbance.

4 Effects of Tokishakuyakusan on Headache [9]

Headache is one of the most common symptoms observed in community and primary care settings, as exemplified by a study revealing that 40 % of the Nordic women in rural communities experience it, indicating that it is more frequent than other somatic symptoms [36]. As expected, headache is included in most of the inventories of menopausal symptom checklists, although the influence of menopause on women's headache depends on the subtypes of headache, such as tension-type headache (TTH) and migraine, which are the two most common ones. More than two-thirds of women with TTH report unchanged or worse status of headache after menopause [37]; on the other hand, migraine improves after menopause, and one of the triggers of migraine is postulated to be the withdrawal of estrogen [38]. The two major types of primary headache mentioned above are, however, often difficult to differentiate in clinical practice and are summarized simply as "headaches" in most of the menopause assessment scales, such as Greene Climacteric Scale and Women's Health Questionnaire.

Headache has been reported to be associated with psychological symptoms. A large-scale study on the Nordic community revealed that depression and anxiety were significantly associated with migraine and nonmigrainous headache and that the former was more strongly associated with psychological symptoms than the latter [39]. A correlation between headache and depression in middle-aged women was also noted in studies conducted in the United States [40] and Japan [41].

In our third study of Kampo medicine for the treatment of menopausal symptoms, we sought to determine the prevalence of headache and its correlates in the Japanese peri- and postmenopausal women and investigate the effect of the Kampo formula Tokishakuyakusan on their headache and concomitant depression. In this retrospective study, we analyzed the records of 345 Japanese peri- and postmenopausal women (age: 40–59 years) who had been enrolled in SHNEP between 2006 and 2010.

The mean ± SD age of the 345 participants was 50.9 ± 4.5 years. The percentages of women who experienced headaches 0–1 time a month, 1–2 times a week, 3–4 times per week, or almost every day were 47.2 %, 27.5 %, 11.6 %, and 13.6 %, respectively. The average age of the women who had headaches almost every day (49.7 ± 4.1) was significantly less (by almost 2 years) than those of the women who experienced the symptom once a month or less frequently (51.6 ± 4.5) ($P < 0.05$, Tukey's test). Additionally, no significant intergroup differences were noted in the ratio of the women in menopause transition to those who were postmenopausal.

Next, we examined the correlations between headaches and other symptoms, namely, vasomotor, depressive, anxious, and insomnia. The scores for the two vasomotor symptoms in the Menopausal Health-Related Quality of Life (MHR-QOL) questionnaire were averaged to generate a vasomotor score. Likewise, the depression score, anxiety score, and insomnia score were calculated from the averages of the scores of four depressive symptoms, two anxious symptoms, and two insomnia symptoms scores, respectively. To determine whether these symptoms were associated with headaches in middle-aged women, we performed a multiple logistic regression analysis by using the presence of headaches once a week or more as the dependent variable and age and the scores for vasomotor symptoms, depression, anxiety, and insomnia as independent variables. Table 3 shows the crude and adjusted ORs for assessing the strength of the relationship between each factor and headaches. Although all the variables included were significantly associated with headaches in the univariate logistic regression analysis, subsequent multiple logistic regression analysis with stepwise variable selection procedure revealed that only age (adjusted OR, 0.92; 95 % CI, 0.88–0.97; $P = 0.0019$) and depression (adjusted

Table 3
Contribution of age, vasomotor symptoms, depression, anxiety, and insomnia to headaches in peri- and postmenopausal women ($N = 345$)

	Crude OR (95 % CI)	*P* value	Adjusted OR (95 % CI)	*P* value
Age	0.93 (0.89–0.98	0.0038	0.92 (0.88–0.97)	0.0019
Vasomotor score	1.31 (1.06–1.63)	0.0136		
Depression score	1.69 (1.36–2.10)	<0.0001	1.73 (1.39–2.16)	<0.0001
Anxiety score	1.51 (1.23–1.86)	<0.0001		
Insomnia score	1.40 (1.16–1.70)	0.0006		

OR, 1.73; 95 % CI, 1.39–2.16; $P < 0.0001$) were significantly associated with headaches after adjustment.

Among the 182 participants who reported having headaches once or more than once a week at their first visits, 37 were treated with either hormone therapy (HT, $N = 17$) or Tsumura Tokishakuyakusan Extract Granules (TJ-23) ($N = 20$); these 37 patients were selected for further analysis.

The percentages of women whose symptom scores decreased after a follow-up period of 147 ± 56 (mean ± SD) days were compared. Significantly more women in the TJ-23 group reported relief from headaches and depression than those in the HT group (headaches, 65 % versus 29 %; depression, 60 % versus 24 %); however, there were no significant intergroup differences in the improvement of vasomotor symptoms, anxiety, and insomnia (Fig. 3).

Finally, an analysis of the association between improvement in headaches and depression in the TJ-23 group showed a significant correlation between the changes in the headache and depression scores with TJ-23 treatment (Fig. 4).

Headache is known to be associated with psychological symptoms and is included in several somatization screening measures, such as Patient Health Questionnaire (PHQ)-15, World Health Organization (WHO)-Social Security Disability (SSD), and Symptom Checklist (SCL)-12. In our study, the presence of headaches once a week or more frequently was found to be associated with depression but not with vasomotor symptoms, anxiety, or insomnia after adjustment. The association between depression and headaches was also confirmed in our previous study [41] and a US population-based study of middle-aged women [40].

The effects of ovarian sex steroids and menopause on headaches appear to differ from the type of headache. TTH is slightly more prevalent in women than in men, and the average of the reported male-to-female ratios is 1:1.30 [37]. This difference is not recognized until children reach puberty, thereby suggesting the involvement of sex steroids in the pathogenesis of TTH [37], although one report suggests that TTH status remains unchanged or becomes worse in 70 % of women with this type of headache after menopause [42]. The sex difference is more marked in the case of migraine: the cumulative lifetime incidence for women is 43 %, while that for men is 18 % [38]. Migraine is known to be affected by hormonal fluctuations, with the effect of estrogen withdrawal being predominant during the perimenopausal period [38]. With the absence of fluctuations in sex hormone levels, the percentage of women reporting migraine after menopause is reduced, as demonstrated by the Penn ovarian aging study [43]. Although HT should be theoretically effective for perimenopausal migraine controlling the hormonal fluctuation, the reports are inconsistent. For example, a large population-based study showed a significant association

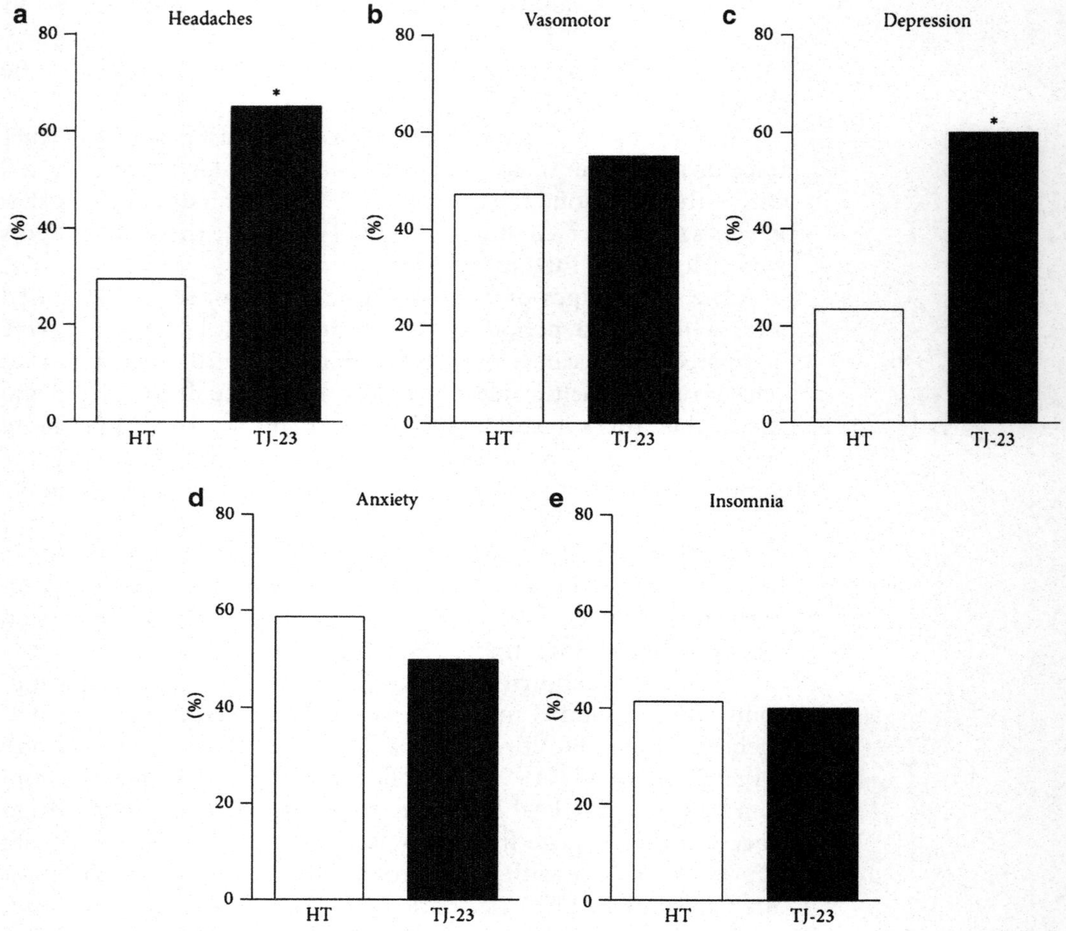

Fig. 3 The percentage of women whose symptom scores decreased after treatment with hormone therapy (HT) or Tokishakuyakusan (TJ-23) $*P < 0.05$ versus HT

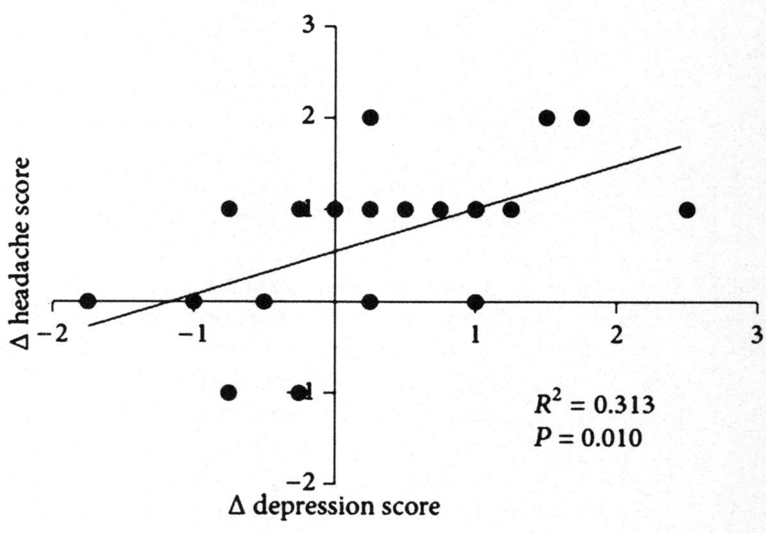

Fig. 4 The association between the improvements in headaches and depression in the Tokishakuyakusan (TJ-23) group

between migraine and nonmigrainous headache with the current use of systemic HT [44]. In the present study, the percentages of women receiving HT whose headache improved, did not change, or worsened were 29 %, 59 %, and 12 %, respectively, which were even better than the percentages indicated in Mueller's report on migraineurs only [45].

The extracts of Ligusticum chuanxiong, a species closely related to the Tokishakuyakusan component Cnidium officinale, have long been used as an analgesic and were shown to alleviate headache [46] and migraine [47] in animal models. Recent reports also indicate that the Chinese equivalent of Tokishakuyakusan, Danggui-Shaoyao-San, exerts antidepressant effects in animal models possibly by suppressing the expression of arginine vasopressin in the pituitary and hypothalamus [48]. The improvements in both headache and depression induced by Tokishakuyakusan could also be attributed to these pharmacological mechanisms. Furthermore, considering the association between headache and depression, it appears that the relieving effect of Tokishakuyakusan on headache may have helped improve the women's mood and vice versa [41].

5 Conclusion

From the results of the recent series of studies of Kampo medicine for the treatment of menopausal symptoms, we reached the following conclusions:

1. Each of the three major Kampo formulae, Tokishakuyakusan, Kamishoyosan, and Keishibukuryogan, was effective in improving sleep disturbances in Japanese peri- and postmenopausal women. Middle-aged women who suffer from difficulties in sleeping but are reluctant to take estrogens or hypnotics due to their unfavorable side effects could be successfully treated by the three Kampo formula as long as the appropriate formula is selected based on each woman's "Sho", or symptom patterns [7].
2. Keishibukuryogan lowered the systolic and diastolic blood pressures, the pulse rate, and the REE of peri- and postmenopausal women with hypertension or high-normal blood pressure. In addition, Keishibukuryogan alleviated menopausal symptoms such as perspiration, headaches/dizziness, and sleep disturbance, and improved the HR-QOL. This Kampo formula could be a therapeutic option for peri- and postmenopausal women with hypertension or high-normal blood pressure who have menopausal symptoms such as vasomotor symptoms and sleep disturbance [8].

3. Headaches in middle-aged women are significantly associated with depression. The Kampo formula Tokishakuyakusan could be an effective treatment for the women with both symptoms.

References

1. Brett KM, Keenan NL (2007) Complementary and alternative medicine use among midlife women for reasons including menopause in the United States: 2002. Menopause 14 (2):300–307
2. van der Sluijs CP, Bensoussan A, Liyanage L, Shah S (2007) Women's health during mid-life survey: the use of complementary and alternative medicine by symptomatic women transitioning through menopause in Sydney. Menopause 14(3):397–403
3. Rossouw JE, Anderson GL, Prentice RL, LaCroix AZ, Kooperberg C, Stefanick ML, Jackson RD, Beresford SA, Howard BV, Johnson KC et al (2002) Risks and benefits of estrogen plus progestin in healthy postmenopausal women: principal results From the Women's Health Initiative randomized controlled trial. JAMA 288(3):321–333
4. Anderson G, Limacher M, Assaf A, Bassford T, Beresford S, Black H, Bonds D, Brunner R, Brzyski R, Caan B et al (2004) Effects of conjugated equine estrogen in postmenopausal women with hysterectomy: the women's health initiative randomized controlled trial. JAMA 291(14):1701–1712
5. Yu F, Takahashi T, Moriya J, Kawaura K, Yamakawa J, Kusaka K, Itoh T, Morimoto S, Yamaguchi N, Kanda A (2006) Traditional Chinese medicine and Kampo: a review from the distant past for the future. J Int Med Res 34 (3):231–239
6. Scheid V, Ward T, Cha W-S, Watanabe K, Liao X (2010) The treatment of menopausal symptoms by traditional East Asian medicines: review and perspectives. Maturitas 66 (2):111–130
7. Terauchi M, Hiramitsu S, Akiyoshi M, Owa Y, Kato K, Obayashi S, Matsushima E, Kubota T (2011) Effects of three Kampo formulae: Tokishakuyakusan (TJ-23), Kamishoyosan (TJ-24), and Keishibukuryogan (TJ-25) on Japanese peri- and postmenopausal women with sleep disturbances. Arch Gynecol Obstet 284(4):913–921
8. Terauchi M, Akiyoshi M, Owa Y, Kato K, Obayashi S, Kubota T (2011) Effects of the Kampo medication keishibukuryogan on blood pressure in perimenopausal and postmenopausal women. Int J Gynecol Obstet 114(2):149–152
9. Terauchi M, Hiramitsu S, Akiyoshi M, Owa Y, Kato K, Obayashi S, Matsushima E, Kubota T (2014) Effects of the kampo formula tokishakuyakusan on headaches and concomitant depression in middle-aged women. Evid-Based Complement Alternat Med 2014:593560
10. Ohayon MM (2002) Epidemiology of insomnia: what we know and what we still need to learn. Sleep Med Rev 6(2):97–111
11. Cappuccio FP, Taggart FM, Kandala N-B, Currie A, Peile E, Stranges S, Miller MA (2008) Meta-analysis of short sleep duration and obesity in children and adults. Sleep 31 (5):619–626
12. Gottlieb DJ, Punjabi NM, Newman AB, Resnick HE, Redline S, Baldwin CM, Nieto FJ (2005) Association of sleep time with diabetes mellitus and impaired glucose tolerance. Arch Intern Med 165(8):863–868
13. Gottlieb DJ, Redline S, Nieto FJ, Baldwin CM, Newman AB, Resnick HE, Punjabi NM (2006) Association of usual sleep duration with hypertension: the sleep heart health study. Sleep 29 (8):1009–1014
14. Hall MH, Muldoon MF, Jennings JR, Buysse DJ, Flory JD, Manuck SB (2008) Self-reported sleep duration is associated with the metabolic syndrome in midlife adults. Sleep 31 (5):635–643
15. Kripke DF, Garfinkel L, Wingard DL, Klauber MR, Marler MR (2002) Mortality associated with sleep duration and insomnia. Arch Gen Psychiatry 59(2):131–136
16. Dennerstein L, Dudley EC, Hopper JL, Guthrie JR, Burger HG (2000) A prospective population-based study of menopausal symptoms. Obstet Gynecol 96(3):351–358
17. Kravitz HM, Ganz PA, Bromberger J, Powell LH, Sutton-Tyrrell K, Meyer PM (2003) Sleep difficulty in women at midlife: a community survey of sleep and the menopausal transition. Menopause 10(1):19–28
18. Health NIo: National Institutes of Health State-of-the-Science Conference statement: management of menopause-related symptoms. Ann Intern Med 2005, 142(12 Pt 1): 1003–1013
19. Ohayon MM (2006) Severe hot flashes are associated with chronic insomnia. Arch Intern Med 166(12):1262–1268

20. Ensrud KE, Stone KL, Blackwell TL, Sawaya GF, Tagliaferri M, Diem SJ, Grady D (2009) Frequency and severity of hot flashes and sleep disturbance in postmenopausal women with hot flashes. Menopause 16(2):286–292
21. Zervas IM, Lambrinoudaki I, Spyropoulou AC, Koundi KL, Voussoura E, Tzavara C, Verdeli H, Aravantinos L, Creatsa M, Paparrigopoulos T (2009) Additive effect of depressed mood and vasomotor symptoms on postmenopausal insomnia. Menopause 16(4):837–842
22. Joffe H, Soares CN, Thurston RC, White DP, Cohen LS, Hall JE (2009) Depression is associated with worse objectively and subjectively measured sleep, but not more frequent awakenings, in women with vasomotor symptoms. Menopause 16(4):671–679
23. Terauchi M, Obayashi S, Akiyoshi M, Kato K, Matsushima E, Kubota T (2010) Insomnia in Japanese peri- and postmenopausal women. Climacteric 13(5):479–486
24. Mizowaki M, Toriizuka K, Hanawa T (2001) Anxiolytic effect of Kami-Shoyo-San (TJ-24) in mice possible mediation of neurosteroid synthesis. Life Sci 69(18):2167–2177
25. Matsumoto K, Kohno S-I, Qjima K, Tezuka Y, Kadota S, Watanabe H (1998) Effects of methylenechloride-soluble fraction of Japanese angelica root extract, ligustilide and butylidenephthalide, on pentobarbital sleep in group-housed and socially isolated mice. Life Sci 62 (23):2073–2082
26. Shinno H, Inami Y, Inagaki T, Nakamura Y, Horiguchi J (2008) Effect of Yi-Gan San on psychiatric symptoms and sleep structure at patients with behavioral and psychological symptoms of dementia. Prog Neuropsychopharmacol Biol Psychiatry 32(3):881–885
27. Thom T, Haase N, Rosamond W, Howard VJ, Rumsfeld J, Manolio T, Zheng Z-J, Flegal K, O'Donnell C, Kittner S et al (2006) Heart disease and stroke statistics–2006 update: a report from the American Heart Association Statistics Committee and Stroke Statistics Subcommittee. Circulation 113(6):e85–e151
28. Burt VL, Whelton P, Roccella EJ, Brown C, Cutler JA, Higgins M, Horan MJ, Labarthe D (1995) Prevalence of hypertension in the US adult population. Results from the Third National Health and Nutrition Examination Survey, 1988-1991. Hypertension 25 (3):305–313
29. Goto H, Shimada Y, Akechi Y, Kohta K, Hattori M, Terasawa K (1996) Endothelium-dependent vasodilator effect of extract prepared from the roots of Paeonia lactiflora on isolated rat aorta. Planta Med 62 (5):436–439
30. Yoo MY, Lee BH, Choi YH, Lee JW, Seo JH, Oh K-S, Koo H-N, Seo HW, Yon GH, Kwon DY et al (2006) Vasorelaxant effect of the root-bark extract of Paeonia moutan on isolated rat thoracic aorta. Planta Med 72(14):1338–1341
31. Yanaga A, Goto H, Nakagawa T, Hikiami H, Shibahara N, Shimada Y (2006) Cinnmaldehyde induces endothelium-dependent and -independent vasorelaxant action on isolated rat aorta. Biol Pharm Bull 29(12):2415–2418
32. Preuss HG, Echard B, Polansky MM, Anderson R (2006) Whole cinnamon and aqueous extracts ameliorate sucrose-induced blood pressure elevations in spontaneously hypertensive rats. J Am Coll Nutr 25(2):144–150
33. Sekiya N, Goto H, Tazawa K, Oida S, Shimada Y, Terasawa K (2002) Keishi-bukuryo-gan preserves the endothelium dependent relaxation of thoracic aorta in cholesterol-fed rabbit by limiting superoxide generation. Phytother Res 16(6):524–528
34. Sekiya N, Tanaka N, Itoh T, Shimada Y, Goto H, Terasawa K (1999) Keishi-bukuryo-gan prevents the progression of atherosclerosis in cholesterol-fed rabbit. Phytother Res 13 (3):192–196
35. Goto H, Shimada Y, Sekiya N, Yang Q, Kogure T, Mantani N, Hikiami H, Shibahara N, Terasawa K (2004) Effects of Keishi-bukuryo-gan on vascular function and hemorheological factors in spontaneously diabetic (WBN/kob) rats. Phytomedicine 11(2/3):188–195
36. Haug TT, Mykletun A, Dahl AA (2004) The association between anxiety, depression, and somatic symptoms in a large population: the HUNT-II study. Psychosom Med 66 (6):845–851
37. Lieba-Samal D, Wöber C (2011) Sex hormones and primary headaches other than migraine. Curr Pain Headache Rep 15 (5):407–414
38. MacGregor EA (2009) Migraine headache in perimenopausal and menopausal women. Curr Pain Headache Rep 13(5):399–403
39. Zwart JA, Dyb G, Hagen K, Ødegård KJ, Dahl AA, Bovim G, Stovner LJ (2003) Depression and anxiety disorders associated with headache frequency. The Nord-Trøndelag Health Study. Eur J Neurol 10(2):147–152
40. Brown JP, Gallicchio L, Flaws JA, Tracy JK (2009) Relations among menopausal symptoms, sleep disturbance and depressive symptoms in midlife. Maturitas 62(2):184–189
41. Terauchi M, Hiramitsu S, Akiyoshi M, Owa Y, Kato K, Obayashi S, Matsushima E, Kubota T (2013) Associations among depression, anxiety and somatic symptoms in peri- and

postmenopausal women. J Obstet Gynaecol Res 39(5):1007–1013

42. Neri I, Granella F, Nappi R, Manzoni GC, Facchinetti F, Genazzani AR (1993) Characteristics of headache at menopause: a clinico-epidemiologic study. Maturitas 17(1):31–37
43. Freeman EW, Sammel MD, Lin H, Gracia CR, Kapoor S (2008) Symptoms in the menopausal transition: hormone and behavioral correlates. Obstet Gynecol 111(1):127–136
44. Aegidius KL, Zwart JA, Hagen K, Schei B, Stovner LJ (2007) Hormone replacement therapy and headache prevalence in postmenopausal women. The Head-HUNT study. Eur J Neurol 14(1):73–78
45. Mueller L (2000) Predictability of exogenous hormone effect on subgroups of migraineurs. Headache 40(3):189–193
46. Peng C, Xie X, Wang L, Guo L, Hu T (2009) Pharmacodynamic action and mechanism of volatile oil from Rhizoma Ligustici Chuanxiong Hort. on treating headache. Phytomedicine 16(1):25–34
47. Wang YH, Liang S, Xu DS, Lin X, He CY, Feng Y, Hong YL (2011) Effect and mechanism of senkyunolide I as an anti-migraine compound from Ligusticum chuanxiong. J Pharm Pharmacol 63(2):261–266
48. Xu F, Peng D, Tao C, Yin D, Kou J, Zhu D, Yu B (2011) Anti-depression effects of Danggui-Shaoyao-San, a fixed combination of traditional Chinese medicine, on depression model in mice and rats. Phytomedicine 18 (13):1130–1136

Chapter 8

Fatigue and Kampo (Japanese Herbal) Medicines: Hochuekkito and Juzentaihoto

Jun-ichi Yamakawa, Junji Moriya, and Junji Kobayashi

Abstract

Together with pain and fever, fatigue is known as one of the living body's three main alarms, an important signal to the body for the maintenance of life and health. The body usually recovers from fatigue with rest, but a feeling of fatigue may persist for a long period. When the symptoms and duration of fatigue exceed the usual fatigued feeling, the body's immune function deteriorates making it prone to psychological disorders such as depression, as well as a range of infectious diseases. Few Western medications are useful for this kind of fatigue. There are, however, many useful formulae among Kampo medications. The introduction below first gives a brief explanation of qi (Ki), blood and fluid (*Kiketsusui*), and the "patterns" of Kampo medical diagnosis before discussing the Kampo medical diagnoses "qi (Ki) deficiency (*Kikyo*), blood deficiency (*Kekkyo*), and dual deficiency of qi (Ki) and blood (*Kiketsu Ryokyo*)" and how fatigue was perceived in olden times. The "Discussion" part focuses on clinical reports on two prominent Kampo medications, hochuekkito (補中益気湯) and juzentaihoto (十全大補湯).

Key words Fatigue, Kampo, Hochuekkito, Juzentaihoto, qi (Ki) deficiency (*Kikyo*), Dual deficiency of qi (Ki), Blood (*Kiketsu Ryokyo*)

1 Introduction

1.1 Fatigue: Definition

Together with pain and fever, fatigue is known as one of the living body's three main alarms, an important signal to the body for the maintenance of life and health. The physiological fatigue that occurs in healthy people can be defined as the condition in which performance has temporarily decreased when the body or mind is stressed. It is usually accompanied by lethargy and the desire for rest. The fatigue that occurs in sick people even with little stress (pathological fatigue) may exhibit chronically decreased performance and lethargy, such as in chronic fatigue syndrome, diabetes, and malignant tumor.

Fatigue is classified as either physiological or pathological. Physiological fatigue occurs in people with no underlying disease when the amount of activity exceeds the level of recuperation and

Akio Inui (ed.), *Herbal Medicines: New Horizons*, Methods in Pharmacology and Toxicology, DOI 10.1007/978-1-4939-4002-8_8,

recovery is possible without intervention. Pathological fatigue occurs with diseases characterized by persistent fatigue, such as chronic fatigue syndrome, when a physical disease such as AIDS or cancer, or a psychological disorder such as depression or sleep disorder is present. Pathological fatigue may also be accompanied by objective symptoms including fever, lymph node swelling, and memory disorder [1, 2].

1.2 Fatigue: Condition

Lack of energy is a clear sign of fatigue. Humans need energy to engage in activity. But when fatigued, activity or movement is not possible. Sleepiness, decreased cognitive ability, lack of concentration, or a feeling of powerlessness appear. Decreased physical activity may also be observed. Fatigue is a condition in which the capacities to accomplish activities such as work and everyday living are diminished, the lack of energy makes engaging in new activities difficult, and sustaining activity becomes harder.

There is also a decrease in action relating to social motivations, which stem variously from physiological needs, curiosity, interests, and concerns. Lassitude, lack of concern, and hypobulia appear and psychological stress may be experienced.

1.3 Pathological Fatigue

The body usually recovers from fatigue with rest. However, a feeling of fatigue may persist for long periods. When the symptoms and duration of fatigue exceed the usual fatigued feeling, the body's immune function deteriorates making it prone to psychological disorders such as depression, as well as a range of infectious diseases [1, 2].

2 Looking at Fatigue from the Kampo Medical Perspective

2.1 The Patterns (Sho) of Kampo Medical DiagnosisKampo medical diagnosis

To obtain a complete response using Kampo treatments for fatigue that does not effectively respond to Western medicine-centered treatments, it is necessary to consider the differences between the Western medical and the Kampo medical perspectives. While Western medicine takes an analytical approach to comprehending local abnormalities (i.e. disease), Kampo medicine characteristically takes a comprehensive approach to general physical disorder (i.e. the sick person). The question therefore arises: how are Kampo medication formulae selected? In turn, this is a matter of understanding the patterns (*Sho*) of Kampo medical diagnosis. What are these patterns? *Patterns* are considered to be "criteria for the use of Kampo medications that have been organized on the basis of Kampo measures for all the subjective and objective symptoms of a sick person; being the "measures" that indicate the relationships between the patient and the illness, patterns are used for differentiating those for whom a medication will or will not be effective and therefore for avoiding unsuitable Kampo medications." Our predecessors wrote about patterns as follows. Keisetsu Otsuka: "Patterns mean evidence or conclusive proof. The kakkonto–pattern (葛根湯証) means the indication for kakkonto, which is the same as calling what is diagnosed as a cold, the aspirin-pattern" [3]. Kunio Matsuda: "Patterns are multiple, unified concepts that become apparent with certain pathological conditions" [4]. Kazuo Tatsuno: "Patterns are the preconditions for a medication to be effective. Patterns mean the clinical pictures representing patients' current conditions" [5]. Katsutoshi Terasawa: "Patterns mean the diagnoses obtained by comprehending the symptoms presented by patients through the basic concepts of qi (*Ki*), blood and fluid; yin and yang; deficiency and excess (*Kyojitsu*); cold and heat (*Kannetsu*); exterior and interior (*Hyori*); the five viscera (*Gozo*); the six stages of disease transformation (*Rokubyoi*), and so on, and they are directions for treatment" [6].

2.2 Patterns in Practice (Qi [Ki], Blood and Fluid [Kiketsusui])

The characteristic features of treatment in Kampo medicine are that it "leads to health by improving physical constitution, without concerning itself with the sickness itself" and that it sustains the human innate balance adjustment mechanism, or homeostasis. In Kampo medicine, three elements in the body, qi (Ki), blood, and fluid, are seen as elements by which normal functioning of organs and tissues as well as the functioning of the mind and body are carried out. Health is sustained on the basis of these three, qi (Ki) and blood and fluid. Blood and fluid (*Shineki*) are first activated by qi (Ki), the motive force, then circulate through the whole body supplying nutrients. Various diseases may occur when this balance is upset. The foundation of this concept came into being in China in the Jin/Yuan Dynasty and the theory of qi (Ki), blood and fluid was established by Nangai Yoshimasu (1750–1813) [7, 8].

Qi (Ki), blood and fluid are the three elements that sustain the body's function and structure. They are thought to represent the environment surrounding the cells for their structural formation and functional expression.

Qi (Ki) is the "Ki" in "*Genki*" (energy, spirit) and "*Kiryoku*" (vitality). It is invisible life energy. "Qi (Ki)" is the term for the mental and functional activities that occur in the body. At the cellular level, qi (Ki) works to activate the metabolism and flow of information within cells and to advance the body's functional expression and structural formation.

The "blood" and the "fluid" both moisten the body and they are the bodily fluids that provide nutrients. The red-colored fluid is the "blood" and the colorless bodily fluids are the "fluid". "Blood" is the blood that flows throughout the body, the blood acting as a lubricant providing oxygen and nutrients by circulating around the body. At the cellular level blood supplies the raw materials needed for the chemical reactions within the cell, and it sustains functional expression and structural formation in the body. "Fluid" is the liquid, meaning the bodily fluids other than blood, such as lymph, digestive fluids, and saliva. At the cellular level, "fluid" sustains intracellular fluid and acts in particular to moisten the skin and membranes, which come in contact with the external world. "Blood and fluid" circulate through the body supporting the action of "qi (Ki)". The Kampo perspective holds that when healthy, the circulation of qi (Ki), blood and fluid is well balanced and that "physical disorders appear when even one of qi (Ki), blood or fluid is deficient or flows poorly".

2.3 Fatigue Means "qi (Ki) Deficiency (Kikyo), Blood Deficiency (Kekkyo), or Dual Deficiency of qi (Ki) and Blood (Kiketsu Ryokyo)"

Qi (Ki) is taken in through food nutrients and breath then supports various actions in the body. It has these five particular actions: (1) promotion action: it promotes internal organ function and blood and fluid flow; (2) warming action: it maintains body temperature, warms internal organs, and promotes their function; (3) defense action: it protects the body's surface to prevent external pathogens entering; (4) qi (Ki) transformation action: it transforms "blood" into energy or vigor, and transforms "fluid" into sweat; (5) fastening action: it regulates the amounts of saliva, menstrual blood, etc. and adjusts excretion of bodily substances. The condition in which there is insufficient "qi (Ki)" is called qi (Ki) deficiency. This condition gives rise to fatigue symptoms such as "a vague feeling of listlessness" and "a lack of desire to do anything". We discuss this further in the "Discussion" part of this paper.

"Blood" means the nutrients produced by digestion of food. The blood thereby produced is sent throughout the body. Having been sent throughout the body, the blood is utilized as a source of nutrients supporting bodily functions, it sustains muscles and bones, as well as skin, hair, and nails. Along with qi (Ki), this blood is the basic substance that supports mental activity and sustains consciousness and mental condition. The condition in which there is insufficient "blood" is called blood deficiency. Dual deficiency of qi (Ki) and blood indicates a condition where there is a combination of both qi (Ki) deficiency and blood deficiency.

Qi (Ki) deficiency means the functions and activities of the entire body diminish while blood deficiency means the blood's moistening and nourishing functions throughout the body are lost. While qi (Ki) gives rise to blood, blood is considered to be the material basis for production of qi (Ki), which means that qi (Ki) deficiency or blood deficiency alone have the tendencies of dual deficiency of qi (Ki) and blood to some extent. In addition, in most advanced cases of either qi (Ki) or blood deficiency, dual deficiency of qi (Ki) and blood develops. Blood deficiency is generally more likely than qi (Ki) deficiency to developing into dual deficiency of qi (Ki) and blood.

Thus, Kampo medicine means thoroughly ascertaining each person's physical constitution and the condition of their illness before selecting the Kampo medications to be used. It could be called a made-to-order method of treatment and when the Kampo medication suitable to the patient is prescribed, the efficacy of treatment is improved. The Kampo medical approach includes the concepts of "same illness, different treatment", whereby different Kampo medications are prescribed for the same Western medical diagnosis, and "different illnesses, same treatment", whereby the same Kampo medication is ultimately prescribed for different Western medical diagnoses. In either case, it is not a matter of addressing the illness by looking at the superficial aspect of the emerged symptoms, but by looking to the more fundamental aspects. Kampo holds that there are various causes for any one phenomenon or event, so, even if two patients have the same fatigue symptoms, the formulae may be completely different, according to the patient.

2.4 The Treatments for Fatigue Devised by Our Predecessors

The backbone of Japanese Kampo medicine is the *ShangHanLun*, a medical text that gathers together the experiences of the ancient Han peoples [9, 10]. It is a "therapeutics" text, a properly organized text with extremely detailed information. There is no other text comparable to it in the world: it is a very important work and also a clinical medicine textbook. The *ShangHanLun* is fundamentally a text that sets out the course and treatments for "acute febrile diseases". However in Japan, many of our predecessors over the years managed to read, digest and absorb the contents of this text, which is written in difficult classical Chinese, though with a concise style, then elaborate on the applications and techniques, and through their researches devise ways for it to be used for "chronic diseases" as well. Thus, Japanese Kampo, with its uniqueness and characteristic features, came into being.

Yet, treatments and formulae for fatigue, the chronic symptom, were devised mainly through the medical thinking of the Chinese in the Jin/Yuan Dynasty [11, 12]. This was a period of war, of meager food and very harsh labor and living conditions. Many people were dying, having been driven to "internal illness" (malnutrition). Medical thinking turned to formulae to supplement the workings of the stomach and intestines by using medications to control the physical stresses. The medications discussed in the "Discussion" part of this paper, hochuekkito and juzentaihoto, were developed at that time. Then the basis for the concept of "nourishing life" emerged. This concept still exists in contemporary Japan.

Here is an example of the practical use of hochuekkito with a description by Gensen Tsuda in his text, *Hyakuho Kuketsushu* (1794) [13]. From *Hochuekkito, Zatsubyo Hassho Mokuteki no Ben* (*Hochuekkito, Identification of the Targets for the 8 Miscellaneous Disease Patterns*): (1) hands and feet feel lifeless, (2) speech has no vigor, (3) eyes lack force, (4) white spittle develops in the mouth, (5) food cannot be tasted, (6) cold things are disliked, hot tea and food are preferred, (7) the navel area palpitates, and (8) the pulse lacks strength. The text states that if symptoms matching even one or two of the above is present, then hochuekkito should be used.

2.5 Effective Formulae for Fatigue—Ginseng (Ninjin) and Astragalus Root (Ogi), the Main Components in Tonifying Formulae

1. For convenience sake, the classification of Kampo formulae calls the group of formulae whose main component is Ginseng and Astragalus Root, *jingizai*. These two crude drugs are contained in almost all Kampo tonifying formulae. Formulae including Ginseng and Astragalus Root are used to improve symptoms presented by patients with chronic disease in physical and mental decline, decreased gastrointestinal functioning and whose main indication is fatigue and listlessness. The ninjin in almost all Kampo tonifying formulae is the root of the Ginseng plant (family Araliaceae): *ninjin* (carrot) the vegetable (family Umbelliferae) is a completely different plant. The clinical effects of Ginseng include activation of digestive and absorption functions and strengthening of the body's nonspecific resistance to various stresses. The saponins contained in Ginseng stimulate protein synthesis and improve metabolism and immunocompetence. It also effectively improves nutritional status and physical weakening due to surgery, etc., anorexia, diminished vitality, and anemia caused by malignant tumors. Other reported effects of Ginseng include prevention of chemotherapy-induced impairment of blood-forming tissue, suppression of immune function decline, and control of cancer cell growth and metastasis [14, 15].

   Astragalus Root is the root of Astragalus membranaceus or Astragalus mongholicus, in the family Fabaceae. The polysaccharides in Astragalus Root have been reported to strengthen immune function and effectively improve resistance to illness in general. It stimulates blood circulation and metabolism at the body surface and improves the skin's nutritional status. It is reported to enhance cellular metabolism and promote DNA synthesis in regenerating liver [16–18].

   Ginseng is suitable for digestive tract weakness (called interior deficiency in Kampo medicine) while Astragalus Root is suitable for weakened resistance at the body surface (or exterior deficiency). While Ginseng works to increase bodily fluid, Astragalus Root works to eliminate excess water. Ingesting a large quantity of Ginseng causes swelling and increased blood pressure, however, combining Astragalus Root, which has a diuretic effect, alleviates the side effects of Ginseng while enhancing the synergistic effect of improving diminished physical strength and resistance. It is therefore the main formula of choice in Kampo medical analeptic therapies.

   Thus, jingizai (formulae combining Ginseng and Astragalus Root) are therapeutic medications for conditions in which there is a deficiency of qi (Ki), the fundamental energy for general biological activity. Hochuekkito, a typical tonifying formula, is used for chronic diseases demonstrating persistent symptoms such as weakness with susceptibility to tiredness, diminished gastrointestinal function, pronounced lassitude in the limbs and anorexia. The effectiveness of juzentaihoto becomes relevant if blood deficiency is also present. Juzentaihoto is used to improve digestive function and for recovery or improvement of physical strength after illness or surgery, however, skin parching and blood deficiency are the particular signs to differentiate it from hochuekkito.

2. Hochuekkito—The predominant formulation for qi (Ki) deficiency

   The pathological condition in which there is a deficiency in the amount of qi (Ki) is called qi (Ki) deficiency. It refers to reduced metabolism, reduced organ function, reduced resistance and decreased life energy, our energy and vital force as living beings. Naturally, most cancer patients who undergo therapies including surgery and anticancer drugs demonstrate symptoms of qi (Ki) deficiency. Surgery and anticancer drugs trigger tissue and organ damage, digestive and absorption functions diminish and anorexia emerges, which in turn further decreases physical strength, creating a vicious cycle. If the condition persists, immunity and recuperative powers also diminish [14, 15].

   Western medical treatments such as digestive drugs, digestive tract prokinetic agents and vitamins do not promise efficacy for this kind of anorexia and decreased physical strength. Kampo treatments to increase the amount of qi (Ki) are effective. To supplement the deficient qi (Ki) and improve qi (Ki) deficiency is to tonify qi (Ki), while increasing the amount of qi (Ki) has the effect of stimulating organ and tissue functioning and lifting one's spirits.

   The predominant qi (Ki) tonifying formula is hochuekkito [12]. It is made from ten crude drugs: Ginseng, Astragalus Root, Atractylodes Rhizome (byakujutsu), Glycyrrhiza (kanzo), Jujube (taiso), Citrus Unshiu Peel (chimpi), Ginger (shokyo), Bupleurum Root (saiko), Cimicifuga Rhizome (shoma), and Japanese Angelica Root (toki). True to name, it is formulated to tonify ("ho") the inside ("chu"), that is, the digestive organs, and to boost energy ("ekki"). It also cures general physical fatigue, supplements lack of good spirits or vitality, and improves the body's vital force. It is used for pathological conditions in which digestive system functioning has decreased, appetite is absent, and energy is lacking. The indications are pronounced susceptibility to tiredness, lack of energy, lack of vitality, orthostatic dizziness, muscle weakness, and lassitude in the limbs.

   It improves lack of tension in smooth and skeletal muscles as well as organ droop and reduced digestive organ motility. Astragalus Root and Japanese Angelica Root stimulate granulation and are effective for skin ulcers and similar conditions that persistently fail to respond. Because of its ability to improve biological defense, including immunologic enhancement, it is also effective when complicating cold or flu and bronchitis. It is commonly used for chronic hepatitis and cirrhosis in people demonstrating deficiency pattern (*Kyosho*), decreased physical strength or general debility induced by infection or malignant tumor, or decreased physical strength after surgery [1, 2, 14, 15].

3. Juzentaihoto—The predominant formulation for dual deficiency of qi (Ki) and blood

   In Kampo medicine, "blood" almost means the same as "blood" in Western medicine; however, Kampo medicine takes a conceptual view of its role, conceiving it to be a biogenic substance found in blood vessels that circulates throughout the body carrying out the roles of nourishing and moistening tissues and organs. Blood deficiency is a pathological change exhibited by excessive bleeding and gives rise to a lack of blood production in the body. It is caused by exhaustion of blood due to degenerative disease, surgical invasion, malignant tumor and the like, or gastrointestinal or atypical genital bleeding.

   Blood deficiency symptoms are the symptoms caused by a decrease in moistening and nourishing by the blood, and they generally reflect poor nutritional status. Blood deficiency also demonstrates symptoms that would suggest autonomic nervous system or endocrine system disorder.

   Common blood deficiency symptoms include poor facial complexion, dull skin, lightheadedness, blurry vision, poor nail color, loss of hair, and hair roughness. Additionally, other characteristic symptoms may appear, depending on which organ is the site of the blood deficiency (i.e., heart blood deficiency or liver blood deficiency).

   In Kampo medicine, the "heart [traditional medical terminology: TM]" sustains the level of consciousness and has the function of regulating the rhythms of wakening and sleep. Accordingly, symptoms such as palpitations, anxiety, impatience, light sleep, insomnia, frequent dreaming, forgetfulness, and decreased cognitive power occur in heart blood deficiency. These are mainly considered symptoms caused by excitability abnormalities in the central nervous system or cerebrum.

   The "liver [TM]" regulates the flow of blood and qi (Ki), stabilizes mental activity, stores blood, provides nutrition to the entire body, and maintains skeletal muscle tension. Accordingly, liver blood deficiency demonstrates symptoms caused by disorders of the autonomic nervous system or endocrine system and the like associated with deficient supplementation of nutrition to organs throughout the body. Early-stage symptoms commonly include dizziness, blurry vision, eye tiredness, feeling of eye dryness, bleary eyes, and other eye symptoms.

This leads to limb numbness, muscle spasm, desensitization, muscle reflex disorder, abnormal sensation, menstrual disorder, delayed menstruation, hypomenorrhea, or amenorrhea.

The crude drugs that have a blood tonifying action (blood tonifying medications) are broadly categorized as medications that tonify either heart blood or liver blood. The crude drugs that primarily tonify heart blood include Longan Aril (ryugan-niku), Polygala Root (onji), Jujube Seed (sansonin), and Salvia Miltiorrhiza Root (tanjin). They fortify the brain's inhibitory processes and demonstrate effectiveness for mental stability and sleep.

The crude drugs that tonify liver blood include Japanese Angelica Root, Peony Root (shakuyaku), Rehmannia Root (jio), Polygonum Root (kashu), Donkey Glue (akyo), and Lycium Fruit (kukoshi). Their primary effects are to improve nutritional status and endocrine system abnormalities by nourishing and moistening.

The main blood tonifying formulation is shimotsuto (四物湯) (Japanese Angelica Root, Peony Root, Cnidium Rhizome [senkyu], and Rehmannia Root). The blood tonifying actions of Japanese Angelica Root, Peony Root, and Rehmannia Root improve the nutritional status of the whole body and have the secondary action of improving endocrine and autonomic system disorders. Cnidium Rhizome and Japanese Angelica Root, which treat blood stasis, stimulate circulation, effectively spreading the tonifying effect to the whole body. They are used for people who have relatively poor physical strength, poor facial complexion, are susceptible to anemia and skin dryness, as well as blood deficiency symptoms such as a fatigued feeling, dizzy sensation, blurry vision, and palpitations.

The predominant formulation used for dual deficiency of qi (Ki) and blood is juzentaihoto. It is made from a combination of ten crude drugs: Ginseng, Atractylodes Rhizome, Poria Sclerotium (bukuryo), Glycyrrhiza, Japanese Angelica Root, Peony Root, Rehmannia Root, Cnidium Rhizome, Astragalus Root, and Cinnamon Bark (keihi). Four of these crude drugs, Ginseng, Atractylodes Rhizome, Poria Sclerotium, and Glycyrrhiza, are the main crude drugs in shikunshito (四君子湯) and improve digestive system function.

The four crude drugs, Japanese Angelica Root, Peony Root, Rehmannia Root, and Cnidium Rhizome, make up the main blood deficiency formulation mentioned above, shimotsuto. Combining the effects of Astragalus Root, which is a qi (Ki) tonifying crude drug, and Cinnamon Bark, which improves blood flow, with the other crude drugs, works to improve both qi (Ki) and blood deficiency. This outlines the basic Kampo medical concepts about fatigue. The discussion below focuses on clinical reports.

2.6 Discussion

Hochuekkito and juzentaihoto are both reported to strengthen immunity and improve nutritional status. They have also been reported to improve QOL when used in clinical practice to alleviate the side effects of cancer chemotherapy and radiation therapy, mainly after surgery.

3 Hochuekkito

Hochuekkito is a tonifying formula that primarily restores vigor in patients with qi (Ki) deficiency and can be expected to improve anorexia, general malaise, and sleep disorder. Similarly to juzentaihoto, there are numerous acknowledged reports on hochuekkito for anorexia and nausea in cancer chemotherapy patients. Abe found that out of 30 malignant tumor patients who underwent chemotherapy after surgery, the efficacy ratio of hochuekkito for improvement of general malaise and anorexia was 83.3 % [19]. A study by Ohara et al. evaluated the clinical effectiveness of hochuekkito or ninjinyoeito (参養栄湯) for patients undergoing chemotherapy (tegafur preparation). They found that it significantly improved subjective symptoms (before–after comparison) including appetite, nausea and vomiting, bowel movement disturbance, and feeling of fatigue and malaise [20]. Ono et al. investigated the clinical effects of hochuekkito and the immune strength of natural killer (NK) cell activity in 35 cases and found that NK cell activity before administration was 24.6 ± 13.7 % and 30.4 ± 14.4 % after administration, which was a significant increase, given a P value of at most 5 % [21]. While its effects on germ discharge count during expectoration and on blood sedimentation in a group receiving concomitant hochuekkito were not clear, it demonstrated significant increases in weight and peripheral blood lymphocyte count and was useful as an adjunct to anti-tuberculosis therapy [22]. Additionally, an administration group demonstrated a significant increase in prognostic nutrition index (PNI = albumin level × 10 + peripheral blood lymphocyte count × 0.005) [23]. In a number of studies, the appetite stimulant effect of hochuekkito restored nutritional status and also improved susceptibility to infection. Apart from chemotherapy, hochuekkito has also been reported to demonstrate significant improvement in gastroptosis symptoms including anorexia, abdominal bloating sensation, nausea and feeling of fatigue and malaise, etc. [24], while it significantly improved symptoms in pediatric orthostatic dysregulation, demonstrating a high disappearance rate for umbilical colic, lassitude, headache, and hypotension, in particular [25]. In addition to numerous such reports, Kuratsune evaluated performance status in chronic fatigue syndrome (CFS), the causes of which remain unexplained and in which sufferers report a particularly persistent and strong sense of fatigue, and found symptomatic improvement in 41.4 % of cases [26].

Hochuekkito improved clinical symptoms and performance status in 12 weeks, a relatively short period, prompting the conclusion that hochuekkito could be the standard therapy for CFS patients, who commonly cannot maintain adequate waking hours due to sleep disorder and everyday life rhythm disorder [27]. In an experiment using animals with CFS, hochuekkito demonstrated improvement in the amount of movement soon after treatment commenced (in 1–2 weeks) and a significant increase in IFN-γ expression in the spleen [28]. A similar experiment found effective improvement in central nervous system disorder, which is thought to be present in CFS [29]. The authors inferred that the pathological condition of CFS includes some kind of immune system abnormality and that the therapeutic effect of hochuekkito lay in its immunostimulatory action. Hochuekkito was also useful for improving the subjective symptoms of snoring, daytime sleepiness, and insomnia in sleep-disordered breathing sufferers [30]. It was effective for improving sperm density and motility in infertile males and demonstrated effective stimulation of spermatogenic function [31]. Hochuekkito was 66.0 % effective for anorexia associated with mild to moderate depression [32]. These and other papers report wide efficacy for pathological conditions considered to be qi (Ki) and/or blood deficiency in oriental medicine.

4 Juzentaihoto

Juzentaihoto is primarily used for prevention of anticancer drug side effects such as queasy, anorexia, lassitude, and bone marrow suppression, and is reported to be useful in clinical practice because of its high safety level. Kurokawa et al. clinically investigated juzentaihoto for anticancer drug side effects in patients after cancer surgery, their investigation of its clinical effects for digestive symptoms as side effects of anticancer drugs in 88 patients after surgery demonstrated improvement in digestive symptoms as side effects of anticancer drugs, with an improvement rate of 83 % for anorexia in particular [33]. Suzuki et al. conducted a randomized controlled trial (envelope method) with 90 participants who had undergone chemotherapy by type of cancer. The administration group took 7.5 g/day of juzentaihoto extract granules for 12 months (17 gastric, 20 colorectal, and 10 breast cancer patients) while the control group took no juzentaihoto (16 gastric, 19 colorectal, and 8 breast cancer patients). Leukocytopenia was evaluated during the observation period. While there was no significant difference between groups for leukocyte count, the administration group delayed onset of leukocytopenia caused by chemotherapy for gastric and for colorectal cancer, and they extended the period from onset of leukocytopenia until lowest score. The trial demonstrated the usefulness of prophylactic administration for gastric and colorectal cancer using juzentaihoto for leukocytopenia, a side effect of cancer chemotherapy [34]. In a study into the effectiveness of juzentaihoto for thrombocytopenia, not just leukocytopenia, Niwa et al. administered juzentaihoto in combination with M-CSF for 31 courses in 20 cases in which blood platelet count dropped below 100,000 after chemotherapy for gynecological cancers. Out of the 31 courses of treatment, 28 courses avoided platelet transfusion, and 3 cases in 3 courses received platelet transfusion. The results suggest that concomitant therapy using juzentaihoto with M-CSF is a useful adjunct therapy for thrombocytopenia during anticancer chemotherapy [35]. Yamada et al. [36] studied its impact on cellular immunity by investigating cellular immunocompetence in 46 esophageal cancer cases, 35 colorectal cancer cases, and 93 gastric cancer cases (total of 174 cases). Participants were divided into a juzentaihoto group and a control group (no administration) using the envelope method. The results showed that hemoglobin and red blood cell counts increased significantly after 2 and 3 months in the juzentaihoto group compared to the control group in cases of concomitant use of total gastric cancer extirpation and anticancer drugs. In cases of concomitant use with anticancer drugs the leukocyte count was prevented from decreasing in the juzentaihoto group for each cancer, NK cell activity was significantly higher in the administration group compared to the control group 1 month after surgery in cases of concomitant use with anticancer drugs for esophageal cancer and total gastric cancer extirpation, thus, juzentaihoto was considered effective in concomitant use with anticancer drugs and for improvement of immunocompetence after surgery. There are numerous reports that juzentaihoto is effective for anticancer drug-induced cytotoxicity, for improvement of subjective symptoms including queasy, lassitude and anorexia, as well as prevention of marrow suppression and immunosuppression [37, 38]; that it improves QOL [39]; and that it extends lifetime [40]. In addition, Tanaka et al. investigated the efficacy and safety of juzentaihoto for alleviating side effect symptoms from cancer radiation therapy. Their study divided 83 patients whose chest or abdomen had been irradiated into a juzentaihoto group ($n = 43$) and a control group (no administration, $n = 40$). The results showed the administration group demonstrating an improvement trend for anorexia in 4–6 weeks and a significant difference in 5 weeks, as well as differences for general malaise in 4 weeks, nausea and vomiting in 5 weeks, and diarrhea in 3–5 weeks. No particular adverse events attributable to juzentaihoto were observed during the administration period. The paper confirmed that the use of juzentaihoto for side effect symptoms associated with radiation therapy for cancer patients presents no safety problems and that it improves or alleviates anorexia, general malaise, nausea and vomiting as well as diarrhea [41]. There are numerous papers on effective examples of juzentaihoto for the various symptoms that occur with cirrhosis and chronic hepatitis, including virogenic cases. One such paper trialed the effects of juzentaihoto as an additional drug in combination with two others, Stronger Neo-Minophagen C (SNMC) and ursodeoxycholic acid (UDCA), for intractable cases of chronic hepatitis C and cirrhosis in which even SNMC and UDCA had not decreased GPT. Juzentaihoto administration demonstrated significant GPT improvement in three out of nine cases (33.3 %) of chronic hepatitis C and in 5 out of 12 cases (41.7 %) of hepatitis C virus-induced cirrhosis. It improved clinical symptoms including general fatigability in 12 out of 20 cases (60.0 %) and anorexia in 10 out of 19 cases (52.6 %) [42]. Another study retrospectively investigated the effect of juzentaihoto on lowering ALT in 67 cases of hepatitis C virus-related chronic liver disease in which IFN therapy was ongoing, mean ALT had not dropped below 80 units, as a rule, even with combined SNMC and UDCA therapy, and the patients complained of fatigue, lassitude or anorexia, which are indications for juzentaihoto. It was effective in 23 out of 40 cases (57.5 %), when effective is deemed to mean a decrease in mean ALT of at least 25 % at every 6 months within 1 year when compared to 6 months before administration [43]. Another study found that juzentaihoto significantly inhibited anemia attributable to IFN plus ribavirin therapy, which has proved effective for hepatitis C virus-related chronic liver disease in recent years but has demonstrated problematic side effects [44]. Many other studies have shown that juzentaihoto suppressed the incidence of liver cancer developing from cirrhosis and significantly increased the survival rate [45], and it significantly increased hemoglobin when used in combination with iron and EPO [45], demonstrating marrow and immunostimulatory effects.

5 Conclusion

Japan is the only country where Western medicine and Kampo medicine can be practiced in an integrated manner. Combining the diagnostic techniques of Western medicine with the clinical practice techniques of Kampo medicine is extremely beneficial. Approximately 150 Kampo formulae are produced as high-quality extract formulations and are covered by health insurance. While Kampo formulations are not considered in the West, traditional medical clinicians in China and Korea do take them into consideration, yet they are mostly decoctions, so there are no data on extract formulations for medical use that can be used in Japan.

The quality of Japanese Kampo formulations is extremely high and evidence based on scientific analysis is distributed. Kampo formulations can be used in the treatment of the state in which laboratory data indicate no abnormality (presymptomatic, *Mibyo*), and their use has spread to the field of preventive medicine. Using affordable Kampo medications promises economic efficiency, an excellent opportunity to redress soaring medical costs. Combining Kampo treatments for cases that do not effectively respond to Western medicine-centered treatments is extremely beneficial.

References

1. Yamakawa J (2012) Efficacy evaluation of kampo medicine in a mouse model of chronic fatigue syndrome. In: Motoo Y (ed) Traditional medicine new research. Nova Science Publishers, Inc, New York, pp 83–122
2. Chen R, Moriya J, Yamakawa J et al (2010) Traditional Chinese medicine for chronic fatigue syndrome. Evid Based Complement Alternat Med 7:3–10
3. Otsuka K, Otsuka Y, Watanabe K (2000) Practical symptom-based kampo therapy (Revised), 5th edn. Nanzando, Tokyo, pp 231–232
4. Matsuda K (1992) Practice of kampo treatment – diagnosis and treatment, 74(11). Shindan To Chiryo Sha Inc, Osaka, pp 2278–2282
5. Tatsuno K (1979) An outline of kampo medicine 1 (1). Yukonsha, Kyoto, pp 12–14
6. Terasawa K (2005) Kampo patterns (Sho): a patient-centered, not disease-centered, diagnostic system. Kagaku 75. Iwanami Shoten Publishers, Tokyo, pp 821–823
7. Matsuda K (1980) "Yoshimasu Nangai", an exposition of his compendium, vol 37. Meicho Shuppan, Osaka, p 16
8. Yoshimasu N Medical Patterns - Modern Kampo Medicine Compendium vol 37 p 134
9. Terasawa K (2006) On the formation of Chinese great classic "shokanron", and its specificity. Kampo Med 57:799–804
10. The Japan Kampo Medicine Association – Academic Committee (2000) Shanhan Zabinglun (Treatise on Cold Damage Disorders), 3rd edn. Toyo Gakujutsu Shuppansha, Chiba
11. Mayanagi M (1989) A bibliographical introduction to Neiwaishangbianhuolun (Treatise on clarification of perplexities about internal and external damage), Piweilun (Treatise on the spleen and stomach), and Lanshimicang (Secret records of the orchid chamber), Kosoto H, Mayanagi M (eds). Wakoku Kanseki Isho Shusei vol 6 Commentary. Enterprise, Tokyo, p 22–36
12. Mayanagi M, Kosoto H (1990) Medical texts in Jin period. J Tradit Sino-Jpn Med 11:495–501
13. Mayanagi M (1995) The history of a Chinese herbal prescription Bu-Zhong-Yi-Qi-Tang. J Tradit Sino-Jpn Med 16:501–507
14. Yamakawa J, Motoo Y, Moriya J et al (2013) Role of kampo medicine in integrative cancer therapy. Evid Based Complement Alternat Med 2013:570848
15. Yamakawa J, Motoo Y, Moriya J et al (2013) Significance of Kampo, traditional Japanese medicine, in supportive care of cancer patients. Evid Based Complement Alternat Med 2013:746486
16. Yamakawa J, Moriya J, Takeuchi K et al (2013) Significance of Kampo, Japanese traditional medicine, in the treatment of obesity: basic and clinical evidence. Evid Based Complement Alternat Med 2013:943075
17. Yamakawa J, Moriya J, Takahashi T et al (2010) A Kampo medicine, Boi-ogi-to, inhibits obesity in ovariectomized rats. Evid Based Complement Alternat Med 7:87–95
18. Abe K (1989) The effects of hochuekkito for side effects of chemotherapy after cancer surgery. Prog Med 9:2916–2922
19. Ohara T, Onda M, Futagawa S et al (1993) Study of the usefulness of combining hochuekkito and ninjinyoeito with Tegafur. Jpn Pharmacol Ther 21:4423–4434
20. Ohno S (1988) Effects of a traditional Chinese medicine "hochuekki-to" on natural killer activity. Arerugi 37:107–114
21. Watanabe A, Hasegawa S (1992) Effect of combined Kampo medicines as adjuvant therapy for pulmonary tuberculosis. Jpn Med J 3553:76–77
22. Suzuki J, Arata S, Sugiyama M (2002) Improvement of immunity and nutrition by hochuekkito in immune-compromised hosts–for the control of MRSA. Prog Med 22:1362–1363
23. Irie K, Tateishi M, Yuu H et al (1992) Clinical effects of hochuekkito on gastroptosis symptoms. J N Remedies Clin 41:423–432
24. Tomita H, Chiba S, Kadowaki J et al (1997) Clinical effects of hochuekkito on pediatric orthostatic disturbance. J Pediatr Pract 60:162–167
25. Kuratsune H, Yamaguchi K, Tokumine Y (1997) Kampo formulations for chronic fatigue syndrome–clinical effects of hochuekkito. Jpn J Clin Exp Med 74:1837–1845

26. Kuratsune H, Nakatomi Y, Kagura M et al (2010) Clinical effectiveness of twice daily hochuekkito for chronic fatigue syndrome patients. Prog Med 30:505–510
27. Moriya J (2006) Establishment of murine model for chronic fatigue syndrome and efficacy of kampo medicine on daily activity. J Kanazawa Med Univ 31:263–268
28. Chen R, Moriya J, Yamakawa J et al (2008) Brain atrophy in a murine model of chronic fatigue syndrome and beneficial effect of Hochu-ekki-to (TJ-41). Neurochem Res 33:1759–1767
29. Matsuzawa K, Nakano H, Oonishi Y (1997) Effects of hochuekkito for sleep-disordered breathing—a preliminary study using pulse oximetry. Jpn J Chest Dis 56:846–849
30. Ping L, Takase K, Mukobayashi M et al (1996) Clinical effects of traditional Chinese herbal medicine "Hochuekkito" on male infertility. Advances Obstet Gynecol 48:406–410
31. Ohara K, Nishimoto M, Miyazato K et al (1994) Effects of hochuekkito (TJ-41) for anorexia. Prog Med 14:1705–1712
32. Kurokawa T, Imai J, Tamakuma M (1989) Improvement of anorexia, nausea and vomiting, and lassitude, side effects of anti-cancer drug administration. "Effects of juzentaihoto in preventing anti-cancer drug side effects–A clinical immunology study". Biotherapy 3:789–795
33. Suzuki S, Abe R, Nomizu T et al (1995) Effect of juzentaihoto (TJ-48) on leukopenia in patients receiving cancer chemotherapy. Prog Med 15:1968–1971
34. Niwa K, Hashimoto M, Tamaya T (2000) Effects of Juzen-taiho-to and M-CSF on thrombocytopenia induced by anti-cancer drugs in gynecologic malignancies. Jpn J Orient Med 51:447–454
35. Yamada T (1992) Clinical study of juzen-taiho-to administration for postoperative esophageal carcinoma, gastric carcinoma, and colorectal carcinoma – Influence of surgical intervention and postoperative chemotherapy on cell mediated immunity. J Med Pharm Soc WAKAN-YAKU 9:157–164
36. Rino Y, Yukawa N, Yamada R et al (2013) Improvement of adverse effects by juzen-taiho-to in the chemotherapy for patients with advanced or recurrent gastric cancer. J Jpn Coll Surg 38:62–66
37. Konno H, Maruo Y, Baba S et al (1997) Improvement of immunocompetence with combined use of juzendaihoto in adjuvant chemotherapy after gastric cancer surgery. Biotherapy 11:193–199
38. Kosaka A, Kamiya T, Sumiyama M et al (1994) Usefulness of TSUMURA Juzentaihoto (TJ-48) for reducing adverse effects of anticancer drugs and improving QOL. Prog Med 14:2259–2264
39. Adachi I (1990) Supporting therapy with Shi Quan Da Bu Tang in advanced breast cancer patients. Biomed Res 11:25–31
40. Tanaka Y, Hashimoto S (1988) Effects of TSUMURA Juzentaihoto on various complaints occurring as adverse reactions during radiotherapy. JAMA 6:70–71
41. Tarao K, Okamoto T, Miyakawa K et al (2003) Effect of Juzen-taiho-to on the serum alanine aminotransferase levels in patients with HCV-associated chronic hepatitis or liver cirrhosis. Jpn J Orient Med 54:191–198
42. Tarao K, Sakamoto Y, Ueno M et al (2010) Juzentaihoto (TJ-48) may be an important and effective anti-inflammatory agent for intractable cases of patients with HCV-associated chronic liver-diseases. Jpn J Orient Med 61:1–8
43. Sho Y, Fujisaki K, Sakashita H et al (2004) Orally administered Kampo medicine, Juzen-taiho-to, ameliorates anemia during interferon plus ribavirin therapy in patients with chronic hepatitis C. J Gastroenterol 39:1202–1204
44. Higuchi K, Shimizu Y, Yasumura S et al (2002) Preventive effect of liver carcinogenesis by juzen-taiho-to in the patients with liver cirrhosis. Kan-Tan-Sui 44:341–346
45. Aoe H, Ota M, Kawahara N et al (2003) Efficacy of using juzentaihoto to augment preoperative autologous blood donation. J Med Technol 47:395–399

Chapter 9

Atopic Dermatitis and Chinese Medicine

Hsiewe Ying Tan and George Binh Lenon

Abstract

Atopic dermatitis (AD) is said to be the most common skin disease among children, which impacts severely on daily life. The etiology has yet to be fully elucidated and current western medicine managements are targeted at symptomatic relief, some of which have unfavorable side effects. According to the traditional Chinese medicine (TCM), AD is said to be related to a congenitally weak constitution, leading to the attack or generation of pathogenic factors. Chinese herbal medicine (CHM) is usually individualized for each and every patient; however, in hope of increasing the scientific evidence of its efficacy and safety in the treatment of AD, several clinical trials have been conducted using non-individualized CHM.

This chapter reviews the findings of clinical and laboratory studies of 4 CHM formulae: Zemaphyte, Pentaherbs Capsule, Hochu-ekki-to, and Xiao Feng San. In clinical studies, Zemaphyte had conflicting results, Pentaherb Capsule and Hochu-ekki-to showed no significant difference in disease severity but found improvement in secondary outcomes, and Xiao Feng San had positive results. All in-vitro studies found potential pharmacological effects that may be beneficial in the management of AD. However, aside from evidence still being deemed insufficient, there were one or more flaws in the clinical study designs, leading to concerns of the credibility of the results. The main concerns identified with studies included the general quality of studies, the suitability of the using a scientific, randomized, control methodology for TCM studies, the lack of pharmacological data of CHM, and the lack of assurance regarding the safety of the intervention. Currently, the treatment of AD with TCM is still highly based on historical and empirical evidence; and as the complete pathophysiology of AD remains unknown, it may be difficult to determine which biochemical and pharmacological properties are required in the CHM to allow it to be deemed a potential pharmacotherapy

Key words Chinese herbal medicine, Traditional Chinese medicine, Atopic dermatitis, Eczema, Review, Clinical studies

1 Introduction

Atopic dermatitis (ADAtopic dermatitis (AD)), also known as atopic eczema, is said to be the most common skin disease among children [1], affecting around 15–30 % of children [2]. However, recent epidemiology studies have shown an unexplained increase in prevalence over the last few decades, especially in industrialized countries [3, 4]. While around 60 % of AD cases tend to resolve in early childhood, more than half experience recurrences into

Akio Inui (ed.), *Herbal Medicines: New Horizons*, Methods in Pharmacology and Toxicology,
DOI 10.1007/978-1-4939-4002-8_9, © Springer Science+Business Media New York 2016

adulthood [5], resulting in an estimated 2–10 % prevalence among adults [6].

The term "atopy" originated from the Greek term "atopos", meaning "out of the way" or "uncommon" and was first used by Coca and Cooke [7] to describe an unusual type of hypersensitivity. According to the World Allergy Organization (WAO), the term "atopy" refers to "a personal and/or familial tendency, usually in childhood or adolescence, to become sensitized and produce IgE antibodies in response to ordinary exposures to allergens, usually proteins. As a consequence, these persons can develop typical symptoms of asthma, rhinoconjunctivitis, or eczema [8]. Despite ongoing debates regarding the involvement of the nomenclature, diagnosis as well as the involvement of IgE-mediated allergy [9, 10], this chronic, inflammatory skin disease is generally characterized by a combination of clinical features such as severe itching, skin redness and dryness, weeping, scaring and lichenification [11, 12], and disease history [13].

AD can cause unbearable frustration, reduced quality of life (QoL), and inconveniences to both the patient and their families or caretaker. The vicious itch-scratch cycle not only disrupts daily activities, such as sleep and work, but also results in reduced work productivity and severe skin damage or disfiguration, leading to low self-esteem or further psychological stress which may, in turn, worsen the condition [1]. Patients may also be subjected to restricted activities, diet and costly therapies, which can amount to several hundred millions of dollars yearly [14]. Furthermore, there is also an increased risk of superinfections by *Staphylococcus aureus* and *Herpes simplex* virus in AD patients [15].

2 Atopic Dermatitis and Western Medicine

It has been hypothesized that the etiology and pathophysiology of AD are a combination of genetic factors as well as environmental factors [12]. Genetic studies showed increased risk of AD in monozygotic twins compared to dizygotic twins [16], as well as in children whose parents have AD compared to children whose parents have asthma or allergic rhinitis [17], have led to the postulation that the eczema phenotype is due to the presence of specific skin genes [18], While researchers have been unsuccessful in completely distinguishing genes that influence the pathophysiology of AD [19], there seems to be a consensus that there is an immunological dysfunction involving IgE-mediated sensitization and T helper type 2-tilted inflammatory response, and skin permeability barrier defects [20–22].

The increase in AD prevalence in general and its prevalence among small families, families of higher socioeconomic status or ethnic groups [15, 23–25] indicates that environmental factors play a role in this condition. Several hypotheses have been proposed regarding the environmental factors of AD, including the "hygiene hypothesis", which states that early exposure to pathogens can protect against atopy [26]. However, there have been inconsistencies among various research findings [25]. AD can also be aggravated by irritants (e.g. detergents, fabrics), allergens (e.g. dust mites, foods), infection, stress, or hormonal changes [12].

Currently, there is no cure for AD; various forms of management available are targeted at symptomatic relief [1]. Based on management guidelines of AD, the ultimate goal is to eliminate or reduce symptoms severity so that it does not affect daily life or require much medication [27, 28]. Management includes recognizing and removing trigger factors, maintain skin hydration, and reduce itching and inflammation [12, 29]. These managements are not always successful because elimination of trigger factors does not guarantee a cure of the condition [28], and the use of emollients, while strongly advocated, has reported a lack of evidence of effectiveness [30]. Furthermore, the commonly used pharmacotherapies such as corticosteroids and calcineurin inhibitors are usually required for long-term use and have been associated with drug tolerance development [31] and adverse effects such as skin atrophy and primary hypothalamic–pituitary–adrenal axis suppression with the former [3] and transient burning sensation upon application and potential malignancy risks with the latter [28, 30].

3 Atopic Dermatitis and Traditional Chinese Medicine

"Failure of conventional therapy" has led to patients seeking assistance from complementary medicine which includes traditional Chinese medicine (TCM) [32]. The use of TCMTraditional Chinese medicine (TCM) has been increasing worldwide for various diseases, including dermatological conditions [33]. As TCM has its unique method of diagnosis to enable targeted treatment, it is expected to contribute to the management of AD. The increasing use of Chinese herbal medicine (CHM) has led researchers to scientifically study this form of ethnobotanical therapy [33]. Furthermore, regulations have been planned or implemented as a safety precaution [34].

Based on TCM theories, the predisposition toward "atopy" suggests that AD patients have a congenitally weak constitution, which in turn, increases susceptibility toward the attack of external pathogenic factors such as wind, dampness, and heat [35]. Some texts have also noted that some babies were born with "fetal heat", which is heat inherited from the mother during pregnancy which can attack the heart or lung, causing AD [36]. Internal pathogenic factors—such as wind and heat generated by emotional disturbances; damp, heat or food stagnation due to either irregular diet

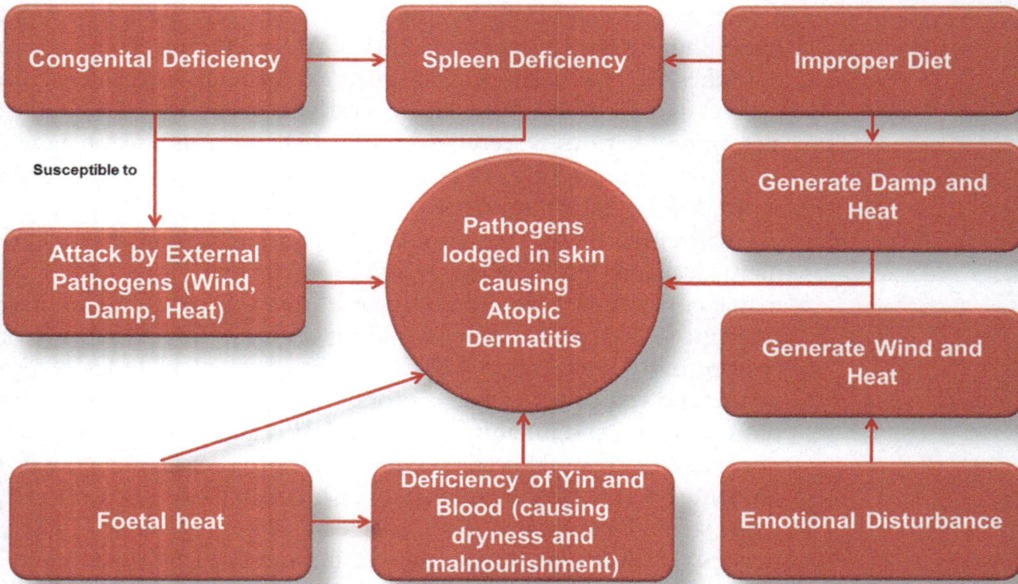

Fig. 1 An illustration of the potential pathogenesis of AD based on Chinese medicine

or Spleen and Stomach deficiency—can also lodge in the skin and result in AD. The recurrent and chronic nature of the disease can injure Yin and Blood, and generate wind and dryness [35]. Figure 1 illustrates the potential pathogenesis of AD based on Chinese Medicine. It is common for AD patients to have a combination of syndromes affecting them.

"Atopic dermatitis" has not been recorded as a disease in historical TCM texts [37]; based on similarities in clinical feature descriptions, the diseases *Si Wan Feng* (四弯风) had been acknowledged as the equivalent of AD [38]. However, there are also other terms which have been or may be used to refer to AD, including the terms *Shi Zhen* (湿疹/溼疹), *Jin Yin Chuang* (浸淫疮), *Shi Chuang* (湿疮), *Shi Lian* (湿敛), *Gan Lian* (干敛), *Ru Xuan* (乳癣), *Nai Xuan* (奶癣), *Tai Xuan* (胎癣), and *Tai Lian Chuang* (胎敛疮) [39, 40].

The treatment principles of AD depend on the syndrome differentiation of the diagnosis. Treatment may include a combination of dietary and lifestyle advice, CHM with or without acupuncture, cupping, and moxibustion. Based on the commonly seen syndromes of AD-like TCM dermatological conditions, there are several proposed formulae, as listed in Table 1.

Generally, all formulae are usually subjected to modifications as CHM treatments are usually individualized, which is a huge challenge when conducting scientific studies. As the popularity of CHM therapy increases, so do the concerns regarding its efficacy

Table 1
Proposed formulae based on the commonly seen syndromes of AD-like TCM dermatological conditions

Syndrome	Formulae	Formula ingredients	Reference
Damp-heat	Modified Long Dan Xie Gan Tang	Long Dan Cao	[39]
		Zhi Zi	
		Huang Qin	
		Sheng Di Huang	
		Xuan Shen	
		Che Qian Cao	
		Ze Xie	
		Mu Tong	
		Bai Xian Pi	
		Di Fu Zi	
		Chan Tui	
		Gan Cao	
	Xiao Feng Dao Chi Tang & Long Dan Xie Gan Tang	Sheng Di Huang	[40]
		Huang Lian	
		Huang Qin	
		Mu Tong	
		Fu Ling	
		Ze Xie	
		Che Qian Zi	
		Jin Yin Hua	
		Bai Xian Pi	
		Gan Cao	
	Li Shi Qing Re Fang and Dan Di Chu Shi Tang	Long Dan Cao	[40]
		Huang Qin	
		Zhi Zi	
		Sheng Di Huang	
		Jin Yin Hua	
		Lian Qiao	
		Fu Ling	
		Ze Xie	
		Mu Tong	
		Che Qian Zi	
		Hua Shi	
		Bai Xian Pi	
	Modified Bi Xie Shen Shi Tang	Bi Xie	[35]
		Huang Bai	
		Fu Ling	
		Mu Dan Pi	
		Sheng Di Huang	
		Ze Xie	
		Hua Shi	
		Yi Yi Ren	
		Gan Cao	

(continued)

Table 1 (continued)

Syndrome	Formulae	Formula ingredients	Reference
	Modified Chu Shi Wei Ling Tang	Cang Zhu Hou Po Chen Pi Zhu Ling Ze Xie Chi Fu Ling Bai Zhu Hua Shi Fang Feng Zhi Zi Gan Cao	[35]
	Modified Xiao Feng Dao Chi San	Jing Jie Fang Feng Cang Zhu Chan Tui Zhi Mu Niu Bang Zi Sheng Di Huang Chi Shao Zhi Zi Deng Xin Cao	[35]
	Modified Bi Xie Fen Qing Yin	Chuan Bi Xie Huang Bai Shi Chang Pu Fu Ling Bai Zhu Lian Zi Dan Shen Che Qian Zi Gan Cao	[35]
	Modified Long Dan Xie Gan Tang or Modified Yin Chen Hao Tang	Long Dan Cao Chai Hu Huang Qin Fu Ling Bai Zhu Yin Chen Hao Che Qian Cao Sheng Di Huang Zhi Zi Gan Cao	[35]

(continued)

Table 1 (continued)

Syndrome	Formulae	Formula ingredients	Reference
	Modified Chu Shi Wei Ling Tang	Fu Ling Pi Chao Huang Bai Chen Pi Ku Shen Zhu Ling Di Fu Zi Bai Xian Pi Huang Qi Yi Yi Ren Chi Xiao Dou Cang Er Zi Chan Tui	[36]
Wind-heat	Xiao Feng San	Niu Bang Zi Sheng Di Huang Ku Shen Cang Zhu Dang Gui Zhi Mu Shi Gao Guan Mu Tong Di Fu Zi Bai Xian Pi Chan Tui Gan Cao	[39]
	Modified Shu Feng Qing Re Yin	Jin Yin Hua Jing Jie Niu Bang Zi Fang Feng Chan Tui Ji Li Huang Qin Zhi Zi Sheng Di Huang Dan Shen Chi Shao Gan Cao	[35]
Wind and damp-heat	Modified Chan Fang Tang	Chan Tui Fang Feng Cang Zhu Ku Shen Huang Bai Lian Qiao Mu Dan Pi Bai Xian Pi	[35]

(continued)

Table 1 (continued)

Syndrome	Formulae	Formula ingredients	Reference
	Modified Xiao Feng San	Jing Jie Fang Feng Cang Zhu Mu Dan Pi Huang Bai Niu Bang Zi Chan Tui Ku Shen Gan Cao	[35]
Wind-dryness	Dang Gui Yin Zi	Dang Gui Dan Shen Bai Shao He Shou Wu Chuan Xiong Huang Qi Fang Feng Bai Ji Li Cang Er Zi Xu Chang Qing Gan Cao	[39]
Wind-dryness due to blood deficiency	Modified Dang Gui Yin Zi or Si Wu Xiao Feng Yin	Dang Gui Bai Shao Qin Jiao Jing Jie Fang Feng Chan Tui Chai Hu Shu Di Huang Sheng Di Huang Bai Xian Pi Hu Ma Ren	[35]
	Modified Dang Gui Yin Zi	Dang Gui Chi Shao Sheng Di Huang Dan Shen He Shou Wu Bai Ji Li Huang Qi Jiang Can Wu Shao She Jing Jie Fang Feng Gan Cao	[35]

(continued)

Table 1 (continued)

Syndrome	Formulae	Formula ingredients	Reference
	Modified Yi Guan Jian	Sheng Di Huang Sha Shen Shu Di Huang Gou Qi Zi Dang Gui Mai Dong Chuan Lian Zi Gan Cao	[35]
Wind-damp	Huo Xue Chu Shi Tang	Fang Feng Chan Yi Dan Shen Ze Lan Wang Bu Liu Xing Chi Shao Chuan Xiong Huang Bai Cang Zhu Jiang Can Di Long	[40]
	Modified Xiao Feng San	Jing Jie Fang Feng Niu Bang Zi Chan Tui Jin Yin Hua Cang Zhu Ku Shen Zhi Mu Shi Gao Sheng Di Huang Hu Ma Ren (Fructus Cannabis) Fu Ling	[35]
Damp stagnation due to spleen deficiency	Chu Shi Wei Ling Tang + Qing Ji Shen Shi Tang	Can Zhu Bai Zhu Chen Pi Fu Ling Yi Yi Ren Ze Xie Hua Shi Zhu Ling Dong Gua Pi Bai Xian Pi	[40]

(continued)

Table 1
(continued)

Syndrome	Formulae	Formula ingredients	Reference
	Modified Si Jun Zi Tang	Dang Shen Fu Ling Bai Zhu Cang Zhu Bai Bian Dou Chen Pi Shan Yao Ze Xie Zhu Ling Dang Gui Da Zao Dan Shen Bai Shao Yi Yi Ren Che Qian Cao	[35]
	Modified Shen Ling Bai Zhu San	Dang Shen Fu Ling Bai Zhu Cang Zhu Bai Bian Dou Chen Pi Shan Yao Yi Yi Ren Gan Cao	[35]
	Modified Shen Ling Bai Zhu San	Fu Ling Shan Yao Tai Zi Shen Sha Ren Bai Zhu Bai Bian Dou Yi Yi Ren Jie Geng Gan Cao Chen Pi	[35]
	Modified Bao He Wan	Shan Zha Gu Ya Mai Ya Chen Pi Ban Xia Fu Ling Lian Qiao Gan Cao	[35]

(continued)

Table 1 (continued)

Syndrome	Formulae	Formula ingredients	Reference
Spleen/stomach deficiency	Jian Pi Chu Shi Tang + Chu Shi Wei Ling Tang	Chao Bai Zhu Cang Zhu Hou Po Chen Pi Fu Ling Ze Xie Liu Yi San (Hua Shi + Gan Cao) Zhu Ling Bai Xian Pi Di Fu Zi	[40]
Spleen dampness and lung-dryness	Modified Qing Zao Jiu Fei Tang + Wei Ling Tang	Sheng Di Huang Pi Pa Ye Sang Ye Shi Gao Mai Dong Fu Ling	[35]
Spleen deficiency and wind-dryness	Modified Bu Pi Run Zao Tang	Huang Qi Chen Pi Bai Shao Fang Feng Gan Cao Dang Gui Dan Shen Ji Xue Teng Bai Sha Shen Shan Yao Bai Bian Dou Fu Ling	[35]
Blood-dryness	Modified Zi Yin Chu Shi Tang	Dang Gui Chao Bai Shao Chai Hu Huang Qin Shu Di Huang Di Gu Pi Yi Mu Cao Chao Zhi Mu Ze Xie Fang Feng He Shou Wu Gan Cao	[36]

(continued)

Table 1 (continued)

Syndrome	Formulae	Formula ingredients	Reference
Yin and blood-dryness	Yang Xue Run Fu Yin + Zi Yin Chu Shi Tang	Dang Gui Shu Di Huang Sheng Di Huang Huang Qi Tian Men Dong Mai Men Dong Tian Hua Fen Tao Ren Hong Gua Dan Shen Bai Xian Pi	[40]
Wind-damp and blood-heat	Xiao Feng San + Liang Xue Chu Shi Tang	Jing Jie Fang Feng Huang Qin Huang Lian Ku Shen Zhi Mu Sheng Di Huang Mu Dan Pi Ze Xie Hua Shi Bai Xian Pi	[40]
Yin deficiency and damp stagnation	Zi Yin Chu Shi Tang	Sheng Di Dang Gui Xuan Shen Dan Shen Fu Ling Ze Xie Bai Xian Pi She Chuang Zi	[40]
Fetal heat	Modified San Xin Dao Chi San	Lian Qiao Xin Gui Zhi Xin Lian Zi Xin Xuan Shen Sheng Di Huang Chi Fu Ling Fu Ling Shan Yao Che Qian Zi Sha Shen Mu Tong	[36]

(continued)

Table 1 (continued)

Syndrome	Formulae	Formula ingredients	Reference
Heart fire	San Xin Dao Chi Tang	Xuan Shen Mu Tong Deng Xin Cao Lian Zi Xin Lian Qiao Xin Sheng Di Huang Zhi Zi Xin Fu Ling Pi Che Qian Zi Che Qian Cao	[35]
Heart fire with damp stagnation	Modified San Xin Dao Chi San	Lian Qiao Xin Zhi Zi Xin Lian Zi Xin Deng Xin Cao Xuan Shen Chan Tui Che Qian Cao Che Qian Zi Sheng Di Huang Gan Cao Shao	[35]
Lung heat	Modified Liang Ge San	Lian Qiao Hu Zhang Shan Zha Huang Qin Jiu Da Huang Jiao Shan Zha Yin Chen Hao Bai Mao Gen Bo He	[35]

and safety, as historical use is insufficient. Regulations have been in place in several countries [33, 41, 42] and the World Health Organization (WHOWorld Health Organization (WHO)) has also been involved in identifying safe and effective herbal medicine [43]. In attempt to validate its efficacy and safety among the scientific world, researchers have been conducting clinical and laboratory studies on CHM.

There are many clinical studies of CHM for the management of AD that have been conducted to date. However, many were seen to be of "poor quality" when compared against the required "gold standard" randomized controlled trials. To date, 4 systematic reviews on CHM for the management of AD had been conducted, all with inconclusive evidence [1, 44–46]. Only a few formulae had undergone a double-blind, randomized, placebo-controlled clinical trial, and several also had further laboratory studies conducted.

4 Zemaphyte

Zemaphyte was a formula that was created by a Chinese medicine practitioner in London for the management of AD [47] and were given as "teabags" consisting of *Glyzyrrhiza uralensis (Gan Cao), Ledebouriella seseloides (Fang Feng), Schizonepeta tenuifolia (Jing Jie), Lophatherum gracile (Dan Zhu Ye), Paeonia lactiflora (Bai Shao), Rehmannia glutinosa (Sheng Di Huang), Anebia clematidis (Chuan Mu Tong), Dictamnus dasycarpus (Bai Xian Pi), Tribulus terrestris (Ji Li), and Potentilla chinensis (Wei Ling Cai)* [48]. Although the formula is no longer being produced due to failure in obtaining a license, it had been tested in three double-blind, randomized, placebo-controlled clinical studies [48–50] and several laboratory studies [51, 52]. Two of the clinical trials were conducted in the United Kingdom, one with adults and one with pediatric participants [48, 50]. Both studies were crossover trials, where patients would take one intervention for 8 weeks, followed by a 4-week washout period, and then taking the other intervention for another 8 weeks. Both studies reported to have significantly better results by Zemaphyte compared to placebo with no reported adverse effects. A 1-year follow-up study was conducted for each of the respective trials showed positive outcomes with no toxicity issues [53, 54]. However, when Zemaphyte was used in a study with a similar protocol in Hong Kong, there was no significant difference except for in one outcome measure (lichenification), although the authors were in agreement regarding the safety of the formula [49]. It was speculated that the contradicting results may be due to "racial variability in drug responsiveness and disposition", as the Hong Kong study consisted exclusively of Chinese patients. Furthermore, based on the lower average weight of the Chinese patients, a lower dose was implemented in the Hong Kong study, which may have affected results.

In-vitro studies have shown that Zemaphyte is able to induce IL-10 and TNF-α, and subsequently reduce the overexpression of CD23 receptors on monocytes and Langerhans cells, as seen in AD patients [55]. Another study showed that Zemaphyte is a potent antioxidant, which can contribute in the downregulation of the inflammatory cells of AD [52].

While clinical and laboratory studies have shown potential benefit of Zemaphyte in the management of AD, there is no information on why the formula failed to obtain a license and has stopped in its manufacture. It may be due to one particular herbal ingredient, *Mu Tong*, as it can be the Chinese name for several herbs, including *Caulis akebiae* and *Clematis armandii*, both of which have been noted to potentially contain aristolochic acid [56]. Another possibility is due certain adverse effects that were seemingly caused by another herbal ingredient, *Bai Xian Pi*, in several other, unrelated occasions [57].

5 Pentaherbs Capsule

The Pentaherbs capsule was first piloted in an open-labeled case series among children [58]. The formulation consists of five herbs: *Herba menthae (Bo He), Flos lonicerae (Jin Yin Hua), Cortex phellodendri (Huang Bai), Rhizoma atractylodis (Cang Zhu)*, and *Cortex moutan (Mu Dan Pi)* [58]. The open-labeled study showed that the formulation had potential benefits and was well tolerated by children; therefore, it was followed by a double-blind, randomized, placebo-controlled clinical study. Children aged 5–21 years old with moderate-to-severe AD had to undergo a 2-week run-in period, 12-week treatment period with either Pentaherbs or placebo capsules and a 4-week follow-up period [59]. The study found no significant difference in disease severity but reported significant improvement in quality of life and reduction in total corticosteroids required by participants in the Pentaherbs group. However, there were significantly more visits to the general medical practitioner by the Pentaherbs group participants with no further elaboration by the authors.

A syrup form of the formulation was subsequently developed and tested in a prospective self-controlled study which reported significant improvement in disease severity and quality of life [60]. The authors, however, noted there was no biochemical evidence of adverse drug reactions despite the withdrawal of two participants with rash during the study.

When subjected to in-vitro experimentation, the Pentaherbs formulation showed that production of AD-related inflammatory mediators such as brain-derived neurotrophic factor, thymus and activation-regulated chemokine, IFN-γ, and TNF-α were suppressed [61]. It was also discovered that the individual herbal ingredients in the formulation had different immune-modulating effects on mast cells: *Cortex Moutan (Mu Dan Pi)* and *Herba Menthae (Bo He)* seem to reduce histamine release and prostaglandin D2 synthesis that had been activated by an anti-IgE and compound 48/80; *Flos Lonicerae (Jin Yin Hua)* and *Rhizoma Atractylodis (Cang Zhu)* inhibited only compound 48/80-released mediators; *Cortex Phellodendri (Huang Bai)* increased only mediator release stimulated by anti-IgE [62]. Nevertheless, it was concluded that the different effects all play a role in the therapeutic effects of the Pentaherbs formulation [62].

6 Hochu-Ekki-To

Hochu-ekki-to is the equivalent of the classical formula, *Bu Zhong Yi Qi Tang*, and consists of *Glycyrrhizae radix (Gan Cao), Ginseng radix (Ren Shen), Atractylodes rhizome (Bai Zhu), Aurantii nobilis*

Pericarpium (Chen Pi), Angelicae radix (Dang Gui), Bupleuri radix (Chai Hu), Zizyphi fructus (Da Zao), Astragali radix (Huang Qi), Zingiberis rhizome (Gan Jiang), and *Cimicifugae rhizome (Sheng Ma)* [63]. The double-blind, randomized, placebo-controlled study included AD patients aged 20–40 years old and was targeted at patients with a *Kikyo* (Qi deficiency) constitution who were asked to undergo a treatment period of 24 weeks [63]. The study did not yield significant difference in improving disease severity, but the authors declared that the treatment group achieved a significantly better prominent efficacy rate (the percentage of patients whose severity score equaled to zero at the end of the trial period) of 19 % compared to the 5 % in the control group. Thus, Hochu-ekki-to can be used as a useful adjunct therapy to reduce the need for topical steroids or calcineurin inhibitors. Only minor adverse effects were reported during the trial, with no significant difference between the intervention and control group.

Although this trial stands out by attempting to include TCM diagnosis and treatment principles by only including patients with *Kikyo* (Qi deficiency) constitution, the treatment strategy, while addressing the Kampo diagnosis (*sho*), did not address the AD condition as per Chinese medicine theory whereby there was no modification to suit individual presentation and the formula only tonified the underlying deficiencies without addressing the potential presence of pathogenic factors.

An in-vitro study of the formula suggested that Hochu-ekki-to is effective in treating hypersensitivity reactions as it is able to reduce serum IgE, IgG, and IL-4 [64], which play a significant role in the inflammation of AD.

7 Xiao Feng San

Xiao Feng San is a classical formula which has been noted to be used for dermatological conditions [35, 39, 40]. It consists of *Glycyrrhiza uralensis (Gan Cao), Saposhnikovia divaricata (Fang Feng), Schizonepeta tenuifolia (Jing Jie), Atractylodes lancea (Cang Zhu), Angelica sinensis (Dang Gui), Rehmannia glutinosa (Sheng Di Huang), Clematis armandii (Chuan Mu Tong), Cryptotympana pustulata (Chan Tui), Linum usitatissimum (Hu Ma Ren), Anemarrhena asphodeloides (Zhi Mu), Gypsum fibrosum (Shi Gao), Sophora flavescens (Ku Shen)*, and *Articum lappa (Niu Bang Zi)* [65]. The double-blind, randomized, placebo-controlled study for this formula included patients with extensive AD and involved an 8-week treatment and 4-week follow-up period [65]. The study found that Xiao Feng San significantly improved symptoms severity when compared to placebo, even after the 4-week follow-up period. Only mild or moderate adverse events were recorded, although there was one case transient elevation of aspartate amino transferase which was resolved after 8 weeks of treatment cessation.

Although Xiao Feng San was reported to be well-tolerated, it contained the herb, *Clematis armandii (Chuan Mu Tong)*, which may potentially contain aristolochic acid [56], as mentioned above. Furthermore, the results of the study need to be interpreted with caution, as the dosage of the formulation used in the trial was significantly higher, with adults taking a total of 27 g of herbal granules a day, compared to the recommended daily dosage of 6–12 g [66].

The authors of the study quoted previous research regarding the pharmacological properties of several of the herbal ingredients of Xiao Feng San, including the anti-inflammatory effects of *Saposhnikovia divaricata* (Fang Feng); the suppression of skin hypersensitivity reaction by *Rehmannia glutinosa* (Sheng Di Huang); and the immuno-modulating functions of *Angelica sinensis* (Dang Gui) and *Glycyrrhiza uralensis* (Gan Cao) [65]. An in-vitro study found that Xiao Feng San significantly suppresses antigen-induced histamine release by IL-3-dependent mouse bone marrow, which may explain its effects in the management of atopic diseases such as asthma and AD [67].

8 Discussion

AD is a condition that has yet to be fully elucidated, making it difficult to find an effective targeted treatment. Furthermore, the presentation and drug reaction of patients are varied, which makes it complicated to come up with a "one for all" treatment. Individualized treatment by CHM, therefore, seems like the perfect solution, if only there were more concrete evidence supporting its use.

While many clinical trials have been conducted in attempt to increase the credibility of the efficacy and safety of CHM treatment for AD, the number of high-quality randomized controlled trials is close to none. Based on the previous systematic reviews, only one study was judged with "low risk" in all risk of bias domains, allowing it to be deemed of high quality [46]. Even so, upon scrutinization, researchers are able to argue against certain aspects of the methodology applied. However, the debate regarding the appropriateness of conducting randomized controlled trials for CHM interventions have been ongoing [68, 69]. One of the commonly identified issues includes the use of standardized treatment for all patients of the same disease, which does not match with the actual practice of Chinese medicine. There have been debates that pragmatic studies are more suited for traditional medicine interventions such as CHM [70]; however, that causes another debate of whether the efficacy of the CHM needs to be established before its effectiveness can be evaluated in pragmatic studies.

Studies on the pharmacological properties of CHM have also been conducted to strengthen the evidence of CHM as a treatment for AD. Research has identified that Chinese herbs possess various pharmacological properties that may be beneficial in the management of AD, including anti-inflammatory, antibacterial, antifungal, and immunosuppressive functions [33]. Pharmacological studies of CHM can be based on the individual herb or on the formula as a whole. However, the pharmacology of the formulae may differ from that of individual herbs due to interaction [71]. Furthermore, in-vitro data do not necessarily reflect the treatment effects seen in humans [72].

Among everything, the main concern regarding CHM for AD is the safety aspect. While most clinical trials, as those mentioned above, all reported no or only mild or moderate adverse events, having poor quality studies and small sample sizes do not allow sufficient credibility of its safety. In addition, CHM is considered as one modality; therefore, if there are any negative reports regarding CHM of any sort, in any condition, it is likely to cause more damage to the reputation of the intervention. Furthermore, in addition to the danger of not knowing the pharmacological properties and chemicals, the herbal contents and quality is variable based on where and how it was cultivated and there might be pollution or adulteration of the herbs [73]. It is also more likely for today's patients to be on polypharmacy, which adds to the concern of drug–herb interactions [73].

9 Conclusion

Currently, there does not seem to be a clear direction on how to increase the credibility of CHM treatment of AD. While there is historical and empirical evidence, there is lack of an appropriate methodology to evaluate it in a way that suits both the Chinese medicine way of practice, as well as the scientific method. Previous systematic reviews have concluded that more evidence is required; it may be a long journey of collecting information until there is enough to fill the gaps. For example, adhering to the scientific method to gather sufficient details of the formula's efficacy before moving on to studies which suit the TCM method. However, with AD, where the complete pathophysiology remains unknown, it may be difficult to determine which biochemical and pharmacological properties are required in the CHM to allow it to be deemed a potential pharmacotherapy.

References

1. Zhang W, Leonard T, Bath-Hextall F, Chambers CA, Lee C, Humphreys R, Williams Hywel C (2004) Chinese herbal medicine for atopic eczema. Cochrane Database Syst Rev (4). doi: 10.1002/14651858.CD002291
2. Bieber T (2008) Atopic dermatitis. N Engl J Med 358(14):1483–1494. doi:10.1056/NEJMra074081
3. Buys LM (2007) Treatment options for atopic dermatitis. Am Fam Physician 75(4):523
4. Möhrenschlager M, Darsow U, Schnopp C, Ring J (2006) Atopic eczema: what's new? J Eur Acad Dermatol Venereol 20(5):503–513. doi:10.1111/j.1468-3083.2006.01580.x
5. Sandstrom Falk MH, Faergemann J (2006) Atopic dermatitis in adults: does it disappear with age? Acta Derm Venereol 86(2):135–139. doi:10.2340/00015555-0040
6. Baron SE, Cohen SN, Archer CB (2012) Guidance on the diagnosis and clinical management of atopic eczema. Clin Exp Dermatol 37(suppl 1):7–12. doi:10.1111/j.1365-2230.2012.04336.x
7. Coca AF, Cooke RA (1923) On the classification of the phenomena of hypersensitiveness. J Immunol 8(3):163–182
8. Johansson SGO, Bieber T, Dahl R, Friedmann PS, Lanier BQ, Lockey RF, Motala C, Ortega Martell JA, Platts-Mills TAE, Ring J, Thien F, Van Cauwenberge P, Williams HC (2004) Revised nomenclature for allergy for global use: report of the nomenclature review Committee of the World Allergy Organization, October 2003. J Allergy Clin Immunol 113(5):832–836
9. Hanifin JM (2012) Atopic dermatitis nomenclature variants can impede harmonization. J Invest Dermatol 132(2):472–473
10. Schmitt J, Flohr C, Williams HC (2012) Outcome measures, case definition, and nomenclature are all important and distinct aspects of atopic eczema: a call for harmonization. J Invest Dermatol 132(2):473–474
11. Chang C, Keen CL, Gershwin ME (2007) Treatment of eczema. Clin Rev Allergy Immunol 33(3):204–225. doi:10.1007/s12016-007-0033-8
12. Feingold S, Huang C, Kristal L, Kalish R, Clark RAF (1998) Eczemas. Curr Probl Dermatol 10(2):41–90. doi:10.1016/s1040-0486(98)90008-4
13. Williams HC, Burney PGJ, Hay RJ, Archer CB, Shipley MJ, Hunter JJA, Bingham EA, Finlay AY, Pembroke AC, Grahambrown RAC, Atherton DA, Lewisjones MS, Holden CA, Harper JI, Champion RH, Poyner TF, Launer J, David TJ (1994) The UK working party diagnostic criteria for atopic dermatitis. I. Derivation of a minimum set of discriminators for atopic dermatitis. Br J Dermatol 131(3):383–396. doi:10.1111/j.1365-2133.1994.tb08530.x
14. Hoare C, Li Wan Po A, Williams H (2000) Systematic review of treatments for atopic eczema. Health Technol Assess 4(37)
15. Ring J, Przybilla B, Ruzicka T (2006) Handbook of atopic eczema. Springer Verlag, New York
16. Schultz Larsen F, Holm NV, Henningsen K (1986) Atopic dermatitis: a genetic-epidemiologic study in a population-based twin sample. J Am Acad Dermatol 15(3):487–494
17. Dold S, Wjst M, Von Mutius E, Reitmeir P, Stiepel E (1992) Genetic risk for asthma, allergic rhinitis, and atopic dermatitis. Arch Dis Child 67(8):1018–1022
18. Brown S, Reynolds NJ (2006) Atopic and non-atopic eczema. Br Med J 332(7541):584–588
19. Weidinger S, Illig T, Baurecht H, Irvine AD, Rodriguez E, Diaz-Lacava A, Klopp N, Wagenpfeil S, Zhao Y, Liao H, Lee SP, Palmer CNA, Jenneck C, Maintz L, Hagemann T, Behrendt H, Ring J, Nothen MM, McLean WHI, Novak N (2006) Loss-of-function variations within the filaggrin gene predispose for atopic dermatitis with allergic sensitizations. J Allergy Clin Immunol 118(1):214–219. doi:10.1016/j.jaci.2006.05.004
20. Hoffjan S, Epplen JT (2005) The genetics of atopic dermatitis: recent findings and future options. J Mol Med 83(9):682–692
21. Paternoster L, Standl M, Chen CM, Ramasamy A, Bøpnnelykke K, Duijts L, Ferreira MA, Alves AC, Thyssen JP, Albrecht E, Baurecht H, Feenstra B, Sleiman PMA, Hysi P, Warrington NM, Curjuric I, Myhre R, Curtin JA, Groen-Blokhuis MM, Kerkhof M, Sääf A, Franke A, Ellinghaus D, Fölster-Holst R, Dermitzakis E, Montgomery SB, Prokisch H, Heim K, Hartikainen AL, Pouta A, Pekkanen J, Blakemore AIF, Buxton JL, Kaakinen M, Duffy DL, Madden PA, Heath AC, Montgomery GW, Thompson PJ, Matheson MC, Le Souëf P, Pourcain BS, Smith GD, Henderson J, Kemp JP, Timpson NJ, Deloukas P, Ring SM, Wichmann HE, Müller-Nurasyid M, Novak N, Klopp N, Rodríguez E, McArdle W, Linneberg A, Menné T, Nohr EA, Hofman A, Uitterlinden AG, Van Duijn CM, Rivadeneira F, De Jongste JC, Van Der Valk RJP, Wjst

M, Jogi R, Geller F, Boyd HA, Murray JC, Kim C, Mentch F, March M, Mangino M, Spector TD, Bataille V, Pennell CE, Holt PG, Sly P, Tiesler CMT, Thiering E, Illig T, Imboden M, Nystad W, Simpson A, Hottenga JJ, Postma D, Koppelman GH, Smit HA, Söderhäll C, Chawes B, Kreiner-Møpller E, Bisgaard H, Melén E, Boomsma DI, Custovic A, Jacobsson B, Probst-Hensch NM, Palmer LJ, Glass D, Hakonarson H, Melbye M, Jarvis DL, Jaddoe VWV, Gieger C, Strachan DP, Martin NG, Jarvelin MR, Heinrich J, Evans DM, Weidinger S (2012) Meta-analysis of genome-wide association studies identifies three new risk loci for atopic dermatitis. Nat Genet 44(2):187–192

22. Saito H (2005) Much atopy about the skin: genome-wide molecular analysis of atopic eczema. Int Arch Allergy Immunol 137 (4):319–325
23. Martin PE, Koplin JJ, Eckert JK, Lowe AJ, Ponsonby AL, Osborne NJ, Gurrin LC, Robinson MN, Hill DJ, Tang MLK, Dharmage SC, Allen KJ (2013) The prevalence and socio-demographic risk factors of clinical eczema in infancy: a population-based observational study. Clin Exp Allergy 43(6):642–651
24. Williams HC (2000) Epidemiology of atopic dermatitis. Clin Exp Dermatol 25(7):522–529
25. Williams HC (2013) Epidemiology of human atopic dermatitis - seven areas of notable progress and seven areas of notable ignorance. Vet Dermatol 24(1):3, e2
26. Strachan DP (1989) Hay fever, hygiene, and household size. Br Med J 299(6710): 1259–1260
27. Leung TNH, Chow CM, Chow MPY, Luk DCK, Ho KM, Hon KL, Sugunan VK (2013) Clinical guidelines on management of atopic dermatitis in children. Hong Kong J Paediatr 18(2):96–104
28. Saeki H, Furue M, Furukawa F, Hide M, Ohtsuki M, Katayama I, Sasaki R, Suto H, Takehara K (2009) Guidelines for management of atopic dermatitis. J Dermatol 36(10):563–577
29. Ring J, Alomar A, Bieber T, Deleuran M, Fink-Wagner A, Gelmetti C, Gieler U, Lipozencic J, Luger T, Oranje AP, Schäfer T, Schwennesen T, Seidenari S, Simon D, Ständer S, Stingl G, Szalai S, Szepietowski JC, Taïeb A, Werfel T, Wollenberg A, Darsow U (2012) Guidelines for treatment of atopic eczema (atopic dermatitis) Part I. J Eur Acad Dermatol Venereol 26 (8):1045–1060. doi:10.1111/j.1468-3083.2012.04635.x
30. NICE (2007) Atopic Eczema in children: management of atopic eczema in children from birth up to the age of 12 years. NICE Clinical Guidelines. RCOG Press, London
31. Hsu C-J, Wang L-F (2007) Emerging treatment of atopic dermatitis. Clin Rev Allergy Immunol 33(3):199–203. doi:10.1007/s12016-007-0043-6
32. Salameh F, Perla D, Solomon M, Gamus D, Barzilai A, Greenberger S, Trau H (2008) The effectiveness of combined Chinese herbal medicine and acupuncture in the treatment of atopic dermatitis. J Altern Complement Med 14(8):1043–1048. doi:10.1089/acm.2008.0162
33. Bedi MK, Shenefelt PD (2002) Herbal therapy in dermatology. Arch Dermatol 138 (2):232–242
34. Kayne SB (2009) Traditional medicine: A global perspective. Pharmaceutical Press, London
35. Chen D, Lu C (2007) The clinical practice of Chinese medicine: eczema & atopic dermatitis (trans: Wang J, Kurtz A). People's Medical Publishing House, Beijing
36. Shen DH, Wu X, Wang N (2007) Manual of dermatology in Chinese medicine. Eastland Press, Seattle, WA
37. Tan HY, Zhang AL, Xue CC, Chen D, Da Costa C, Lenon GB (2013) Evaluation of the efficacy and safety of a Chinese herbal formula (RCM-106) for atopic dermatitis: study protocol for a randomised, double-blind, placebo-controlled trial in children. BMJ Open 3(12): e003906. doi:10.1136/bmjopen-2013-003906
38. State Administration of Traditional Chinese Medicine of the People's Republic of China (1994) Criteria of diagnosis and therapeutic effect of diseases and syndromes in traditional Chinese medicine, vol ZY/T001.1-94. Chinese Medicine Profession Standards of the People's Republic of China
39. Li L, Zhao C (1991) Dermatology. The English-Chinese Encyclopedia of Practical Traditional Chinese Medicine. Higher Education Press, Beijing
40. Lin L (1995) Practical traditional Chinese dermatology (trans: Tai W), 1st edn. Hai Feng Publishing, Hong Kong
41. Barnes J (2003) Quality, efficacy and safety of complementary medicines: fashions, facts and the future. Part I Regulation and quality. Br J Clin Pharmacol 55(3):226–233
42. Watanabe K, Matsuura K, Gao P, Hottenbacher L, Tokunaga H, Nishimura K, Imazu Y, Reissenweber H, Witt CM (2011) Traditional Japanese Kampo medicine: clinical research between modernity and traditional medicine - The state of research and methodological suggestions for the future. Evid Based

Complement Alternat Med 2011:513842. doi:10.1093/ecam/neq067

43. Arun G, Chandra K (2012) Evaluation of efficacy and safety of herbal/ayurvedic medicines. In: The Modern Ayurveda. CRC Press, p 317–336. doi:10.1201/b11722-12
44. Armstrong NC, Ernst E (1999) The treatment of eczema with Chinese herbs: a systematic review of randomized clinical trials. Br J Clin Pharmacol 48(2):262–264. doi:10.1046/j.1365-2125.1999.00004.x
45. Gu S, Yang Angela WH, Xue Charlie CL, Li Chun G, Pang C, Zhang W, Williams Hywel C (2013) Chinese herbal medicine for atopic eczema. Cochrane Database Syst Rev (9). doi:10.1002/14651858.CD008642.pub2
46. Tan HY, Zhang AL, Chen D, Xue CC, Lenon GB (2013) Chinese herbal medicine for atopic dermatitis: a systematic review. J Am Acad Dermatol 69(2):295–304
47. Atherton DJ, Sheehan MP, Rustin MHA, Whittle B, Guy G (1992) Treatment of atopic eczema with traditional Chinese medicinal plants. Pediatr Dermatol 9(4):373–375
48. Sheehan MP, Atherton DJ (1992) A controlled trial of traditional Chinese medicinal plants in widespread non-exudative atopic eczema. Br J Dermatol 126(2):179–184
49. Fung AYP, Look PCN, Chong LY, But PPH, Wong E (1999) A controlled trial of traditional Chinese herbal medicine in Chinese patients with recalcitrant atopic dermatitis. Int J Dermatol 38(5):387–392. doi:10.1046/j.1365-4362.1999.00732.x
50. Sheehan MP, Rustin MHA, Atherton DJ, Buckley C, Harris DJ, Brostoff J, Ostlere L, Dawson A (1992) Efficacy of traditional Chinese herbal therapy in adult atopic dermatitis. Lancet 340(8810):13–17
51. Banerjee P, Xu XJ, Poulter LW, Rustin MHA (1998) Changes in CD23 expression of blood and skin in atopic eczema after Chinese herbal therapy. Clin Exp Allergy 28(3):306–314. doi:10.1046/j.1365-2222.1998.00233.x
52. Chung LY (2008) Antioxidant profiles of a prepared extract of Chinese herbs for the treatment of atopic eczema. Phytother Res 22(4):493–499. doi:10.1002/ptr.2350
53. Sheehan MP, Atherton DJ (1994) One-year follow up of children treated with Chinese medicinal herbs for atopic eczema. Br J Dermatol 130(4):488–493. doi:10.1111/j.1365-2133.1994.tb03383.x
54. Sheehan MP, Stevens H, Ostlere LS, Atherton DJ, Brostoff J, Rustin MHA (1995) Follow-up of adult patients with atopic eczema treated with Chinese herbal therapy for 1 year. Clin Exp Dermatol 20(2):136–140
55. Latchman YE, Xu XJ, Poulter LW, Rustin MHA, Atherton DJ, Brostoff J (2002) Chinese medical herbs in the treatment of atopic dermatitis. Allergy Clin Immunol Int 14(1):4–9
56. TGA (2001) Aristolochia alert for practitioners. http://www.tga.gov.au/safety/alerts-medicine-aristolochia-010723.htm.
57. Blackwell R (1996) Adverse events involving certain Chinese herbal medicines and the response of the profession. J Chin Med 50:12–22
58. Hon KLE, Leung TF, Wong Y, Lam WKC, Guan DQB, Ma KC, Sung YTR, Fok TF, Leung PC (2004) A pentaherbs capsule as a treatment option for atopic dermatitis in children: an open-labeled case series. Am J Chin Med 32(6):941–950. doi:10.1142/s0192415x04002545
59. Hon KLE, Leung TF, Ng PC, Lam MCA, Kam WYC, Wong KY, Lee KCK, Sung YT, Cheng KF, Fok TF, Fung KP, Leung PC (2007) Efficacy and tolerability of a Chinese herbal medicine concoction for treatment of atopic dermatitis: a randomized, double-blind, placebo-controlled study. Br J Dermatol 157(2):357–363. doi:10.1111/j.1365-2133.2007.07941.x
60. Hon KL, Lo W, Cheng WKF, Leung TF, Chow CM, Lau CBS, Fok TF, Ng PC, Leung PC (2012) Prospective self-controlled trial of the efficacy and tolerability of a herbal syrup for young children with eczema. J Dermatol Treat 23(2):116–121. doi:10.3109/09546634.2010.514893
61. Leung TF, Wong KY, Wong CK, Fung KP, Lam CWK, Fok TF, Leung PC, Hon KLE (2008) In vitro and clinical immunomodulatory effects of a novel Pentaherbs concoction for atopic dermatitis. Br J Dermatol 158(6):1216–1223. doi:10.1111/j.1365-2133.2008.08502.x
62. Chan BCL, Hon KLE, Leung PC, Sam SW, Fung KP, Lee MYH, Lau HYA (2008) Traditional Chinese medicine for atopic eczema: pentaherbs formula suppresses inflammatory mediators release from mast cells. J Ethnopharmacol 120(1):85–91. doi:10.1016/j.jep.2008.07.034
63. Kobayashi H, Ishii M, Takeuchi S, Tanaka Y, Shintani T, Yamatodani A, Kusunoki T, Furue M (2010) Efficacy and safety of a traditional herbal medicine, hochu-ekki-to in the long-term management of Kikyo (Delicate Constitution) patients with atopic dermatitis: A 6-month, multicenter, double-blind, randomized, placebo-controlled study. Evid Based Complement Alternat Med 7(3):367–373. doi:10.1093/ecam/nen003
64. Nakada T, Watanabe K, Matsumoto T, Santa K, Triizuka K, Hanawa T (2002) Effect of orally

administered Hochu-ekki-to, a Japanese herbal medicine, on contact hypersensitivity caused by repeated application of antigen. Int Immunopharmacol 2(7):901–911. doi:10.1016/s1567-5769(02)00027-9

65. Cheng HM, Chiang LC, Jan YM, Chen GW, Li TC (2011) The efficacy and safety of a Chinese herbal product (Xiao-Feng-San) for the treatment of refractory atopic dermatitis: a randomized, double-blind, placebo-controlled trial. Int Arch Allergy Immunol 155(2):141–148. doi:10.1159/000318861
66. Scheid V, Bensky D, Ellis A, Barolet R (2009) Chinese herbal medicine formulas and strategies, 2nd edn. Eastland Press, Seattle
67. Shichijo K, Saito H (1997) Effect of Chinese herbal medicines and disodium cromoglycate on IgE- dependent histamine release from mouse cultured mast cells. Int J Immunopharmacol 19(11–12):677–682. doi:10.1016/s0192-0561(97)00097-0
68. Bansal D, Hota D, Chakrabarti A (2010) Research methodological issues in evaluating herbal interventions. Open Access J Clin Trials 2:15–21
69. Cardini F, Wade C, Regalia AL, Gui S, Li W, Raschetti R, Kronenberg F (2006) Clinical research in traditional medicine: priorities and methods. Complement Ther Med 14(4):282–287. doi:10.1016/j.ctim.2006.07.003
70. Carter B (2003) Methodological issues and complementary therapies: researching intangibles? Complement Ther Nurs Midwifery 9(3):133–139. doi:10.1016/s1353-6117(03)00042-8
71. Yuan R, Lin Y (2000) Traditional Chinese medicine: an approach to scientific proof and clinical validation. Pharmacol Ther 86(2):191–198. doi:10.1016/s0163-7258(00)00039-5
72. Kobayashi M, Davis SM, Utsunomiya T, Pollard RB, Suzuki F (1999) Antiviral effect of gingyo-san, a traditional Chinese herbal medicine, on influenza a2 virus infection in mice. Am J Chin Med 27(1):53–62
73. Byard RW (2010) A review of the potential forensic significance of traditional herbal medicines. J Forensic Sci 55(1):89–92. doi:10.1111/j.1556-4029.2009.01252.x

Chapter 10

Rikkunshito and Ghrelin

Hiroshi Takeda, Shunsuke Ohnishi, Koji Nakagawa, Naoto Okubo, Chihiro Yamada, Chiharu Sadakane, Yayoi Saegusa, Miwa Nahata, and Tomohisa Hattori

Abstract

Rikkunshito is a kampo herbal medicine which is widely used in Japan for the treatment of the upper gastrointestinal symptoms of patients with functional dyspepsia (FD), gastroesophageal reflux disease (GERD), dyspeptic symptoms of postgastrointestinal surgery patients, and chemotherapy-induced dyspepsia in cancer patients. Recently, very unique characteristics of rikkunshito have been unveiled; oral administration of rikkunshito potentiates orexigenic action of ghrelin through several different mechanisms. In addition, several lines of evidence obtained from both animal and human studies indicate that rikkunshito can be an attractive and promising therapeutic option for the anorectic conditions including cisplatin-induced dyspepsia, anorexia of aging, stress-induced hypophagia, cancer cachexia-anorexia syndrome, and drug-related anorexia. We will highlight what is known about the orexigenic effect of rikkunshito with a special focus on an interaction with ghrelin signaling system.

Key words Rikkunshito, Ghrelin, GHSR1a, Serotonin 2B-receptor, Serotonin 2C-receptor, Phosphodiesterase 3, Anorexia

1 Introduction

Rikkunshito is a kampo herbal medicine which is prepared by compounding eight herbal medicines: *Atractylodis lanceae rhizoma, Ginseng radix, Pinelliae tuber, Poria, Zizyphi fructus, Aurantii nobilis pericarpium, Glycyrrhizae radix, and Zingiberis rhizoma*. Rikkunshito is widely used in Japan for the treatment of the upper gastrointestinal symptoms of patients with functional dyspepsia (FD)Functional dyspepsia (FD) and gastroesophageal reflux disease (GERD)Gastroesophageal reflux disease (GERD) and dyspeptic symptoms of postgastrointestinal surgery patients [1–3].

Clinical efficacy of rikkunshito for functional gastrointestinal disorders has been considered to be owing to its prokinetic activity [1–3]. Recently, novel pharmacological action of rikkunshito has emerged [4–7]. Oral administration of rikkunshito stimulates

Akio Inui (ed.), *Herbal Medicines: New Horizons*, Methods in Pharmacology and Toxicology,
DOI 10.1007/978-1-4939-4002-8_10, © Springer Science+Business Media New York 2016

secretion of ghrelin, an orexigenic hormone secreted from the stomach, in rodents and human [8, 9]. More recent evidence suggests that rikkunshito enhances ghrelin's orexigenic effect by several additional mechanisms [10–13]. We will summarize the currently available evidence regarding the clinical efficacy of rikkunshito from a pharmacological point of view with a special attention to an interaction with ghrelin signaling system.

2 Pharmacology of Rikkunshito

2.1 Rikkunshito as a Prokinetic Agent

Rikkunshito was reported to promote gastric emptying in both animal and human studies [14, 15] (Fig. 1). Hesperidin and l-arginine were identified as two of the active ingredients contributing to facilitate gastric emptying [16]. Rikkunshito stimulates gastric myoelectric activity [17], and direct effects of rikkunshito on gastrointestinal smooth muscle cells were also reported [18–20].

The effects of rikkunshito on gastric adaptive relaxation have been reported in isolated guinea pig stomachs [21], conscious dogs [22], and isolated fundus smooth muscle from *Suncus murinus* [23] and diabetic neuropathic rats with gastric dysmotility [20]. Rikkunshito not only increased gastric adaptive relaxation at the basal level but also ameliorated inhibited relaxation by the nitric oxide synthase inhibitor [20]. Improvement in gastric accommodation was also reported in virtual reality stress-imposed healthy humans [24].

Rikkunshito was reported to stimulate gastrointestinal contractions in the interdigestive state and gastric emptying in conscious dogs through cholinergic neurons and serotonin type-3 receptors [25]. The prokinetic effect of rikkunshito by 5-HT3 receptor

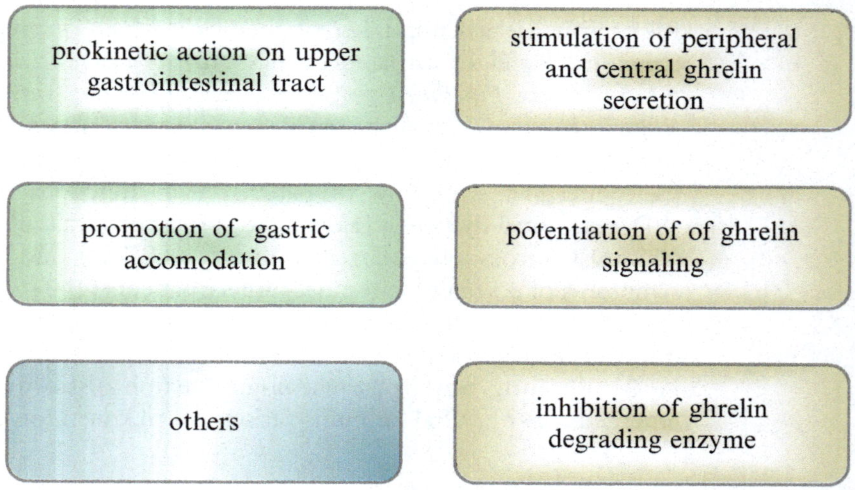

Fig. 1 Summary of mechanism of action of rikkunshito focusing on the ghrelin signaling system

antagonism was also reported in delayed gastric emptying induced by either nitric oxide synthase inhibitor [16] or serotonin [26].

Recently, Herbrechter et al. [27] analyzed the antagonistic effects of the rikkunshito constituents at heterologously expressed 5-HT3A receptors using the two-electrode voltage-clamp technique. They showed that ethanol tinctures from *Aurantii, Ginseng, Zingiberis, Atractylodis,* and *Glycyrrhiza* inhibited the 5-HT3A receptor response; among them, the strongest antagonism was found for *Glycyrrhiza*. Liquiritigenin, glabridin, and licochalcone A from *Glycyrrhiza* and hesperetin which are the aglycone of hesperidin from *Aurantii* were found to be the most effective inhibitors of the 5-HT-induced currents in the screening.

2.2 Rikkunshito as a Ghrelin Enhancer

Ghrelin is a peripherally active orexigenic gut hormone consisting of 28 amino acids, and the third N-terminal amino-acid serine (Ser) residue is octanoylated [28, 29]. Ghrelin is involved in the hypothalamic regulation of energy homeostasis by increasing food intake and reducing fat utilization [30, 31]. Plasma levels of ghrelin rise during fasting, and fall upon eating, which has led to the suggestion that ghrelin is a meal-initiating hormone [32]. Plasma levels of ghrelin are inversely correlated with body weight in humans and rise after weight loss Cummings et al. [33]. Besides the regulation of energy homeostasis, ghrelin mediates an increase in gastric motility, induces a positive inotropic effect on the heart, and causes vasodilatation [28, 34, 35].

Rikkunshito increases plasma ghrelin levels both in humans and in animals [9, 25] and was also reported to restore the decreased plasma ghrelin levels induced by stress or cisplatinum [8, 36].

The induction of ghrelin secretion by rikkunshito is supposed to be based on the 5-HT2B/2C–receptor antagonism owing to multiple active ingredients (Table 1). We screened 33 compounds contained in rikkunshito and found that 13 out of 33 compounds

Table 1
Potential target molecules for pharmacological actions of rikkunshito

Target molecules	References
GHSR1a receptor	[13]
5-HT2B receptor	[8]
5-HT2C receptor	[8]
5-HT3 receptor	[27]
α2 adrenergic receptor	[38]
PDE3	[86]
CES, BuChE	[12]

showed antagonistic activity against binding to any of 5-HT 1A, 1B/D, 2A, 2B, 2C, 3, 4, 6, and 7 receptors [5, 6, 8]. Among them, 3,3′,4′,5,6,7,8-heptamethoxyflavone (HMF), nobiletin, and tangeretin contained in *Aurantii nobilis pericarpium* had potent 5-HT2B–receptor antagonistic activity. The inhibitory activity of hesperidin against the 5-HT2B receptor was weak, but the concentration of hesperidin in rikkunshito is the highest among the ingredients tested. In addition, isoliquiritigenin, which is an ingredient of *Glycyrrhizae radix*, had the most potent activity against the 5-HT2C receptor binding. Our study indicated that the administration of HMF, isoliquiritigenin, and hesperidin attenuated the decrease in plasma ghrelin level, while tangeretin, nobiletin, and 8-shogaol did not. Rikkunshito, hesperidin, and isoliquiritigenin ameliorated reduced hypothalamic ghrelin secretion and reduction in GHS-R signal transduction in the hypothalamus via 5-HT2CR antagonism [8, 37]. This suggested that the ingredients that inhibit 5-HT2B /5-HT2C–receptor binding are likely to be effective in vivo.

Recently, rikkunshito was shown to alleviate urocortin 1 (UCN1)-induced inhibition of circulating ghrelin levels in rats by α2 adrenergic receptor (AR) antagonism [38, 39]. It was found that several components, namely, glycycoumarin, 6- and 8-shogaol, 10-gingerol, and eudesmol, functioned as α2-AR antagonists. These results suggest that the effects of rikkunshito on decreased food intake in response to ICV UCN1 administration may be induced through the α2-AR antagonist property of some of its specific components.

The potentiating effects on ghrelin signaling in vitro were also demonstrated in GHS-R-expressing cells, showing significantly sustained increase in intracellular Ca^{2+} levels induced by ghrelin, mediated by the increased binding ability of ghrelin to its receptor following pretreatment by rikkunshito or its one of the active components, atractylodin (*Atractylodis lanceae rhizoma*) [20]. Rikkunshito's unique action as a ghrelin signaling enhancer was demonstrated in rat GERD model [40] and mouse restraint stress model [41].

Finally, an inhibitory effect of rikkunshito on ghrelin metabolizing enzymes, which inactivate ghrelin to deacylated form, was shown [12]. Several components of rikkunshito, such as glycycoumarin (*Glycyrrhizae radix*) and pachymic acid (*Hoelen*), were reported to show inhibitory activity against ghrelin-deacylating enzyme, butyrylcholinesterase [12].

2.3 Pharmacokinetics of Rikkunshito

Recently, Kitagawa et al. [42] investigated the pharmacokinetics of the ingredients of rikkunshito in healthy volunteers. They found that 18 or 21 of 32 typical ingredients were detected in plasma or urine after oral treatment with rikkunshito. Specifically, pharmacokinetic parameters of nine ingredients derived from rikkunshito

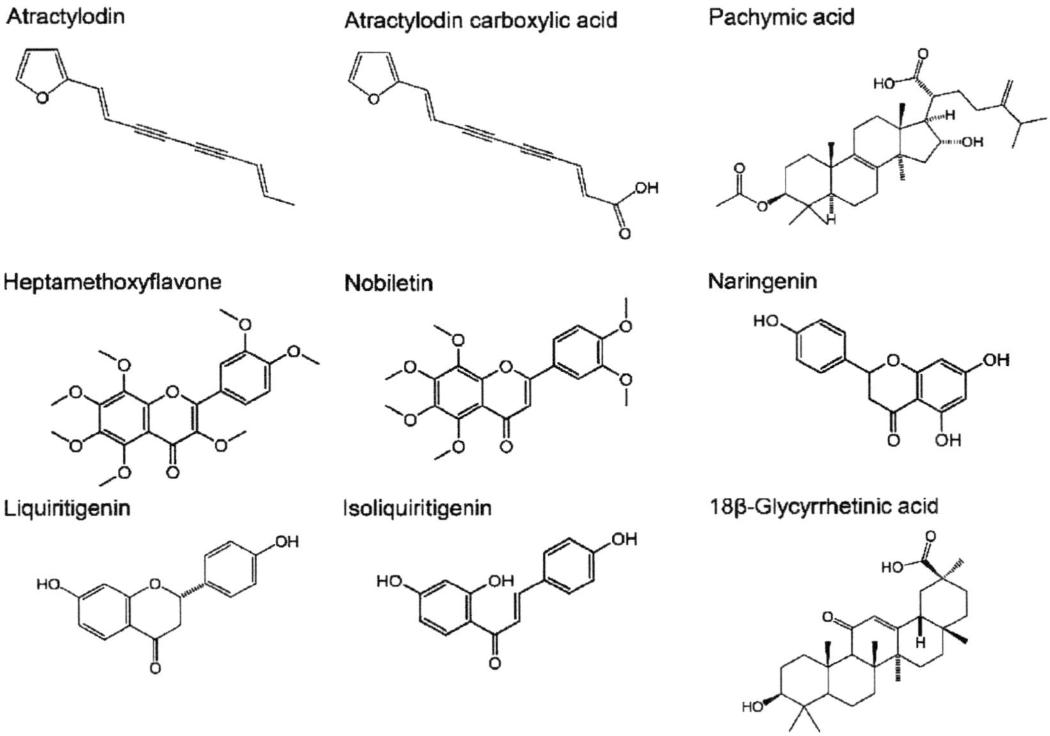

Fig. 2 Chemical structures of nine ingredients derived from rikkunshito which were shown to be detected in human circulation after oral administration (Adopted from Kitagawa H, et al., PLoS One. 2015;10:e0133159)

(atractylodin, atractylodin carboxylic acid, pachymic acid, HMF, naringenin, nobiletin, liquiritigenin, isoliquiritigenin, and 18β-glycyrrhetinic acid) were determined (Fig. 2). This study clearly shown that multiple ingredients of rikkunshito were absorbed into the human body and suggests that the pharmacological effect of rikkunshito is likely to be mediated by multiple ingredients acting successively on a target molecule.

3 Functional Dyspepsia

3.1 Functional Dyspepsia and Ghrelin

Functional dyspepsia (FD) is a common functional gastrointestinal disorder. FD is characterized by chronic recurrent epigastric symptoms including pain, burning, and postprandial fullness [43]. The exact cause of FD remains unclear, but several pathophysiological mechanisms have been indicated as possible etiological factors, such as delayed gastric emptying, impaired proximal gastric accommodation, and visceral hypersensitivity [43].

Although it remains controversial whether the plasma ghrelin levels of patients with FD increase or decrease [44–51], plasma ghrelin levels have been reported to be correlated with the FD symptom score. In addition, ghrelin affects gastric motility and gastric acid secretion, which are strongly related to the pathogenesis of FD [45].

Futagami et al. [52] asked whether single nucleotide polymorphisms (SNPs) of preproghrelin gene might contribute to early phase of gastric emptying in FD patients. They found a correlation between the preproghrelin 3056TT genotype and low acylated-ghrelin levels in *Helicobacter pylori (H. pylori)*-negative FD patients [52]. They also reported that Leu72Met (408C > A), which has been linked to obesity-related phenotypes, was significantly associated with early phase of gastric emptying in FD patients [53].

Akamizu et al. [54] attempted to evaluate the clinical response to repeated ghrelin administration in patients with anorexia caused by functional disorders including six FD patients. Ghrelin administration tended to increase daily food intake in comparison to levels before and after completion of treatment, although this difference did not reach statistical significance. Hunger sensation was significantly elevated at the end of drip infusion. No severe adverse effects were observed.

3.2 Functional Dyspepsia and Rikkunshito

Several clinical studies have demonstrated the effectiveness of rikkunshito in the treatment of functional dyspepsia. In a double-blinded, randomized, placebo-controlled trial of rikkunshito, gastric emptying and gastrointestinal symptoms were evaluated in 42 patients with FD [14]. Subjects were randomized to receive either oral treatment with 2.5 g rikkunshito three times daily or placebo. Gastric emptying was measured by the acetaminophen absorption method. After 7 days of treatment, gastric emptying was significantly accelerated, and gastrointestinal symptoms were significantly reduced in patients treated with rikkunshito, indicating that rikkunshito has a prokinetic action on gastric emptying and may be useful in treating FD.

A comparative clinical study of 235 patients with dysmotility-like dyspepsia was conducted [55]. Rikkunshito-treated patients were given 2.5 g of rikkunshito three times a day for 2 weeks, and placebo-treated patients were given 2.5 g of placebo, including 2.5 % rikkunshito, as control. As a result, the dysmotility-like dyspepsia generalized improvement rate (DDGI) was significantly higher in the rikkunshito-treated group than in the placebo group.

Arai et al. [56] conducted a randomized controlled study to compare the effects of rikkunshito and domperidone on upper gastrointestinal symptoms as well as plasma acylated-ghrelin levels in patients with FD. Although the changes in dyspeptic symptoms scores were comparative in both groups, elevation of plasma acylated-ghrelin level was noted only in rikkunshito-treated group. Of particular interest, the improvement of dyspeptic symptoms by rikkunshito was correlated with an increase of plasma ghrelin level.

Recently, a multicenter, randomized, placebo-controlled, parallel-group trial of rikkunshito in 247 patients with functional dyspepsia was conducted [57]. The administration of rikkunshito for 8 weeks reduced dyspepsia; epigastric pain was significantly improved and postprandial fullness tended to improve compared to the placebo treatment group. There were no severe adverse events in either groups. In a post hoc analysis of the same study, Togawa et al. [58] demonstrated that a low baseline level of plasma des-acyl-ghrelin was an independently associated factor for the efficacy of rikkunshito against FD especially in *H. pylori*-negative population.

4 Gastroesophageal Reflux Disease (GERD)

4.1 GERD and Ghrelin

Gastroesophageal reflux disease (GERD) is defined as a condition that develops when the reflux of gastric acidic content causes troublesome symptoms such as heartburn or complications like esophageal mucosal injury [59].

GERD is often associated with decreased upper gastrointestinal motility [60]. Because ghrelin is an appetite-stimulating hormone known to increase gastrointestinal motility, changes in ghrelin kinetics may be related to the pathogenesis of GERD. However, there have been very few data concerning the relationship between ghrelin and GERD so far.

Rubenstein et al. [61] conducted a case–control study in 822 men undergoing colorectal cancer screening who were recruited to also undergo upper endoscopy. They found that serum ghrelin was inversely associated with GERD but positively associated with Barrett's esophagus. Shindo et al. [62] also showed that acylated-ghrelin levels were significantly lower in nonerosive reflux disease (NERD) patients than in healthy volunteers.

Using a rat model, Nahata et al. [63] investigated whether ghrelin signaling is impaired in rats with GERD and studied its involvement in upper gastrointestinal motility. They found that impaired ghrelin signaling is involved in gastrointestinal dysmotility in GERD rats. Moreover, rikkunshito improves gastrointestinal motility by enhancing the decreased response to ghrelin. Nahata et al. also showed that aberrantly increased secretion of peripheral ghrelin and decreased ghrelin responsiveness may occur in GERD rats [63]. These results suggest that although GERD rats have higher plasma ghrelin levels, ghrelin signaling in GERD rats may be suppressed due to reduced MCH and/or orexin synthesis in the hypothalamus.

4.2 GERD and Rikkunshito

The therapeutic effects of rikkunshito were reported in proton pump inhibitor (PPI)- refractory patients with GERD or NERD. In children with symptomatic GERD, rikkunshito relieved symptoms and reduced distal esophageal acid exposure through improved esophageal acid clearance [64, 65]. Although rikkunshito did not change the number of acid reflux events, it reduced the esophageal acid clearance time. The mechanism underlying the improved esophageal clearance capacity with rikkunshito remains unknown.

Tominaga et al. [66] compared the efficacies of rikkunshito combined with rabeprazole (RPZ) and a double dose of RPZ in a prospective randomized multicenter trial in PPI-refractory GERD patients. One hundred and four patients with GERD symptoms remaining after 4-week treatment with RPZ were enrolled. Four-week treatment with rikkunshito combined with RPZ significantly decreased FSSG (the frequency scale for the symptoms of GERD) score similar to that seen on treatment with a double dose of RPZ. In the subgroup analysis, the improvement rate of male nonerosive GERD patients in the rikkunshito group was significantly greater than that of such patients in the other group. From these results, it was concluded that rikkunshito combined with standard-dose RPZ therapy may be a useful new strategy for PPI-refractory GERD patients. In a randomized, placebo-controlled, double-blind clinical trial for 242 patients with PPI-refractory NERD, treatment for 4 or 8 weeks with rikkunshito (7.5 g/day) improved their mental component summary (MCS) scores in the Short-Form Health Survey-8 (SF-8), which was especially more effective in patients with a low body mass index (<22). Moreover, rikkunshito significantly improved the acid-related dysmotility symptoms of FSSG in female and elderly patients (≥65 years) [67, 68].

Rikkunshito was also reported to improve globus sensation in patients with PPI-refractory laryngopharyngeal reflux (LPR). This was, at least in part, due to the stimulation of gastric emptying suggesting that rikkunshito is an effective treatment option for PPI-refractory LPR [69].

5 Stress

5.1 Stress and Ghrelin

Stress and negative emotions have been associated with both increased and decreased food intake. The mechanism underlying this opposed behavioral responses to similar stressors has not been determined, but high stress levels appear to lead to decreased eating [70].

Conflicting data are available regarding the effect of stress on ghrelin secretion [71]. In animal studies, elevations in plasma ghrelin have been observed in response to various psychological/environmental stressors, including a tail pinch stress, a water avoidance stress, chronic exposure to cold, repeated restraint stress, and chronic social defeat stress. In contrast, exposure to immune, visceral, or strenuous physical stressors causes reduction of plasma ghrelin level. In humans, acute psychosocial stress or cold exposure increased plasma ghrelin levels. However, there are several reports showing that plasma ghrelin level did not change or even decreased by an exposure to stresses. Collectively, these findings support the idea that acute or severe stress causes a reduction of circulating ghrelin level resulting in the suppression of appetite, whereas mild or chronic repeated stress causes an upregulation of ghrelin secretion as an adaptation to stress [71, 72]. In support of this notion, Lutter et al. [73] found that increased ghrelin levels produced anxiolytic and antidepressant responses in mice suggesting that increased ghrelin in response to stress protects against depressive reactions to stress and helps them cope with stress.

Corticotropin-releasing factor (CRFCorticotropin-releasing factor (CRF)) and its family peptides, urocortin1 (Ucn1), urocortin2 (Ucn2), and urocortin3 (Ucn3), play an important role in the control of food intake [74]. Among the CRF family peptides, Ucn1 was shown to have the most potent inhibitory effect on the food intake in mice. Ucn1 has been identified in the brain and has a higher affinity for CRF2 receptors (CRFR2) than for CRF1 receptors (CRFR1); hence, it is believed that CRFR2 plays the major role in satiety. Activation of CRFR1 in the brain can suppress feeding independently of CRFR2-mediated mechanisms. CRF1 and CRF2 receptor-mediated anorexia appear to exhibit different time courses; in rats, ICV administration of CRFR1 agonists elicited rapid-onset anorexia with short duration, while CRFR2 agonists caused delayed-onset, prolonged anorexia [74].

There are several reports showing that administration of Ucn1 to humans and rodents reduces plasma ghrelin concentrations [75]. In addition, Ucn1-induced reduction of plasma ghrelin and food intake were restored by CRFR2 but not CRFR1 [75]. However, much less information is available on the relationship between ghrelin and CRFR1.

Novelty stress model, where animals are removed from their home cage and placed somewhere they have never been before, has been used to estimate the levels of anxiety and depression [76, 77]. Using novelty stress model, we found that 3h after stress loading, appetite reduction was associated with a decrease in plasma ghrelin level, reduced levels of neuropeptide Y/agouti-related peptide mRNA, and increased levels of proopiomelanocortin mRNA in the hypothalamus [78]. Administering a CRF1R selective antagonist, but not a CRF2R antagonist, resolved the reduction in food intake 3 h after the novelty stress by enhancing circulating ghrelin concentrations. Interestingly, 5-HT1B/2CR antagonist and melanocortin-4 receptor (MC4R) antagonist alleviated the novelty stress-induced hypophagia and the reduction in circulating ghrelin level [36]. We hypothesized that acute appetite suppression due to CRF1R activation after a novelty stress is caused by a chain reaction of appetite control mechanisms mediated by 5-HT1B/2CR in ARC to MC4R system in paraventricular nucleus (PVN), causing lowered peripheral ghrelin secretion.

We recently reported that restraint stress causes a significant elevation of plasma des-acyl-ghrelin levels only, whereas plasma acylated-ghrelin levels remain unaffected [41]. We found that novelty stress causes a decrease in food intake, which is associated with decreased plasma ghrelin levels after stress [36]. However, increased plasma ghrelin levels with fasting were not observed in a young mouse novel stress model [78–80]. Exogenous acylated-ghrelin ameliorated the decreased food intake by temporarily increasing plasma acylated-ghrelin levels above the physiological concentration [36]. Thus, the transmission of ghrelin signals to the hypothalamic feeding center may be abnormal under novelty stress. A few studies have investigated a possible relationship between corticotropin-releasing factor (CRFCorticotropin-releasing factor (CRF)) receptors and plasma ghrelin dynamics.

We reported that novelty stress and CRF administration reduced plasma ghrelin levels and food intake and that a CRF1 receptor antagonist but not a CRF2 receptor antagonist prevented these decreases [36]. Interestingly, we also found that a selective 5-HT2C or 5-HT1B receptor antagonist and a melanocortin-4 (MC4) receptor antagonist prevented the decreased plasma acylated-ghrelin levels in novelty stressed mice [36]. We hypothesized that the acute appetite loss and the decrease in plasma ghrelin levels occurred via CRF1 receptors, the effects of which were mediated through 5-HT2C/1B and MC4 receptor systems.

We showed that, compared with normal mice, intracerebroventricular administration of mCPP induced a significant decrease in food intake in novelty stressed mice [36]. Administration of 5-HT2C/1B receptor antagonists ameliorated the decrease in food intake and plasma acylated-ghrelin levels [36]. Thus, an increase in 5-HT2C/1B receptor activity may occur after novelty stress, resulting in anorexia or reduced plasma ghrelin levels.

In addition, we showed that peripheral administration of SB215505 and SB204741, selective 5-HT2B receptor antagonists, prevented the decrease in food intake in novelty stressed mice [79].

5.2 Effect of Rikkunshito on Stress

Rikkunshito has recently been evaluated for its clinical usefulness in stress and depression [81]. This medicine has modulatory effects on the hypothalamo–pituitary–adrenal (HPA) axis and autonomic nervous function. It regulates adrenocorticotropic hormone (ACTH) and cortisol levels in plasma to normal ranges in FD [81]. Some abnormalities of gastrointestinal function are presumed to result from changes in hormone levels. Moreover, the herbal components of rikkunshito, *P. tuber* and *Zingiberis rhizome*, have modulatory effects on human plasma adrenocorticotropic hormone (ACTH) and cortisol levels with continual stress exposure [81].

Oral administration of rikkunshito inhibited the reduction of food intake at 1 and 3 h in mice exposed to the novelty stress, and coadministration of the ghrelin receptor antagonist [D-Lys3]

GHRP-6 with rikkunshito abolished this effect [36]. Rikkunshito also increased plasma acyl-ghrelin concentrations at 1 and 3 h after the novelty stress, suggesting that blocking the decrease in endogenous peripheral ghrelin in mice exposed to the novelty stress also acts to sustain feeding behavior. We found that the oral administration of glycycoumarin and isoliquiritigenin inhibited the reduction in food intake in mice exposed to the novelty stress [36]. We have previously shown that glycycoumarin and isoliquiritigenin potently inhibit 5-HT2C receptor ligand binding and that orally administering rikkunshito abolishes the decrease in food intake in mCPP-treated rats [8]. These findings support the notion that rikkunshito improved hypophagia and decreased plasma ghrelin levels via 5-HT2C receptor antagonism-like action in mice exposed to the novelty stress.

Rikkunshito ameliorated the novelty stress-induced decreases in food intake and plasma ghrelin levels in young mice [36, 79] and in aged mice [78, 80], and co-administering [D-Lys3]-GHRP-6 abolished the effects of rikkunshito [36]. Rikkunshito completely ameliorated the decreased food intake in young and aged mice after mCPP injection [30]. Rikkunshito administration attenuated the hyperactivation of the HPA axis and the decreased food intake induced by novelty stress, which was similar to the effects of SB242084 [36].

We and others reported that rikkunshito had an antagonistic effect on 5-HT2C receptors in vivo [8, 13]. In addition, the results of in vitro radiobinding assays revealed that components in rikkunshito, such as isoliquiritigenin, exhibited 5-HT2B/2C receptor binding inhibitory activity [8].

6 Aging

6.1 Anorexia of Aging and Ghrelin

In the elderly subjects, the reduction in energy intake often exceeds energy expenditure resulting in weight loss and protein energy malnutrition [82]. Protein energy malnutrition in the elderly is a frequent and clinically important problem, which leads to increased morbidity, mortality, disability, and health costs in this growing population. One of the most important causes of the reduction in energy intake is anorexia. The causes of the anorexia of aging have not yet been fully defined, and they are probably multifactorial and include sensory impairment, social isolation, and psychological and physiologic factors, in addition to the presence of disease [82, 83].

Although many peripheral anorexigenic hormones including cholecystokinin, leptin, and insulin have been found to rise with increased age, findings for ghrelin are controversial [71, 82]. Several lines of animal studies also have revealed mixed results. The reason for these conflicting data seems to be owing to the differences in their experimental conditions under which the plasma ghrelin concentration was measured. Indeed, our group found that plasma ghrelin in aged C57BL/6 mice does not increase under fasted conditions, but is higher than that in young mice under freely fed conditions [71]. This suggests that regulation of ghrelin secretion from the stomach may be disturbed in older mice. In agreement with this, recent clinical studies have suggested that disturbance of regulation of ghrelin secretion and reduced production during hunger and satiety may cause "anorexia of aging" in elderly people [71].

In a previous study, Ariyasu et al. [84] reported that subcutaneous injection of ghrelin (360 μg/kg twice a day) enhanced food intake in 72-h fasted and aged mice and restored the decrease in body weight caused by fasting. Contrary to their data, we found that much lower dose of ghrelin (33 μg/kg) failed to increase food intake in 75-week-old mice, whereas the same dose of ghrelin had an orexigenic effect in young mice [85], suggesting that aging is associated with attenuation of endogenous ghrelin signaling. Collectively, it seems that dysregulation of ghrelin secretion as well as ghrelin resistance in the appetite control system is occurring in aged mice.

Although the detailed mechanisms of disturbed ghrelin dynamics remain unclear, one of the possible causes seems to be leptin. We have found that plasma leptin and insulin levels in aged mice are significantly higher compared to those in young ones [85]. Leptin and insulin are reported to inhibit ghrelin secretion from the stomach into the circulation [86]; hence, elevated leptin and insulin in the elderly may contribute to inhibition of secretion of ghrelin during fasting, resulting in prolonged satiety and inhibition of hunger sensation. Moreover, the activation of phosphoinositide 3-kinase (PI3K)-phosphodiesterase 3 (PDE3) pathway was recently proposed as a mechanism by which leptin blocks ghrelin signaling in neuropeptide Y (NPY) neurons, and it may counteract the adenylate cyclase-cAMP-protein kinase A system implicated in the effect of ghrelin [87]. Other studies showed that the effect of leptin was abolished by the administration of either PDE3 inhibitor [88] or PI3K inhibitor [89]. We demonstrated that the plasma leptin level in aged mice was greatly increased under both feeding and fasting conditions. Furthermore, we found that administration of either a PI3K inhibitor LY-294002 or the PDE3 inhibitor cilostamide improved anorexia in aged mice [85]. These results suggest that plasma leptin, which increases with age, may induce resistance to ghrelin reactivity via camp downregulation.

6.2 Effect of Rikkunshito on Anorexia of Aging

Utumi et al. [90] carried out oral administration of rikkunshito to elderly dementia patients with appetite loss and examined its effects on food intake. Food intake, weight, total protein, albumin, and potassium in plasma were examined before and after the administration of rikkunshito for 4 weeks. Food intake was significantly improved after the administration of rikkunshito in the six elderly dementia patients. Other parameters, such as body weight and albumin in plasma, did not change significantly during the examination, although they slightly increased in some patients.

We demonstrated that the administration of rikkunshito improve anorexia of aging [85]. In addition, we found that rikkunshito increased the reactivity of ghrelin by inhibiting PDE3 activity. The components of rikkunshito (nobiletin, isoliquiritigenin, and HMF) had inhibitory effects against PDE3 activity. These results suggest that dysregulation of ghrelin secretion and ghrelin resistance in the appetite control system occurred in aged mice and that rikkunshito ameliorated aging-associated anorexia via inhibition of PDE3 [85].

7 Cisplatin-Induced Anorexia

7.1 Cisplatin-Induced Anorexia and Ghrelin

Patients with cancer being treated with cytotoxic drugs such as cisplatin often experience a number of undesirable side effects which include acute and delayed nausea, vomiting, anorexia, dyspepsia, and disrupted gastrointestinal function.

Recent evidence has demonstrated the relationship between chemotherapy-induced gastrointestinal disorders and ghrelin in both clinical and animal studies. In human studies, one report has demonstrated that an increase in plasma ghrelin concentrations was observed after the start of anticancer chemotherapy [91], but more recent studies revealed that the plasma concentration of acylated ghrelin was decreased during the treatment with anticancer drugs [92–96]. In animal studies, we and others reported that circulating ghrelin concentrations were reduced in cisplatin-treated rats until 6 h during the early stage of anorexia [8, 10].

Intraperitoneal injection of 5-HT decreased 24-h food intake as well as plasma acylated-ghrelin level in a dose-dependent manner [8]. This result suggests that the cisplatin-induced reduction in the plasma level of acylated ghrelin may be mediated via a release of 5-HT from the gastrointestinal tract mucosa triggered by cisplatin. Indeed, a 5-HT2B–receptor agonist BW723C86 and a 5-HT2C agonist m-chlorophenylpiperazine HCl (mCPP) markedly decreased plasma acylated-ghrelin levels and increased intragastric ghrelin content suggesting that 5-HT2B/2C–receptor stimulation inhibits the release of gastric ghrelin into the circulation [8]. In contrast, 5-HT3 and 5-HT4 agonists had no effect on ghrelin dynamics. 5-HT2B and 5-HT2C antagonists suppressed the cisplatin- induced decrease of plasma acylated-ghrelin level and food intake. These results strongly imply that activation of 5-HT2B and 5-HT2C–receptors, but not 5-HT3 and 5-HT4 receptors, play an important role in the decrease in plasma ghrelin level in cisplatin-induced anorexia. Of note, granisetron used in this study clearly inhibited delayed gastric emptying after cisplatin treatment, but it failed to improve cisplatin-induced anorexia [8, 10].

Peripheral administration of exogenous ghrelin ameliorates anorexia [8, 95] and vomiting [96] induced by cisplatin. Administration of exogenous ghrelin has been shown to have the potential to reduce each of these symptoms in relevant animal models treated with cisplatin as an cytotoxic agent: emesis in the ferret [96] and anorexia in the rat and mouse [95].

Yakabi et al. [10] examined the changes of hypothalamic ghrelin secretion in cisplatin-treated rats to elucidate the mechanism underlying chemotherapy-induced delayed anorexia. Although ghrelin secretion in the hypothalamus did not decrease within 24 h of cisplatin administration, it started to decline significantly after 24 h and continued to decrease at least until 48 h, while their plasma ghrelin levels were comparable. They also showed that hypothalamic 5-HT2C receptor gene expression increased significantly in cisplatin- treated rats and the administration of mCPP inhibited hypothalamic ghrelin secretion [10]. Intracerebroventricular (ICV)-administered 5-HT2C antagonist SB242084 prevented a decrease in secretion of hypothalamic ghrelin in cisplatin-treated rats, but granisetron, a 5-HT3 antagonist did not [8]. These results indicate that the reduced ghrelin secretion in the hypothalamus secondary to 5-HT2C receptor activation may be involved in cisplatin-induced anorexia.

In another study, Yakabi et al. [11] demonstrated that hypothalamic GHS-R1a gene expression was significantly reduced after cisplatin or mCPP treatment, and this change was reversed by the treatment with 5-HT2C receptor antagonist, SB242084, but not with 5-HT3 receptor antagonists. 5-HT2C receptor antagonist also suppressed cisplatin-induced delayed anorexia. ICV injection of GHS-R1a antagonist to saline- or cisplatin-treated rats significantly reduced food intake compared with those injected with saline alone, and this inhibitory effect was abolished by the coadministration of 5-HT2C receptor antagonist. From these results, it was suggested that delayed-onset anorexia induced by cisplatin may be partly mediated by the activation of the hypothalamic 5-HT2C receptor and the resultant suppression of hypothalamic GHS-R1a gene expression as well as decreased ghrelin secretion in the hypothalamus.

7.2 Effect of Rikkunshito on Cisplatin-Induced Anorexia

Clinical trials have been conducted to investigate the effect of rikkunshito on chemotherapy-induced anorexia. Ohno et al. [94] performed a crossover clinical trial using rikkunshito involving ten patients with unresectable or recurrent gastric cancer treated with S-1 and cisplatin. They reported that rikkunshito attenuated the decrease in plasma acyl-ghrelin levels, increased food intake during chemotherapy, and reduced the degree of anorexia caused by chemotherapy. Seike et al. [97] evaluated the effect of rikkunshito in 19 patients with advanced esophageal cancer treated with docetaxel, 5- FU, and cisplatin. They reported that rikkunshito ameliorated chemotherapy-induced nausea and vomiting and improved the quality-of-life (QOL) score, particularly for mood and daily activity.

Rikkunshito ameliorated the decrease in circulating ghrelin concentration and this effect was abolished by coadministration of a GHS-R1a antagonist, [D-Lys3]-GHRP-6 [8]. This finding suggests that the mechanism of improvement of anorexia by rikkunshito may involve ghrelin receptor activation. Moreover, Yakabi et al. [10] found that rikkunshito reversed the decrease in hypothalamic ghrelin secretion and the decrease in GHS-R1a gene expression 24 h after cisplatin treatment. ICV injection of the GHS-R1a antagonist impedes the rikkunshito-mediated improvement in cisplatin-induced anorexia [10]. Hence, it seems likely that rikkunshito ameliorates cisplatin-induced anorexia by restoring ghrelin secretion and GHS-R1a expression in the hypothalamus. Collectively, rikkunshito suppressed cisplatin-induced anorexia by improving ghrelin signal transduction system by both the peripheral and the central mechanisms.

The induction of ghrelin secretion by rikkunshito is supposed to be based on the 5-HT2B/2C–receptor antagonism owing to multiple active ingredients. We screened 33 compounds contained in rikkunshito and found that 13 out of 33 compounds showed antagonistic activity against binding to any of 5-HT 1A, 1B/D, 2A, 2B, 2C, 3, 4, 6, and 7 receptors [8]. Among them, HMF, nobiletin, and tangeretin contained in *Aurantii nobilis pericarpium* had potent 5-HT2B–receptor antagonistic activity. The inhibitory activity of hesperidin against the 5-HT2B receptor was weak, but the concentration of hesperidin in rikkunshito is the highest among the ingredients tested. In addition, isoliquiritigenin, which is an ingredient of *Glycyrrhizae radix*, had the most potent activity against the 5-HT2C receptor binding. Our study indicated that the administration of HMF, isoliquiritigenin, and hesperidin attenuated the decrease in plasma ghrelin level, while tangeretin, nobiletin, and 8-shogaol did not. This suggested that the ingredients that inhibit 5-HT2B /5-HT2C–receptor binding are likely to be effective in vivo.

8 Cancer Anorexia–Cachexia Syndrome

8.1 Cancer Anorexia–Cachexia Syndrome and Ghrelin

Cancer anorexia–cachexia syndrome is characterized by decreased food intake, weight loss, muscle tissue wasting, and psychological distress and a lower quality of life [98, 99]. In advanced-stage cancer, up to 85 % of patients experience this syndrome which contributes to at least 20 % of cancer deaths overall [100]. The weight loss experienced by patients can be severe and is associated with a worsened prognosis, poorer response to chemotherapy, and increased morbidity [101]. In addition to metabolic changes, cachexia is often associated with anorexia. But the lack of nutrients alone cannot explain the metabolic changes seen in cachexia. In clinical trials, nutritional supplementation and dietary counseling failed to increase body weight [102]. Only limited treatment options exist for patients with clinical cancer cachexia. Corticosteroids improve the sensation of well-being and lead to increased food intake, but this effect lasts only a few weeks [98]. Progesterone such as megestrol acetate causes weight gain [100, 103], but this gain is resulted only from increased body fat and fluid, with no change in lean body mass [100]. Moreover, therapy with progesterone increases the frequency of thromboembolic events [99, 104]. Hence a better understanding of the underlying mechanisms of this syndrome should be very important in the development of new therapies to improve quality of life and potentially to prolong survival in patients with cancer-induced anorexia–cachexia.

Accumulating evidence suggests that anorexia–cachexia is caused predominantly by cytokines that are either produced by cancer cells or released by the host immune system in response to the cancer [98–100]. Pro-inflammatory cytokines including IL-1β, IL-6, and TNF-α can be produced by tumor cells, as well as from the host response to tumor [98–100]. Up to 50 % of cancer patients exhibit evidence of elevated inflammation at diagnosis, and the associated increase in cytokines is strongly implicated in producing anorexia, at least partly due to action at the central melanocortin system [105].

CRF is a mediator of the endocrine, autonomic, and immune responses to stress, including anorexia and anxiety-related behavior [106]. The central 5-HT system has been implicated in the processes of meal satiation and satiety, and hypothalamic 5-HT and CRF activities are stimulated by pro-inflammatory cytokines [107]. On the basis of these findings, it is probable that 5-HT and CRF might have a role in the pathogenesis of cancer anorexia–cachexia by modulating central and peripheral mechanisms as part of the stress response.

Although one recent study reported reduced plasma ghrelin concentrations in cancer patients [108], cachexia is more frequently associated with increased circulating ghrelin levels compared to healthy control subjects or non-cachectic patients with the same underlying diseases [109, 110]. Increased plasma ghrelin concentrations in cachectic patients could be a compensatory response to tissue wasting. Alternatively, it might reflect a state of ghrelin resistance.

Recently, Fujitsuka et al. [20] found that plasma acyl-ghrelin concentrations in tumor-bearing rats were higher than that in free-fed normal rats, but lower than that in pair-fed normal rats. This indicates that the compensatory responses to cachectic state including upregulation of ghrelin secretion are attenuated in tumor-bearing rats.

Use of ghrelin and other GHS-R1a agonists has been tested in animal models of cancer cachexia [103] and has demonstrated an increase in food intake, weight gain, and reversal of lean and fat mass losses [110–112]. Early trials in cancer patients demonstrated that administering ghrelin increased appetite [112–114]. Phases I and II clinical trials with the orally available, synthetic ghrelin mimetic RC-1291 have demonstrated increases in body weight and lean body mass in healthy subjects [115] and in cancer patients [116], without any dose-limiting side effects.

Recent studies have demonstrated that CRF decreased the plasma level of acyl-ghrelin [20, 70]. Fujituska et al. [20] found that CRF receptor antagonist, a-helical CRF, improved cancer anorexia–cachexia syndrome in tumor-bearing rats. They also found that the administration of 5-HT2C receptor antagonist SB242084 decreased hypothalamic CRF level and improved anorexia, gastrointestinal dysmotility, and body weight loss in tumor-bearing rats with cachexia [20]. In earlier studies, 5-HT concentration in the hypothalamus was reported to be increased in humans and animals with cancer [117, 118]. CRF neurons are involved in 5-HT-regulated ghrelin secretion and this pathway has a major role in cancer anorexia–cachexia.

Peripheral ghrelin administration stimulates food intake in cancer patients [93].

8.2 Cancer Anorexia–Cachexia Syndrome and Rikkunshito

In animal model of cancer cachexia, rikkunshito was found to reduce hypothalamic CRF levels and improve anorexia, gastrointestinal dysmotility, muscle wasting, and anxiety-related behavior [13]. It was also shown that Orikkunshito activated the efferent vagus nerve, which may be mediated by both the vagal afferent nerve and the direct central action. Of particular interest, rikkunshito and its active component, atractylodin, prolonged survival in these animals [13]. In vitro, ghrelin-induced cellular signaling in GHS-R-expressing cells was enhanced by pretreatment with rikkunshito and atractylodin which enhance ghrelin/GHS-R binding activity. In contrast to the effect of rikkunshito, either 5-HT2C receptor antagonist or exogenous ghrelin failed to prolong survival [13]. This suggests that the sensitizing effect on ghrelin signaling pathway may be essential for ameliorating anorexia–cachexia and the prolongation of survival. These findings are compatible with the idea that the physiological functions of endogenous ghrelin are enhanced by the dual actions of rikkunshito, which involve the stimulation of ghrelin secretion and the activation of GHS-R activity [119, 120].

Terawaki et al. recently developed a novel peritoneal dissemination-derived 85As2 rat cachexia model [121]. Using that model, they showed that oral administration of rikkunshito substantially ameliorated cancer cachexia-related anorexia and body composition changes. By using bleomycin (BLM)-induced lung fibrosis-associated cachexia model, Tsubouchi et al. asked whether rikkunshito administration could ameliorate pulmonary cachexia [122]. They indicated that rikkunshito administration exerts protective effects on pulmonary cachexia by ameliorating skeletal muscle wasting and food intake reduction as mediated by the ghrelin system and, thus, highlights rikkunshito as a potential therapeutic agent for the management of lung fibrosis. Of interest, rikkunshito was reported to exert ameliorating effects against acute lung injury by protecting the alveolar epithelial cells and regulating lung inflammation in a same model, but this effect was independently of the ghrelin system [123].

9 Gastrectomy

9.1 Gastrectomy and Ghrelin

Loss of body weight is a common complication of gastrectomy. It impairs patient's quality of life, increases risks of various diseases including infection, and affects long-term prognosis. Because the fundic glands of the stomach produce the large proportion of ghrelin, plasma ghrelin decreases to 10–30 % of the preoperative level after total gastrectomy and 50–70 % after distal gastrectomy [124]. Ghrelin concentrations recover relatively soon after surgery, and the ghrelin concentrations of patients with distal gastrectomy were 51–88 % of preoperative levels [124]. Chronic gastritis due to *Helicobacter pylori* infection and vagotomy are additional factors that perturb the ghrelin secretion of gastric cancer patients after gastrectomy. In the rodent, vagotomy alone has led to the significant reduction of the baseline of fasting plasma ghrelin [125]. After radical esophagectomy for esophageal cancers (which includes truncal vagotomy and reconstruction of the whole gastric tube), ghrelin secretion in human patients was reduced by one-half compared to preoperative levels and gradually recovered within a few years [126]. Vagotomy also perturbs the normal ghrelin secretion response (i.e., significant decline immediately after oral food intake).

A randomized clinical trial that revealed that recombinant ghrelin administration successfully increased both food intake and appetite and ameliorated weight loss after total gastrectomy [127]. Ghrelin administration could thus be a promising strategy to transiently improve the nutritional status of patients who have undergone gastrectomy, but its effect in the long term remains unclear.

9.2 Gastrectomy and Rikkunshito

Yagi et al. [17] evaluated the effect of rikkunshito on symptoms and gastric myoelectric activity in dyspeptic pediatric patients whose symptoms persisted for over 1 year after gastrointestinal surgery. With the administration of rikkunshito, all patients exhibited symptomatic relief and a significant decrease in mean symptom scores that were sustained over a 1-month period. The coordinating and stimulating effect of rikkunshito on the gastric myoelectric activity therefore seems to play an important role in the reduction of dyspeptic symptoms.

Pylorus-preserving gastrectomy (PPG) is now being applied to early gastric cancer to avoid the dumping syndrome and to reduce bile reflux and maintain normal mucosal integrity of the remnant stomach [128]. The patients with PPG had been reported to have better QOL than those with distal gastrectomy because of a decrease in dumping related symptoms. However, some patients still suffer from dyspeptic symptoms such as epigastric fullness, nausea, and vomiting due to delayed gastric emptying. Although prokinetic agents including erythromycin, cisapride, metoclopramide, and domperidone theoretically accelerate gastric emptying and alleviate symptoms after PPG, these drugs lack supporting evidence of positive effect. Takahashi et al. [129] examined the clinical effects of rikkunshito on patients who were to undergo PPG. The results indicated that rikkunshito accelerated emptying of solid meals from the remnant stomach and decreased postoperative stasis-related symptoms. Thus, rikkunshito may improve the postoperative QOL of patients undergoing PPG.

Recently, Takiguchi et al. [130] demonstrated a significant improvement of GI symptoms after treatment with rikkunshito for 4 weeks in 25 patients who had undergone gastrectomy. They reported that the mean ratio of the acyl-ghrelin /total ghrelin concentration was increased after rikkunshito administration. Gunji et al. [131] conducted an open-label, prospective, single-arm study performed to investigate the long-term QOL of 19 patients who underwent proximal gastrectomy (PG) for early-stage gastric cancer >6 months before the present study and to determine the pharmacologic effects, efficacy, and safety of rikkunshito in those patients. The patients' body weight increased significantly after the administration of rikkunshito. However, neither their appetite nor plasma acylated and deacylated ghrelin levels were significantly affected.

10 Critically Ill

10.1 Critically Ill Patients and Ghrelin

In the critically ill patients, abnormalities in gastrointestinal motor function have recently been emerged as one of the most important cause of food intolerance and aspiration pneumonia [132]. The tone of the lower esophageal sphincter was markedly reduced in critically ill patients and is likely to increase the risk of aspiration and ventilator-associated pneumonia. Feed intolerance occurs in up to 50 % of critically ill patients, predominately due to delayed gastric emptying, and is considered a risk factor for adverse sequelae, such as inadequate nutrition [132]. The motor function of both the proximal and/or distal stomach is disordered in ~50 % of critically ill patients and underlies the delayed gastric emptying. Usually, the proximal stomach acts as a reservoir for liquid feed. In critical illness, however, the usual relaxation that occurs in response to the presence of nutrient is delayed and reduced [132]. The coordination, magnitude, and frequency of contractions in the proximal and distal stomach are reduced, leading to decreased transpyloric flow of chyme. Furthermore, in the critically ill, inhibitory small intestinal feedback on gastric emptying appears to be substantially enhanced [132].

Fasting plasma ghrelin concentrations are markedly reduced in the early phase of critical illness [133]. The reduction in ghrelin secretion may play a role in delayed gastric emptying, weight loss, and decreased appetite that all occur frequently in the critically ill patients. Up to now, ghrelin administration (either physiological replacement or pharmacological doses) has not yet been evaluated as a therapy in critically ill patients.

10.2 Critically Ill Patients and Rikkunshito

Hayakawa et al. [134] conducted a randomized prospective study to compare the effects of rikkunshito with that of metoclopramide in critically ill patients who were projected to require intragastric tube feeding for more than 7 days. All patients were undergoing mechanical ventilation at the time of enrollment. The rikkunshito group reached 50 % of the target amount of enteral feeding significantly earlier than the metoclopramide group. An increase in the plasma level of active ghrelin in rikkunshito group was greater than that of metoclopramide treatment group. This suggests that rikkunshito treatment may be useful in a critical care setting.

11 Drug Adverse Events: SSRI, Pirfenidone, and Levodopa

11.1 Selective Serotonin Reuptake Inhibitors (SSRI)-Induced Dyspepsia

Selective serotonin reuptake inhibitors (SSRIs) are commonly prescribed to patients with major depression. Upper gastrointestinal symptoms such as nausea and vomiting are one of the most common adverse events, and for some patients, dyspeptic symptoms become critical issues that impair their quality of life and may result in discontinuation of SSRI therapy [135].

By using a freely moving conscious rat model equipped with force transducers, Fujitsuka et al. [136] found that intraperitoneal administration of SSRIs, fenfluramine, or fluvoxamine decreased plasma level of acyl-ghrelin and changed upper gastrointestinal motility from a fasted-like pattern to fed-like motor activities similar to those seen after feeding. These effects on ghrelin and gastrointestinal motility were blocked by 5-HT2C receptor antagonist. Neither melanocortin 4 nor the 3/4 receptor antagonists blocked this motor effect, although they restored the anorexia induced by

SSRIs suggesting that SSRI-induced anorexia is dependent on a melanocortin system [136]. From these results, it was concluded that SSRIs have inhibitory effects on acyl-ghrelin and gastrointestinal motor activities via an activation of 5-HT2C receptors.

Upper gastrointestinal symptoms such as nausea and vomiting are common adverse events associated with selective serotonin reuptake inhibitors (SSRIs) and may result in discontinuation of drug therapy in patients with depressive disorders. Oka et al. [137] conducted a randomized controlled study to determine if rikkunshito reduces gastrointestinal symptoms in depressed patients treated with fluvoxamine. Fifty patients with depressive disorder were randomly assigned for the treatment with fluvoxamine alone or fluvoxamine in combination with rikkunshito for 8 weeks. The number of patients who complained of gastrointestinal adverse events was significantly lower in the fluvoxamine plus rikkunshito group than that in the control group. This suggests that rikkunshito reduces fluvoxamine-induced adverse events, especially nausea, and improves quality of life (QOL) of the patients.

Concomitant oral administration of rikkunshito with an SSRI suppressed the decrease in plasma acylated ghrelin, changed the fed-like motor activity to fasted activity, improved anorexia, and enhanced gastric emptying [136]. These effects of rikkunshito were abolished by coadministration of a ghrelin receptor antagonist and were mimicked by its active ingredient hesperidin. Given that hesperidin was shown to interact with 5-HT2C and 5-HT2B receptors [8], it makes sense that appetite-stimulating effect of rikkunshito may be attributed to its 5-HT2C receptor antagonism.

11.2 Pirfenidone

Pirfenidone is an antifibrotic agent for patients with idiopathic pulmonary fibrosis (IPF), but this drug has adverse gastrointestinal (GI) effects. Shimazu et al. [138] performed a randomized controlled trial on 17 IPF patients to evaluate the ameliorating effect of add-on treatment with rikkunshito compared to pirfenidone monotherapy. Rikkunshito improved GI symptoms to the level prior to pirfenidone therapy. Plasma levels of des-acyl-ghrelin and acyl-ghrelin /des-acyl-ghrelin ratio changed significantly at 8 weeks compared to 2 weeks, although GI adverse events due to PFD were most severe in the first 2 weeks of treatment. The authors concluded that rikkunshito contributed to improvement of GI symptoms, but plasma ghrelin levels did not reflect the improvement of GI symptoms.

11.3 Levodopa

Oral administration of l-dopa (levodopa) is the first-line therapy for Parkinson's disease (PD). The oral administration of l-dopa/carbidopa (LD/CD) given in the fasting state or before a low protein meal inhibits gastric emptying in healthy volunteers or in PD patients who have already developed delayed solid gastric emptying [139]. Wang et al. [140] showed that the administration of

LD/CD impaired gastric propulsive motor function in naïve rats and 6-OHDA PD models in rats. Pretreatment with rikkunshito prevented LD/CD inhibitory effect through an action that in part medicated through increased ghrelin signaling as well as other unknown mechanisms.

In a clinical study, effects of rikkunshito on gastroparesis in Parkinson's disease patients were reported by Doi et al. [141]. Twenty patients with mild gastrointestinal symptoms were enrolled; 14 of the 20 patients had constipation. Sixteen patients were taking levodopa/ carbidopa, two were taking dopamine agonists, and the others were not treated yet. Twelve weeks after rikkunshito administration, 67 % of patients reported improvement of their gastrointestinal symptoms, particularly appetite loss and bloating. Rikkunshito significantly shortened the gastric emptying time in these patients measured by the 13C-sodium acetate expiration breath test, without any adverse effects, except for its bitter taste.

12 Summary

Because kampo (Japanese herbal) medicines contain multiple active ingredients, it is usually difficult to disclose its precise mechanism of action. However, recent progress in our knowledge about the unique characteristics of rikkunshito as a powerful orexigenic drug prompted us to investigate the potential mechanism action much further. From the clinical point of view, currently available clinical evidence showing the efficacy of kampo medicine is very limited. Well-designed randomized, placebo-controlled studies are warranted to disclose the merit for the usage of kampo medicine in a clinical setting.

References

1. Suzuki H, Inadomi JM, Hibi T (2009) Japanese herbal medicine in functional gastrointestinal disorders. Neurogastroenterol Motil 21:688–696
2. Tominaga K, Arakawa T (2015) Clinical application of kampo medicine (rikkunshito) for common and/or intractable symptoms of the gastrointestinal tract. Front Pharmacol 6:7
3. Mochiki E, Yanai M, Ohno T, Kuwano H (2010) The effect of traditional Japanese medicine (Kampo) on gastrointestinal function. Surg Today 40:1105–1111
4. Oka T, Okumi H, Nishida S, Ito T, Morikiyo S, Kimura Y, Murakami M, JOPM-EBM Working Team (2014) Effects of Kampo on functional gastrointestinal disorders. Biopsychosoc Med 8:5
5. Takeda H, Muto S, Nakagawa K, Ohnishi S, Sadakane C, Saegusa Y, Nahata M, Hattori T, Asaka M (2012) Rikkunshito as a ghrelin enhancer. Methods Enzymol 514:333–351
6. Saegusa Y, Hattori T, Nahata M, Yamada C, Takeda H (2015) A new strategy using rikkunshito to treat anorexia and gastrointestinal dysfunction. Evid Based Complement Alternat Med 2015:364260
7. Mogami S, Hattori T (2014) Beneficial effects of rikkunshito, a Japanese kampo medicine, on gastrointestinal dysfunction and anorexia in combination with Western drug: a systematic review. Evid Based Complement Alternat Med 2014:519035
8. Takeda H, Sadakane C, Hattori T, Katsurada T, Ohkawara T, Nagai K, Asaka M (2008)

Rikkunshito, an herbal medicine, suppresses cisplatin-induced anorexia in rats via 5-HT2 receptor antagonism. Gastroenterology 134:2004–2013

9. Matsumura T, Arai M, Yonemitsu Y, Maruoka D, Tanaka T, Suzuki T, Yoshikawa M, Imazeki F, Yokosuka O (2010) The traditional Japanese medicine Rikkunshito increases the plasma level of ghrelin in humans and mice. J Gastroenterol 45:300–307
10. Yakabi K, Sadakane C, Noguchi M, Ohno S, Ro S, Chinen K, Aoyama T, Sakurada T, Takabayashi H, Hattori T (2010) Reduced ghrelin secretion in the hypothalamus of rats due to cisplatin-induced anorexia. Endocrinology 151:3773–3782
11. Yakabi K, Kurosawa S, Tamai M, Yuzurihara M, Nahata M, Ohno S, Ro S, Kato S, Aoyama T, Sakurada T, Takabayashi H, Hattori T (2010) Rikkunshito and 5-HT2C receptor antagonist improve cisplatin-induced anorexia via hypothalamic ghrelin interaction. Regul Pept 161:97–105
12. Sadakane C, Muto S, Nakagawa K, Ohnishi S, Saegusa Y, Nahata M, Hattori T, Asaka M, Takeda H (2011) 10-Gingerol, a component of rikkunshito, improves cisplatin-induced anorexia by inhibiting acylated ghrelin degradation. Biochem Biophys Res Commun 412:506–511
13. Fujitsuka N, Asakawa A, UezonoY MK, Yamaguchi T, Niijima A, Yada T, Maejima Y, Sedbazar U, Sakai T, HattoriT KY, Inui A (2011) Potentiation of ghrelin signaling attenuates cancer anorexia–cachexia and prolongs survival. Transl Psychiatry 1:e23
14. Tatsuta M, Iishi H (1993) Effect of treatment with liu-jun-zi-tang (TJ-43) on gastric emptying and gastrointestinal symptoms in dyspeptic patients. Aliment Pharmacol Ther 7:459–462
15. Kusunoki H, Haruma K, Hata J, Ishii M, Kamada T, Yamashita N et al (2010) Efficacy of rikkunshito, a traditional Japanese medicine (Kampo), in treating functional dyspepsia. Intern Med 49:2195–2202
16. Kido T, Nakai Y, Kase Y et al (2005) Effects of rikkunshi-to, a traditional Japanese medicine, on the delay of gastric emptying induced by N (G)-nitro-L-arginine. J Pharmacol Sci 98:161–167
17. Yagi M, Homma S, Kubota M, Iinuma Y, Kanada S, Kinoshita Y, Ohtaki M, Yamazaki S, Murata H (2004) The herbal medicine rikkunshi-to stimulates and coordinates the gastric myoelectric activity in post-operative dyspeptic children after gastrointestinal surgery. Pediatr Surg Int 19:760–765
18. Sakai Y, Nobe K, Maruyama Y, Momose K, Homma I (2004) A traditional herbal medicine, rikkunshi-to (TJ-43), prevents intracellular signaling disorders in gastric smooth muscle of diabetic rats. Am J Chin Med 32:245–256
19. Ozaki M, Nagatomo T, Maeda T, Kishioka S, Yamamoto H (2006) Pharmacological differences between Liu-Jun-Zi-Tang, a traditional Chinese herbal medicine, and domperidone on isolated guinea-pig ileum. Biol Pharm Bull 29:1349–1354
20. Kito Y, Suzuki H (2010) Properties of rikkunshi-to (TJ-43)-induced relaxation of rat gastric fundus smooth muscles. Am J Physiol Gastrointest Liver Physiol 298: G755–G763
21. Hayakawa T, Arakawa T, Kase Y et al (1999) Liu-Jun-Zi-Tang, a Kampo medicine, promotes adaptive relaxation in isolated guinea pig stomachs. Drugs Exp Clin Res 25:211–218
22. Furukawa N, Manabe N, Kase Y, Hattori T, Imamura H, Kusunoki H, Haruma K (2013) Intragastric infusion of rikkunshito (kampo) induces proximal stomach relaxation in conscious dogs. Auton Neurosci 179:14–22
23. Mondal A, Takehara A, Aizawa S, Tanaka T, Fujitsuka N, Hattori T, Sakai T, Sakata I (2015) Rikkunshito induces gastric relaxation via the β-adrenergic pathway in Suncus murinus. Neurogastroenterol Motil 27:875–884
24. Shiratori M, Shoji T, Kanazawa M, Hongo M, Fukudo S (2011) Effect of rikkunshito on gastric sensorimotor function under distention. Neurogastroenterol Motil 23:323–329
25. Yanai M, Mochiki E, Ogawa A, Morita H, Toyomasu Y, Ogata K, Tabe Y, Ando H, Ohno T, Asao T, Aomori T, Fujita Y, Kuwano H (2013) Intragastric administration of rikkunshito stimulates upper gastrointestinal motility and gastric emptying in conscious dogs. J Gastroenterol 48:611–619
26. Tominaga K, Kido T, Ochi M, Sadakane C, Mase A, Okazaki H, Yamagami H, Tanigawa T, Watanabe K, Watanabe T, Fujiwara Y, Oshitani N, Arakawa T (2011) The traditional Japanese medicine rikkunshito promotes gastric emptying via the antagonistic action of the 5-HT3 receptor pathway in rats. Evid Based Complement Alternat Med 2011:248481
27. Herbrechter R, Ziemba PM, Hoffmann KM, Hatt H, Werner M, Gisselmann G (2015) Identification of glycyrrhiza as the rikkunshito constituent with the highest antagonistic potential on heterologously expressed 5-HT3A receptors due to the action of flavonoids. Front Pharmacol 6:130

28. Kojima M, Hosoda H, Date Y, Nakazato M, Matsuo H, Kangawa K (1999) Ghrelin is a growth-hormone-releasing acylated peptide from stomach. Nature 402:656–660
29. Kojima M, Kangawa K (2005) Ghrelin: structure and function. Physiol Rev 85:495–522
30. Nakazato M, Murakami N, Date Y, Kojima M, Matsuo H, Kangawa K, Matsukura S (2001) A role for ghrelin in the central regulation of feeding. Nature 409:194–198
31. Tschöp M, Smiley DL, Heiman ML (2000) Ghrelin induces adiposity in rodents. Nature 407:908–913
32. Cummings DE, Purnell JQ, Frayo RS, Schmidova K, Wisse BE, Weigle DS (2001) A preprandial rise in plasma ghrelin levels suggests a role in meal initiation in humans. Diabetes 50:1714–1719
33. Cummings DE, Weigle DS, Frayo RS, Breen PA, Ma MK, Dellinger EP, Purnell JQ (2002) Plasma ghrelin levels after diet-induced weight loss or gastric bypass surgery. N Engl J Med. 346:1623–1630
34. Chen CY, Asakawa A, Fujimiya M, Lee SD, Inui A (2009) Ghrelin gene products and the regulation of food intake and gut motility. Pharmacol Rev 61:430–481
35. Müller TD, Nogueiras R, Andermann ML, Andrews ZB, Anker SD, Argente J, Batterham RL, Benoit SC, Bowers CY, Broglio F, Casanueva FF, D'Alessio D, Depoortere I, Geliebter A, Ghigo E, Cole PA, Cowley M, Cummings DE, Dagher A, Diano S, Dickson SL, Diéguez C, Granata R, Grill HJ, Grove K, Habegger KM, Heppner K, Heiman ML, Holsen L, Holst B, Inui A, Jansson JO, Kirchner H, Korbonits M, Laferrère B, LeRoux CW, Lopez M, Morin S, Nakazato M, Nass R, Perez-Tilve D, Pfluger PT, Schwartz TW, Seeley RJ, Sleeman M, Sun Y, Sussel L, Tong J, Thorner MO, van der Lely AJ, van der Ploeg LH, Zigman JM, Kojima M, Kangawa K, Smith RG, Horvath T, Tschöp MH (2015) Ghrelin. Mol Metab 4:437–460
36. Saegusa Y, Takeda H, Muto S, Nakagawa K, Ohnishi S, Sadakane C, Nahata M, Hattori T, Asaka M (2011) Decreased plasma ghrelin contributes to anorexia following novelty stress. Am J Physiol Endocrinol Metab 301: E685–E696
37. Arai T, Maejima Y, Muroya S, Yada T (2013) Rikkunshito and isoliquiritigenin counteract 5-HT-induced 2C receptor-mediated activation of pro-opiomelanocortin neurons in the hypothalamic arcuate nucleus. Neuropeptides 47:225–230
38. Yakabi K, Harada Y, Takayama K, Ro S, Ochiai M, Iizuka S, Hattori T, Wang L, Taché Y (2014) Peripheral α2-β1 adrenergic interactions mediate the ghrelin response to brain urocortin 1 in rats. Psychoneuroendocrinology 50:300–310
39. Harada Y, Ro S, Ochiai M, Hayashi K, Hosomi E, Fujitsuka N, Hattori T, Yakabi K (2015) Ghrelin enhancer, rikkunshito, improves postprandial gastric motor dysfunction in an experimental stress model. Neurogastroenterol Motil 27:1089–1097
40. Nahata M, Muto S, Oridate N, Ohnishi S, Nakagawa K, Sadakane C, Saegusa Y, Hattori T, Asaka M, Takeda H (2012) Impaired ghrelin signaling is associated with gastrointestinal dysmotility in rats with gastroesophageal reflux disease. Am J Physiol Gastrointest Liver Physiol 303:G42–G53
41. Nahata M, Saegusa Y, Sadakane C, Yamada C, Nakagawa K, Okubo N, Ohnishi S, Hattori T, Sakamoto N, Takeda H (2014) Administration of exogenous acylated ghrelin or rikkunshito, an endogenous ghrelin enhancer, improves the decrease in postprandial gastric motility in an acute restraint stress mouse model. Neurogastroenterol Motil 26:821–831
42. Kitagawa H, Munekage M, Matsumoto T, Sadakane C, Fukutake M, Aoki K, Watanabe J, Maemura K, Hattori T, Kase Y, Uezono Y, Inui A, Hanazaki K (2015) Pharmacokinetic profiles of active ingredients and its metabolites derived from rikkunshito, a ghrelin enhancer, in healthy Japanese volunteers: a cross-over, randomized study. PLoS One 10: e0133159
43. Tack J, Talley NJ, Camilleri M et al (2006) Functional gastroduodenal disorders. Gastroenterology 130:1466–1479
44. Ogiso K, Asakawa A, Amitani H et al (2011) Ghrelin: a gut hormonal basis of motility regulation and functional dyspepsia. J Gastroenterol Hepatol 26(suppl 3):67–72
45. Shinomiya T, Fukunaga M, Akamizu T et al (2005) Plasma acylated ghrelin levels correlate with subjective symptoms of functional dyspepsia in female patients. Scand J Gastroenterol 40:648–653
46. Takamori K, Mizuta Y, Takeshima F et al (2007) Relation among plasma ghrelin level, gastric emptying, and psychologic condition in patients with functional dyspepsia. J Clin Gastroenterol 41:477–483
47. Shindo T, Futagami S, Hiratsuka T et al (2009) Comparison of gastric emptying and plasma ghrelin levels in patients with functional dyspepsia and non-erosive reflux disease. Digestion 79:65–72

48. Yagi T, Asakawa A, Ueda H, Miyawaki S, Inui A (2013) The role of ghrelin in patients with functional dyspepsia and its potential clinical relevance (Review). Int J Mol Med 32:523–531
49. Kim YS, Lee JS, Lee TH et al (2012) Plasma levels of acylated ghrelin in patients with functional dyspepsia. World J Gastroenterol 18:2231–2237
50. Hijaz NM, Friesen CA, Schurman JV, Pearce RE, Abdel-Rahman SM (2015) Plasma ghrelin and liquid gastric emptying in children with functional dyspepsia consistent with post-prandial distress syndrome. Neurogastroenterol Motil 27:1120–1126
51. Kazemi M, Eshraghian A, Hamidpour L, Taghavi S (2015) Changes in serum ghrelin level in relation to meal-time in patients with functional dyspepsia. United European Gastroenterol J 3:11–16
52. Futagami S, Shimpuku M, Kawagoe T, Izumi N, Ohishi N, Yamawaki H, Shindo T, Nagoya H, Horie A, Kodaka Y, Gudis K, Itoh T, Sakamoto C (2013) The preproghrelin 3056 TT genotype is associated with the feeling of hunger and low acylated ghrelin levels in Japanese patients with Helicobacter pylori-negative functional dyspepsia. Intern Med 52:1155–1163
53. Yamawaki H, Futagami S, Shimpuku M, Shindo T, Maruki Y, Nagoya H, Kodaka Y, Sato H, Gudis K, Kawagoe T, Sakamoto C (2015) Leu72Met408 polymorphism of the ghrelin gene is associated with early phase of gastric emptying in the patients with functional dyspepsia in Japan. J Neurogastroenterol Motil 21:93–102
54. Akamizu T, Iwakura H, Ariyasu H, Hosoda H, Murayama T, Yokode M, Teramukai S, Seno H, Chiba T, Noma S, Nakai Y, Fukunaga M, Nakai Y, Kangawa K, FD Clinical Study Team (2008) Repeated administration of ghrelin to patients with functional dyspepsia: its effects on food intake and appetite. Eur J Endocrinol 158:491–498
55. Harasawa S, Miyoshi A, Miwa T, Masamune O, Matsuo Y, Mori H et al (1998) Double-blind multicenter post-marketing clinical trial of TJ-43 TSUMURAR ikkunshi-to for the treatment of dysmotility-like dyspepsia. J Clin Exp Med 187:207–229
56. Arai M, Matsumura T, Tsuchiya N, Sadakane C, Inami R, Suzuki T, Yoshikawa M, Imazeki F, Yokosuka O (2012) Rikkunshito improves the symptoms in patients with functional dyspepsia, accompanied by an increase in the level of plasma ghrelin. Hepatogastroenterology 59:62–66
57. Suzuki H, Matsuzaki J, Fukushima Y, Suzaki F, Kasugai K, Nishizawa T, Naito Y, Hayakawa T, Kamiya T, Andoh T, Yoshida H, Tokura Y, Nagata H, Kobayakawa M, Mori M, Kato K, Hosoda H, Takebayashi T, Miura S, Uemura N, Joh T, Hibi T, Tack J, Rikkunshito study group (2014) Randomized clinical trial: rikkunshito in the treatment of functional dyspepsia–a multicenter, double-blind, randomized, placebo-controlled study. Neurogastroenterol Motil 26:950–961
58. Togawa K, Matsuzaki J, Kobayakawa M, Fukushima Y, Suzaki F, Kasugai K, Nishizawa T, Naito Y, Hayakawa T, Kamiya T, Andoh T, Yoshida H, Tokura Y, Nagata H, Mori M, Kato K, Hosoda H, Takebayashi T, Miura S, Uemura N, Joh T, Hibi T, Suzuki H (2015) Association of baseline plasma des-acyl ghrelin level with the response to rikkunshito in patients with functional dyspepsia. J Gastroenterol Hepatol. doi:10.1111/jgh.13074 [Epub ahead of print]
59. Vakil N, van Zanten SV, Kahrilas P, Dent J, Jones R, Group GC (2006) The montreal definition and classification of gastroesophageal reflux disease: a global evidence-based consensus. Am J Gastroenterol 101: 1900–1920
60. Penagini R, Bravi I (2010) The role of delayed gastric emptying and impaired oesophageal body motility. Best Pract Res Clin Gastroenterol 24:831–845
61. Rubenstein JH, Morgenstern H, McConell D, Scheiman JM, Schoenfeld P, Appelman H, McMahon LF Jr, Kao JY, Metko V, Zhang M, Inadomi JM (2013) Associations of diabetes mellitus, insulin, leptin, and ghrelin with gastroesophageal reflux and Barrett's esophagus. Gastroenterology 145:1237–1244
62. Shindo T, Futagami S, Hiratsuka T, Horie A, Hamamoto T, Ueki N, Kusunoki M, Miyake K, Gudis K, Tsukui T, Iwakiri K, Sakamoto C (2009) Comparison of gastric emptying and plasma ghrelin levels in patients with functional dyspepsia and non-erosive reflux disease. Digestion 79:65–72
63. Nahata M, Saegusa Y, Harada Y, Tsuchiya N, Hattori T, Takeda H (2013) Changes in ghrelin-related factors in gastroesophageal reflux disease in rats. Gastroenterol Res Pract 2013:504816
64. Kawahara H, Kubota A, Hasegawa T, Okuyama H, Ueno T, Ida S et al (2007) Effects of rikkunshito on the clinical symptoms and esophageal acid exposure in children with symptomatic gastroesophageal reflux. Pediatr Surg Int 23:1001–1005

65. Kawahara H, Okuyama H, Nose K, Nakai H, Yoneda A, Kubota A, Fukuzawa M (2010) Physiological and clinical characteristics of gastroesophageal reflux after congenital diaphragmatic hernia repair. J Pediatr Surg 45:2346–2350
66. Tominaga K, Iwakiri R, Fujimoto K, Fujiwara Y, Tanaka M, Shimoyama Y, Umegaki E, Higuchi K, Kusano M, Arakawa T, GERD 4 Study Group (2012) Rikkunshito improves symptoms in PPI-refractory GERD patients: a prospective, randomized, multicenter trial in Japan. J Gastroenterol 47:284–292
67. Tominaga K, Kato M, Takeda H, Shimoyama Y, Umegaki E, Iwakiri R, Furuta K, Sakurai K, Odaka T, Kusunoki H, Nagahara A, Iwakiri K, Furuta T, Murakami K, Miwa H, Kinoshita Y, Haruma K, Takahashi S, Watanabe S, Higuchi K, Kusano M, Fujimoto K, Arakawa T, G-PRIDE Study Group (2014) A randomized, placebo-controlled, double-blind clinical trial of rikkunshito for patients with non-erosive reflux disease refractory to proton-pump inhibitor: the G-PRIDE study. J Gastroenterol 49:1392–1405
68. Sakata Y, Tominaga K, Kato M, Takeda H, Shimoyama Y, Takeuchi T, Iwakiri R, Furuta K, Sakurai K, Odaka T, Kusunoki H, Nagahara A, Iwakiri K, Furuta T, Murakami K, Miwa H, Kinoshita Y, Haruma K, Takahashi S, Watanabe S, Higuchi K, Fujimoto K, Kusano M, Arakawa T, G-PRIDE study group (2014) Clinical characteristics of elderly patients with proton pump inhibitor-refractory non-erosive reflux disease from the G-PRIDE study who responded to rikkunshito. BMC Gastroenterol 14:116
69. Tokashiki R, Okamoto I, Funato N, Suzuki M (2013) Rikkunshito improves globus sensation in patients with proton-pump inhibitor-refractory laryngopharyngeal reflux. World J Gastroenterol 19:5118–5124
70. Stone A, Brownell K (1994) The stress-eating paradox: multiple daily measurements in adult males and females. Psychol Health 9:425–436
71. Takeda H, Muto S, Nakagawa K, Ohnishi S, Asaka M (2012) Rikkunshito and ghrelin secretion. Curr Pharm Des 18:4827–4838
72. Ochi M, Tominaga K, Tanaka F, Tanigawa T, Shiba M, Watanabe T, Fujiwara Y, Oshitani N, Higuchi K, Arakawa T (2008) Effect of chronic stress on gastric emptying and plasma ghrelin levels in rats. Life Sci 82:862–868
73. Lutter M, Sakata I, Osborne-Lawrence S, Rovinsky SA, Anderson JG, Jung S, Birnbaum S, Yanagisawa M, Elmquist JK, Nestler EJ, Zigman JM (1998) The orexigenic hormone ghrelin defends against depressive symptoms of chronic stress. Nat Neurosci 11:752–753
74. Richard D, Lin Q, Timofeeva E (2002) The corticotropin-releasing factor family of peptides and CRF receptors: their roles in the regulation of energy balance. Eur J Pharmacol 440:189–197
75. Yakabi K, Noguchi M, Ohno S, Ro S, Onouchi T, Ochiai M, Takabayashi H, Takayama K, Harada Y, Sadakane C, Hattori T (2011) Urocortin 1 reduces food intake and ghrelin secretion via CRF(2) receptors. Am J Physiol Endocrinol Metab 301:E72–E82
76. Fone KC, Shalders K, Fox ZD, Arthur R, Marsden CA (1996) Increased 5-HT2C receptor responsiveness occurs on rearing rats in social isolation. Psychopharmacology (Berl) 123:346–352
77. Miura H, Qiao H, Ohta T (2002) Influence of aging and social isolation on changes in brain monoamine turnover and biosynthesis of rats elicited by novelty stress. Synapse 46:116–124
78. Nahata M, Muto S, Nakagawa K, Ohnishi S, Sadakane C, Saegusa Y, Iizuka S, Hattori T, Asaka M, Takeda H (2013) Serotonin 2C receptor antagonism ameliorates novelty-induced hypophagia in aged mice. Psychoneuroendocrinology 38:2051–2064
79. Yamada C, Saegusa Y, Nakagawa K, Ohnishi S, Muto S, Nahata M, Sadakane C, Hattori T, Sakamoto N, Takeda H (2013) Rikkunshito, a Japanese Kampo medicine, ameliorates decreased feeding behavior via ghrelin and serotonin 2B receptor signaling in a novelty stress murine model. BioMed Res Int 2013:792940
80. Yamada C, Sadakane C, Nahata M, Saegusa Y, Nakagawa K, Okubo N, Ohnishi S, Hattori T, Takeda H (2015) Serotonin 2C receptor contributes to gender differences in stress-induced hypophagia in aged mice. Psychoneuroendocrinology 55:81–93
81. Naito T, Itoh H, Takeyama M (2003) Some gastrointestinal function regulatory kampo medicines have modulatory effects on human plasma adrenocorticotropic hormone and cortisol levels with continual stress exposure. Biol Pharm Bull 26:101–104
82. Morley JE (2013) Pathophysiology of the anorexia of aging. Curr Opin Clin Nutr Metab Care 16:27–32
83. Di Francesco V, Fantin F, Omizzolo F, Residori L, Bissoli L, Bosello O, Zamboni M (2007) The anorexia of aging. Dig Dis 25:129–137
84. Ariyasu H, Iwakura H, Yamada G, Nakano K, Kangawa K, Akamizu T (2008) Efficacy of

ghrelin as a therapeutic approach for age-related physiological changes. Endocrinology 149:3722–3728

85. Takeda H, Muto S, Hattori T, Sadakane C, Tsuchiya K, Katsurada T, Ohkawara T, Oridate N, Asaka M (2010) Rikkunshito ameliorates the aging-associated decrease in ghrelin receptor reactivity via phosphodiesterase III inhibition. Endocrinology 151:244–252
86. Barazzoni R, Zanetti M, Stebel M, Biolo G, Cattin L, Guarnieri G (2003) Hyperleptinemia prevents increased plasma ghrelin concentration during short-term moderate caloric restriction in rats. Gastroenterology 24:1188–1192
87. Kohno D, Nakata M, Maekawa F, Fujiwara K, Maejima Y, Kuramochi M, Shimazaki T, Okano H, Onaka T, Yada T (2007) Leptin suppresses ghrelin-induced activation of neuropeptide Y neurons in the arcuate nucleus via phosphatidylinositol 3-kinase-andphosphodiesterase 3-mediated pathway. Endocrinology 148:2251–2263
88. Niswender KD, Morton GJ, Stearns WH, Rhodes CJ, Myers MG Jr, Schwartz MW (2001) Intracellular signalling. Key enzyme in leptininduced anorexia. Nature 413:794–795
89. Zhao AZ, Huan JN, Gupta S, Pal R, Sahu A (2002) A phosphatidylinositol 3-kinase phosphodiesterase 3B-cyclic AMP pathway in hypothalamic action of leptin on feeding. Nat Neurosci 5:727–728
90. Utumi Y, Iseki E, Murayama N, Nozawa M, Kumagai R, Matsubara Y, Ichimiya Y, Arai H (2011) Effect of rikkunshi-to on appetite loss found in elderly dementia patients: a preliminary study. Psychogeriatrics 11:34–39
91. Shimizu Y, Nagaya N, Isobe T, Imazu M, Okumura H, Hosoda H, Kojima M, Kangawa K, Kohno N (2003) Increased plasma ghrelin level in lung cancer cachexia. Clin Cancer Res 9:774–778
92. Hiura Y, Takiguchi S, Yamamoto K, Kurokawa Y, Yamasaki M, Nakajima K, Miyata H, Fujiwara Y, Mori M, Doki Y (2012) Fall in plasma ghrelin concentrations after cisplatin-based chemotherapy in esophageal cancer patients. Int J Clin Oncol 17:316–323
93. Hiura Y, Takiguchi S, Yamamoto K, Takahashi T, Kurokawa Y, Yamasaki M, Nakajima K, Miyata H, Fujiwara Y, Mori M, Kangawa K, Doki Y (2012) Effects of ghrelin administration during chemotherapy with advanced esophageal cancer patients: a prospective, randomized, placebo-controlled phase 2 study. Cancer 118:4785–4794
94. Ohno T, Yanai M, Ando H, Toyomasu Y, Ogawa A, Morita H, Ogata K, Mochiki E, Asao T, Kuwano H (2011) Rikkunshito, a traditional Japanese medicine, suppresses cisplatin-induced anorexia in humans. Clin Exp Gastroenterol 4:291–296
95. Seike J, Sawada T, Kawakita N, Yamamoto Y, Yuasa Y, Yamai H, Takachi H, Yoshida T, Tangoku A (2011) A new candidate supporting drug, rikkunshito, for the QOL in advanced esophageal cancer patients with chemotherapy using docetaxel/5-FU/CDDP. Int J Surg Oncol 2011:715623
96. Liu YL, Malik NM, Sanger GJ, Andrews PL (2006) Ghrelin alleviates cancer chemotherapy-associated dyspepsia in rodents. Cancer Chemother Pharmacol 58:326–333
97. Rudd JA, Ngan MP, Wai MK, King AG, Witherington J, Andrews PL, Sanger GJ (2006) Anti-emetic activity of ghrelin in ferrets exposed to the cytotoxic anti-cancer agent cisplatin. Neurosci Lett 392:79–83
98. Tisdale MJ (2009) Mechanisms of cancer cachexia. Physiol Rev 89:381–410
99. Inui A (2002) Cancer anorexia–cachexia syndrome: current issues in research and management. CA Cancer J Clin 52:72–91
100. Argilés JM, Busquets S, Stemmler B, López-Soriano FJ (2014) Cancer cachexia: understanding the molecular basis. Nat Rev Cancer 14:754–762
101. Fearon KC, Glass DJ, Guttridge DC (2012) Cancer cachexia: mediators, signaling, and metabolic pathways. Cell Metab 16:153–166
102. Loprinzi CL, Schaid DJ, Dose AM, Burnham NL, Jensen MD (1993) Body-composition changes in patients who gain weight while receiving megestrol acetate. J Clin Oncol 11:152–154
103. Gagnon B, Bruera E (1998) A review of the drug treatment of cachexia associated with cancer. Drugs 55:675–688
104. DeBoer MD (2011) Ghrelin and cachexia: will treatment with GHSR-1a agonists make a difference for patients suffering from chronic wasting syndromes? Mol Cell Endocrinol 340:97–105
105. Smagin GN, Dunn AJ (2000) The role of CRF receptor subtypes in stress-induced behavioura responses. Eur J Pharmacol 405:199–206
106. Inui A (1999) Feeding and body-weight regulation by hypothalamic neuropeptides-mediation of the actions of leptin. Trends Neurosci 22:62–67

107. Legakis I, Stathopoulos J, Matzouridis T, Stathopoulos GP (2009) Decreased plasma ghrelin levels in patients with advanced cancer and weight loss in comparison to healthy individuals. Anticancer Res 29:3949–3952
108. Takahashi M, Terashima M, Takagane A et al (2009) Ghrelin and leptin levels in cachectic patients with cancer of the digestive organs. Int J Clin Oncol 14:315–320
109. Nagaya N, Uematsu M, Kojima M et al (2001) Elevated circulating level of ghrelin in cachexi associated with chronic heart failure: relationships between ghrelin and anabolic/catabolic factors. Circulation 104:2034–2038
110. Hanada T, Toshinai K, Kajimura N, Nara-Ashizawa N, Tsukada T, Hayashi Y, Osuye K, Kangawa K, Matsukura S, Nakazato M (2003) Anti-cachectic effect of ghrelin in nude mice bearing human melanoma cells. Biochem Biophys Res Commun 301:275–279
111. Wang W, Andersson M, Iresjo BM, Lonnroth C, Lundholm K (2006) Effects of ghrelin on anorexia in tumor-bearing mice with eicosanoid-related cachexia. Int J Oncol 28:1393–1400
112. DeBoer MD, Zhu XX, Levasseur P, Meguid MM, Suzuki S, Inui A, Taylor JE, Halem HA, Dong JZ, Datta R, Culler MD, Marks DL (2007) Ghrelin treatment causes increased food intake and retention of lean body mass in a rat model o cancer cachexia. Endocrinology 148:3004–3012
113. Neary NM, Small CJ, Wren AM, Lee JL, Druce MR, Palmieri C, Frost GS, Ghatei MA, Coombes RC, Bloom SR (2004) Ghrelin increases energy intake in cancer patients with impaired appetite: acute, randomized, placebo-controlled trial. J Clin Endocrinol Metab 89:2832–2836
114. Strasser F, Lutz TA, Maeder MT, Thuerlimann B, Bueche D, Tschop M, Kaufmann K, Holst B, Brandle M, von Moos R, Demmer R, Cerny T (2008) Safety, tolerability and pharmacokinetics of intravenous ghrelin for cancer-related anorexia/cachexia: a randomised, placebo-controlled, double-blind, double-crossover study. Br J Cancer 98:300–308
115. Garcia JM, Polvino WJ (2007) Effect on body weight and safety of RC-1291, a novel, orally available ghrelin mimetic and growth hormone secretagogue: results of a phase I, randomized, placebocontrolled, multiple-dose study in healthy volunteers. Oncologist 12:594–600
116. Garcia JM, Graham C, Kumor K, Polvino W (2007) A Phase II, randomized, placebo-controlled, double blind study of the efficacy and safety of RC-1291 for the treatment of cancer-cachexia. J Clin Oncol 25:9133
117. Wang W, Danielsson A, Svanberg E, Lundholm K (2003) Lack of effects by tricyclic antidepressant and serotonin inhibitors on anorexia in MCG 101 tumor bearing mice with eicosanoid-related cachexia. Nutrition 19:47–53
118. Makarenko IG, Meguid MM, Gatto L, Goncalves CG, Ramos EJ, Chen C et al (2005) Hypothalamic 5- HT1B-receptor changes in anorectic bearing rats. Neurosci Lett 376:71–75
119. Suzuki H, Asakawa A, Amitani H, Fujitsuka N, Nakamura N, Inui A (2013) Cancer cachexia pathophysiology and translational aspect of herbal medicine. Jpn J Clin Oncol 43:695–705
120. Fujitsuka N, Uezono Y (2014) Rikkunshito, a ghrelin potentiator, ameliorates anorexia-cachexia syndrome. Front Pharmacol 5:271
121. Terawaki K, Sawada Y, Kashiwase Y, Hashimoto H, Yoshimura M, Suzuki M, Miyano K, Sudo Y, Shiraishi S, Higami Y, Yanagihara K, Kase Y, Ueta Y, Uezono Y (2014) New cancer cachexia rat model generated by implantation of a peritoneal dissemination-derived human stomach cancer cell line. Am J Physiol Endocrinol Metab 306:E373–E387
122. Tsubouchi H, Yanagi S, Miura A, Mogami S, Yamada C, Iizuka S, Hattori T, Nakazato M (2014) Rikkunshito ameliorates cachexia associated with bleomycin-induced lung fibrosis in mice by stimulating ghrelin secretion. Nutr Res 34:876–885
123. Tsubouchi H, Yanagi S, Miura A, Iizuka S, Mogami S, Yamada C, Hattori T, Nakazato M (2014) Rikkunshito ameliorates bleomycin-induced acute lung injury in a ghrelin-independent manner. Am J Physiol Lung Cell Mol Physiol 306:L233–L245
124. Takiguchi S, Takata A, Murakami K, Miyazaki Y, Yanagimoto Y, Kurokawa Y, Takahashi T, Mori M, Doki Y (2014) Clinical application of ghrelin administration for gastric cancer patients undergoing gastrectomy. Gastric Cancer 17:200–205
125. Hosoda H, Kangawa K (2008) The autonomic nervous system regulates gastric ghrelin secretion in rats. Regul Pept 146:12–18
126. Doki Y, Takachi K, Ishikawa O et al (2006) Ghrelin reduction after esophageal substitution and its correlation to postoperative body

weight loss in esophageal cancer patients. Surgery 139:797–805

127. Adachi S, Takiguchi S, Okada K et al (2010) Effects of ghrelin administration after total gastrectomy: a prospective, randomized, placebo-controlled phase II study. Gastroenterology 138:1312–1320
128. Imada T, Rino Y, Takahashi M et al (1998) Postoperative functional evaluation of pylorus-preserving gastrectomy for early gastric cancer compared with conventional distal gastrectomy. Surgery 123:165–170
129. Takahashi T, Endo S, Nakajima K, Souma Y, Nishida T (2009) Effect of rikkunshito, a chinese herbal medicine, on stasis in patients after pylorus-preserving gastrectomy. World J Surg 33:296–302
130. Takiguchi S, Hiura Y, Takahashi T et al (2013) Effect of rikkunshito, a Japanese herbal medicine, on gastrointestinal symptoms and ghrelin levels in gastric cancer patients after gastrectomy. Gastric Cancer 16:167–174
131. Gunji S, Ueda S, Yoshida M, Kanai M, Terajima H, Takabayashi A (2013) Effects of rikkunshito, a kampo medicine, on quality of life after proximal gastrectomy. J Surg Res 185:575–580
132. Deane A, Chapman MJ, Fraser RJ, Horowitz M (2010) Bench-to-bedside review: The gut as an endocrine organ in the critically ill. Crit Care 14:228
133. Nematy M, O'Flynn JE, Wandrag L, Brynes AE, Brett SJ, Patterson M, Ghatei MA, Bloom SR, Frost GS (2006) Changes in appetite related gut hormones in intensive care unit patients: a pilot cohort study. Crit Care 10:R10
134. Hayakawa M, Ono Y, Wada T, Yanagida Y, Sawamura A, Takeda H, Gando S (2014) Effects of rikkunshito (traditional Japanese medicine) on enteral feeding and the plasma ghrelin level in critically ill patients: a pilot study. J Intensive Care 2:53
135. Ueda N, Yoshimura R, Shinkai K, Sakata Y, Nakamura J (2003) Higher plasma 5-hydroxyindoleacetic acid levels are associated with SSRI-induced nausea. Neuropsychobiology 48:31–34
136. Fujitsuka N, Asakawa A, Hayashi M, Sameshima M, Amitani H, Kojima S, Fujimiya M, Inui A (2009) Selective serotonin reuptake inhibitors modify physiological gastrointestinal motor activities via 5-HT2c receptor and acyl ghrelin. Biol Psychiatry 65:748–759
137. Oka T, Tamagawa Y, Hayashida S, Kaneda Y, Kodama N, Tsuji S (2007) Rikkunshi-to attenuates adverse gastrointestinal symptoms induced by fluvoxamine. Biopsychosoc Med 1:21
138. Shimizu Y, Shimoyama Y, Kawada A, Kusano M, Hosomi Y, Sekiguchi M, Kawata T, Horie T, Ishii Y, Yamada M, Dobashi K, Takise A (2014) Gastrointestinal symptoms in idiopathic pulmonary fibrosis patients treated with pirfenidone and herbal medicine. J Biol Regul Homeost Agents 28:433–442
139. Marrinan S, Emmanuel AV, Burn DJ (2014) Delayed gastric emptying in Parkinson's disease. Mov Disord 29:23–32
140. Wang L, Mogami S, Karasawa H, Yamada C, Yakabi S, Yakabi K, Hattori T, Taché Y (2014) Preventive effect of rikkunshito on gastric motor function inhibited by L-dopa in rats. Peptides 55:136–144
141. Doi H, Sakakibara R, Sato M, Hirai S, Masaka T, Kishi M, Tsuyusaki Y, Tateno A, Tateno F, Takahashi O, Ogata T (2014) Dietary herb extract rikkunshi-to ameliorates gastroparesis in Parkinson's disease: a pilot study. Eur Neurol 71:193–195

Chapter 11

Daikenchuto and GI Disorders

Toru Kono, Mitsuo Shimada, Masahiro Yamamoto, and Yoshio Kase

Abstract

This overview of herbal medicine use in Japan was designed to provide a review of the accumulating scientific evidence of the mechanism and clinical action of daikenchuto (DKT). Use of traditional Japanese medicines, including DKT, has a relatively "short" history of 500 years of clinical use. Only in the last 30 years has the Japanese government officially recognized herbal medicine as a valid form of treatment alongside the typical Western medicines.

There has been a recent surge in scientifically robust data from basic and clinical studies for DKT, including placebo-controlled double-blind studies for various gastrointestinal disorders, and absorption, distribution, metabolism, and excretion studies have been conducted or are in the process of being conducted in both Japan and the USA. Clinical studies suggest that DKT is beneficial for postoperative ileus. Basic studies indicate that the effect of DKT is a composite of numerous actions mediated by multiple compounds supplied via multiple routes. In addition to known mechanisms of action via enteric/sensory nerve stimulation, novel mechanisms via the TRPA1 channel and two pore domain potassium channels have recently been elucidated. DKT compounds target these channels with and without absorption, both before and after metabolic activation by enteric flora, with different timings and possibly with synergism.

Key words Daikenchuto, Kampo, CGRP, Adrenomedullin, TRPA1, KCNK, Hydroxy-α-sanshool, 6-shogaol, Ginsenoside Rb1, Postoperative ileus, Crohn's disease

1 Introduction

Kampo, a distinctively unique Japan's traditional herbal medicine, is fully integrated into the modern health care system in Japan [1], it is neither a folk remedy nor alternative therapy in Japan. Kampo medicines are dispensed at all the university, national, and foundation hospitals as prescription drugs, frequently in combination with Adrenomedullin (ADM)western drugs. Rooted in Chinese medicine, the knowledge of Kampo formulae have been transmitted for 1500 years, but due to the difficulty of cultivating and procuring identical species of some of the herbs in the Chinese formulae and the quandary of maritime commerce at the time, Kampo followed a decidedly unique path of development in Japan [2]. Inevitably, there are stark differences between Japanese and Chinese herbal formulae.

Akio Inui (ed.), *Herbal Medicines: New Horizons*, Methods in Pharmacology and Toxicology,
DOI 10.1007/978-1-4939-4002-8_11,

Until recently, the safety of traditional medicines made from natural resources being comparable to that of modern drugs has been unfathomable. This preconceived idea has been overturned by the establishment of a robust quality control system for Kampo prescriptions, which ensures that the cultivation and harvest of botanical raw materials are in accord with WHO good agricultural and collection practices (GACP) guidelines for medicinal plants and that the final products are manufactured in accord with both the Japanese Good Manufacturing Process (GMP) and Kampo GMP guidelines, the former provided by the law and the latter by the self-imposed standards by the industrial association. In addition, at least for the top selling Kampo products, which comprise over 80 % of the market share, extensive component analysis and quality inspection for residual agrichemicals, heavy metals, aflatoxin, microbials, and other contaminants at critical steps in the manufacturing process assure the manufacture of safe, high-quality, and standardized Kampo products [2]. Since 1967 when the Japanese government initially approved four prescriptions, the number of approved Kampo prescriptions has been steadily increasing, and at present 148 Kampo prescriptions (Japan Pharmaceutical Information Center (JAPIC) Kampo extract granules for ethical use 2014) are covered by the national health insurance and are officially registered by the Japanese Ministry of Health as multicomponent remedies containing extracts derived mainly from plant- and mineral-based substances. As prescription drugs, Kampo is considered to be in the same class as western drugs. On the other hand, there are Western-trained physicians in every country who continue to deprecate herbal medicines, owing to a lack of understanding about the fundamental differences between Kampo and western drugs [2]. As described in Table 1, the ideal drug in western medicine is a magic bullet with a single target, which frequently acts on unintended targets producing unwanted side effects. By contrast, Kampo contains multiple components which act synergistically and cooperatively on multiple targets, resulting in a substantially lowered risk of developing side effects [3]. Another major

Table 1
Differences between western and Kampo medicines

Western (allopathic medicines)	Single compound	Single target (magic bullet)	High selectivity no side effects
		Unintended multiple targets	Efficacious but with serious side effects
Kampo medicines	Compatible compound groups	Intended multiple targets	Efficacious with few side effects

difference is that a candidate, novel compound in western medicine can take anywhere from 10 to 15 years to verify its efficacy in pharmacokinetic and basic studies and placebo-controlled clinical trials before it is approved as a pharmaceutical drug for the market. On the contrary, Kampo has been clinically used in humans and its content refined empirically for approximately 1500 years [4]. Given that rigorous scientific investigations of Kampo have only commenced in the last few decades, allopathic physicians have necessarily been skeptical about their use. Fortunately, however, several Kampo products are currently subjected to stringent scientific analyses commensurate with those employed for conventional new drug development.

2 What is Daikenchuto?

Since 1986 DKT (Dai-ken-chu-to), a Kampo medicine has been prescribed for the treatment of two symptoms: abdominal bloating and cold sensation in the abdomen and Japanese government insurance started to cover the medical fee of DKT. DKT is the most frequently prescribed as Kampo medicine in Japan, especially in the field of gastroenterology. Dai-ken-chu-to translate as, "to reconstruct strongly the diseased gastrointestinal tract to the health." The "Da" implies maximal effect, "(ken)" connotes reconstruction, "(chu)" denotes gastrointestinal tract, and "(to)" character of DKT indicates water solubility [2]. Approximately 500 million DKT sachets (2.5 g/sachet) are prescribed annually in Japan, and major adverse events have not been reported to date.

The formulation of DKT is composed of extract granules of *Japanese pepper*, *processed ginger*, *ginseng radix*, and *maltose powder*. In a typical case of the representative product manufactured by Tsumura & Co., DKT extract powder is made as an aqueous extract from the mixture of these medicinal plants at the weight ratio of 2:5:3. 1.25 g of DKT extract powder is mixed with 10 g maltose and some excipient providing 15 g of the final product. Maltose confers a sweet taste and improves the palatability of the formulation. Other benefits of high maltose (a disaccharide) content include low calorie and controlled sweetness to approximately 1/3 of comparable, sweetened products. The standard dosage of DKT is 15 g/day, and the water-soluble nature of DKT, due to its high maltose content, makes this dosage possible.

As shown in Fig. 1, the main ingredients of DKT include hydroxy-α-sanshool (*Japanese pepper*), [6]-shogaol (*processed ginger*), ginsenoside Rb_1 (*ginseng radix*), and maltose, which have been identified by three-dimensional high-performance liquid chromatography. Contamination studies have certified DKT to be free of unexpected pharmaceutical ingredients, toxins, pesticides, microbes, and heavy metals.

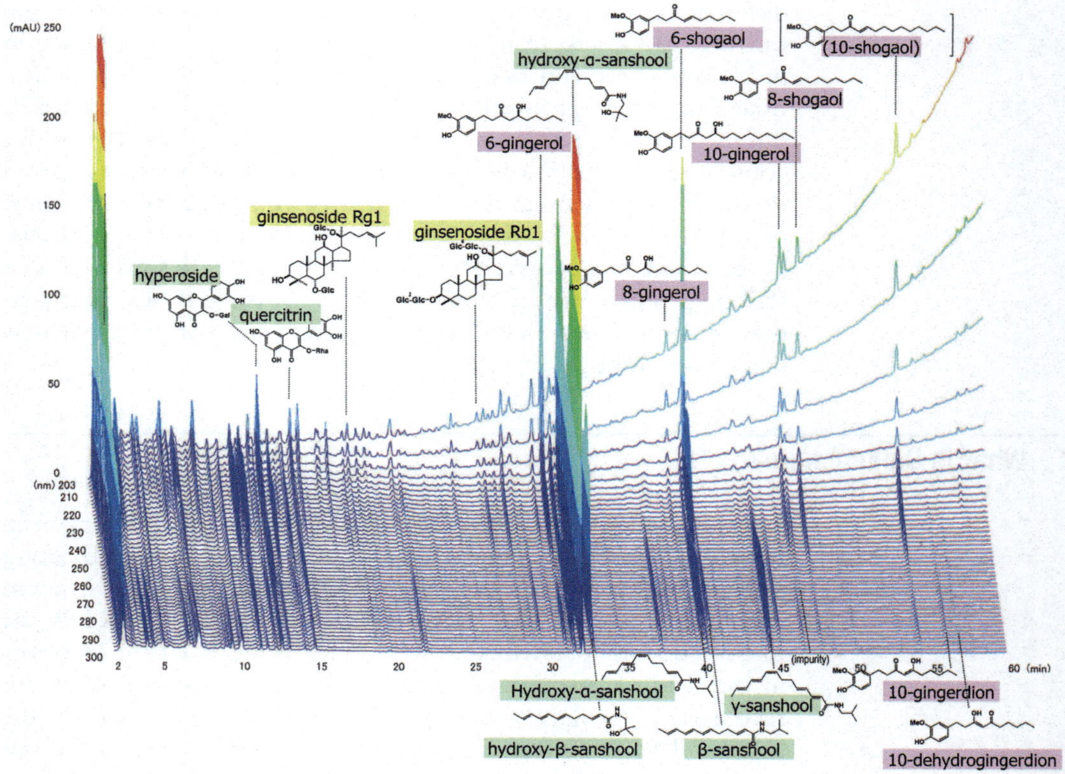

Fig. 1 Three-dimensional high-performance liquid chromatography of daikenchuto. Three-dimensional high-performance liquid chromatography are used as characteristic markers (hydroxy-α-sanshool, [6]-shogaol, ginsenoside Rb1) for quality control

Recent mechanistic studies are increasingly demonstrating the prokinetic effect of DKT [5]. However, ingredient analysis and pharmacokinetic studies, which are considered indispensable in conventional drug development, have been sparse until now because of the conundrum of tracking multiple ingredients. Nonetheless, scientific breakthrough occurred with the pharmacokinetic study of DKT [6, 7] made possible by the advent of technologies such as liquid chromatography–mass spectrometry (LC–MS/MS) for the identification of ingredients and characterization of their kinetics with greater accuracy and precision. The use of 3D-HPLC has helped identify the multiple ingredients in DKT, but the pharmacokinetic data has revealed for the first time that these ingredients are absorbed and metabolized at different rates. For instance, the main active ingredients of Japanese pepper, namely, hydroxy-α-sanshool (HASHydroxy-α-sanshool (HAS)) and hydroxy-β-sanshool (HBS)Hydroxy-β-sanshool (HBS), produce transient peaks, indicating their rapid absorption at high concentrations (HAS in the order of μM) as well as their rapid elimination over a few hours. The main active ingredients of processed ginger ([6]-shogaol and

[6]-gingerol) are also absorbed, but are rapidly metabolized and conjugated after absorption, therefore, their plasma concentrations are less than 1 % compared with that of the Japanese pepper ingredients. By contrast, most of the ginseng ingredients remain virtually unabsorbed. Moreover, pharmacokinetic analysis of luminal content after administration revealed that Japanese pepper ingredients are rapidly absorbed before reaching the colonic lumen; processed ginger ingredients are transformed into various metabolites in the upper small intestine and liver with some ingredients returning to the intestine via bile duct; and ginseng ingredients reach the colon intact and are absorbed only after they are metabolized by the enteric microbiota. Among the bacterial metabolites of ginseng ingredients, some have been found to have antitumor and anti-inflammatory properties such as compound K [8, 9]. Taken together, one of the key findings from the pharmacokinetic study is that the ingredients are absorbed at different rates and act accordingly on various target cells. The significance of this finding will be elaborated after the explanation of one of the important pharmacologic effects of DKT.

3 How to Work: Basic Evidence of Daikenchuto

The objective of this section is to introduce the experimental evidence-based information of DKT.

As mentioned earlier, DKT is primarily prescribed for the treatment of abdominal bloating and cold sensation in the abdomen, and the latter has been previously attributed to its effect in improving intestinal blood flow [5]. The critical players responsible for vasodilatory effects are the two peptides, calcitonin gene-related peptide (CGRPCalcitonin gene-related peptide (CGRP)) and adrenomedullin (ADM) [10–14]. CGRP is one of the most potent mediators of microvascular vasodilation in the human body, and its vasodilatory effects following stimulated release from the extrinsic sensory innervation are considered to serve as an important protective mechanism for maintaining mucosal integrity [15–18]. Because blood flow has to meet the relatively high metabolic needs of the gastrointestinal tract as well as provide both valuable buffering and a pathway for removal of toxins that may have entered tissue [19]. Therefore, maintaining or increasing blood flow is thought to be a central element in protecting the gastrointestinal tract and even in the prevention of intestinal adhesions resulting from inflammation [20, 21].

Neuropeptides are important for the regulation of gastrointestinal blood flow. A number of neuropeptides such as CGRP, VIP, and SP have been localized immunohistochemically in sensory nerves innervating various viscera, including the gastrointestinal tract [22–24]. Intraduodenal or intracolonic administration of

DKT to normal rats increased small and large intestinal blood flow in a dose-dependent manner [13, 25]. The pharmacological study suggests that DKT-induced hyperemia of the rat intestine is mediated by CGRP, but neither by VIP nor SP release. Moreover, the results from the study by RT-PCR revealed that DKT had an up-regulatory effect on CGRP.

Another important factor for understanding the mechanism of action of DKT is through study of the receptors involved.

A receptor with seven transmembrane domains [26, 27], the calcitonin receptor-like receptor (CRLR), can function as either a CGRP receptor or an ADM receptor. The CRLR is an "immature" receptor, depending on which members of receptor activity-modifying proteins (RAMPs) are expressed. RAMPs are required to transport CRLR to the plasma membrane.

The CRLR can be the CGRP receptor through the binding of RAMP1 and can be the ADM receptor through the RAMP2 [28]. The RAMP3 can be altered by both CGRP and ADM receptor (Fig. 2).

Therefore, to confirm the existence of CGRP and/or ADM receptor, it is necessary to determine the existence of not only CRLR but also RAMPs. Our RT-PCR study revealed that DKT had an up-regulatory effect on CRLR and RAMPs [13]. These lines indicated that when DKT stimulates CGRP and ADM,

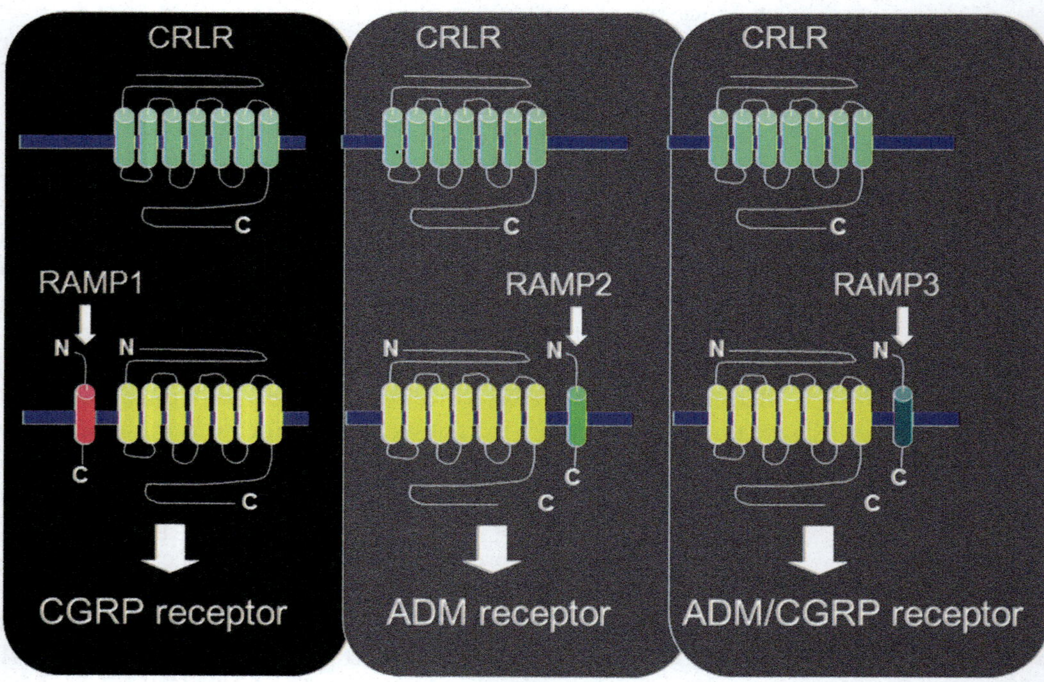

Fig. 2 Association of CRLR with a RAMP dictates the specificity of ligand binding

simultaneously up-regulates CRLR and RAMPs, and develops up-regulation of CGRP and ADM receptors. Thus, DKT can be used as an endogenous CGRP, ADM, and their receptors up-regulator for intestine.

ADM belongs to the same peptide family as CGRP and has potent vasodilatory effects in the microvascular system [29]. ADM is ubiquitous in the GI tract and plays important roles in the regulation of microcirculation, angiogenesis, antifibrosis, antibiosis, and down-regulation of proinflammatory cytokines.

The main difference between the microvascular activities of ADM and CGRP is their comparative potencies. The potency of ADM is less than that of CGRP, 1/3- to 1/10-fold less in rat skin [30], and approximately 1/300-fold less in mouse mesentery [31]. CGRP is the primary vasodilator in physiologic conditions and acts peripherally.

The major difference between the production cells of ADM and CGRP is that the former is not produced by neuronal cells but rather by epithelial and smooth muscle cells and other nonneuronal tissues [32].

One of the characteristics of the small and large intestines is the production of ADM by the intestinal epithelial cells in human, rat, and mouse. Like CGRP, ADM has anti-inflammatory and powerful anticytokine effects, and is especially noted for its ability to inhibit TNFα [14, 33].

Both ADM and CGRP are key peptides for understanding the mechanism of vasodilatory actions of DKT. DKT contains TRPV1-stimulating ingredients such as HAS, shogaols, and gingerols, and previous studies indicated the involvement of TRPV1 activation in its prokinetics activity and CGRP release. One of the frequently asked questions is whether DKT is equivalent to capsaicin. We have discovered that this is not the case because DKT-induced increase in blood flow is not abrogated by the inhibitors of transient receptor potential vanilloid receptor 1 (TRPV1)Transient receptor potential vanilloid receptor 1 (TRPV1), a capsaicin receptor [12]. Another common point of contention is whether an augmentation of blood flow will aggravate preexisting inflammation. Our results from the experimental colitis model have shown that blood flow increases in areas of poor circulation, while it remains unchanged in regions of high levels of inflammation. This is likely due to the mobilization and exhaustion of the two primary targets of DKT, i.e., CGRP and ADM, in inflamed areas and that DKT remedy itself is neither CGRP nor ADM. In addition, mechanistic probing of ADM production has revealed that DKT induces ADM release from the IECs in a dose- and time-dependent manner largely via its active ingredient, [6]-shogaol. Furthermore, [6]-shogaol appears to stimulate a type of Ca^{2+}channel called the transient receptor potential ankyrin 1 (TRPA1) to promote ADM release from the IECs as well [12].

Besides CGRP, several important neurally mediated mechanisms have been suggested as mediating the increased effective intestinal motility of DKT [34, 35]. First, DKT accelerates acetylcholine (Ach) release from cholinergic myenteric neurons mediated by activation of 5-HT receptors (5-HT3 and 5-HT4) [35, 36], and smooth muscles contract due to the released ACh through stimulation of muscarinic receptors (M2R and M3R). Second, it has been reported that DKT raises plasma levels of motilin, a gastrointestinal polypeptide hormone, and this improves morphine-induced constipation in patients and canines [37, 38]. Third, DKT induces the release of substance P from primary sensory nerves through the TRPV1 on intramucosal terminal sensory nerves, and this contracts smooth muscle [34, 39]. Recent report revealed that the DKT up-regulates the activation of nicotinic acetylcholine receptors [40].

4 Synergistic Effects with Multitargets

Pharmacokinetics studies have shown that, when TU-100 is administered orally, HAS and HBS are rapidly absorbed in the gut and reaches to the high concentrations in the blood (approximately 1 μM in human and rats) within 15 min [6, 7]. On the other hand, the plasma concentration of [6]-shogaol is low and does not correspond with the effective dose observed in in vitro studies, but such a dose would likely be considered high in the lumen. In addition, we have confirmed that DKT administered directly using a long tube is clinically effective in patients. In subsequent studies, we analyzed the kinetics of Japanese pepper ingredients, HAS and HBS, which are known agonists of TRPA1 and TRPV1 receptors (actions resembling those of processed ginger ingredients) and antagonists of two-pore-domain potassium channels, KCNK. KCNK channels exist in cell membranes of excitatory cells such as neurons and muscles as highly regulated, K^+-selective leak channels [41, 42]. They are fundamental to maintaining the resting potential and regulating cellular excitability. In the neurons, KCNK channels regulate the opening of voltage-gated Na^+ channels which generate action potentials. Recent studies have shown that HAS and HBS accelerate colonic motility by inhibiting KCNK3 and KCNK9 channels in the intestinal smooth muscle and neuronal cells. In light of these findings combined with the pharmacokinetic data, we postulated as follows [5]: DKT administration causes an initial blockade of KCNK channels in the intestinal smooth muscle and neuronal cells by the Japanese pepper ingredients, which leads to increased membrane sensitivity, i.e., decreased threshold for additional exogenous stimuli, in this case the subsequent exposure to ginger and ginseng ingredients (Fig. 3). In short, these results

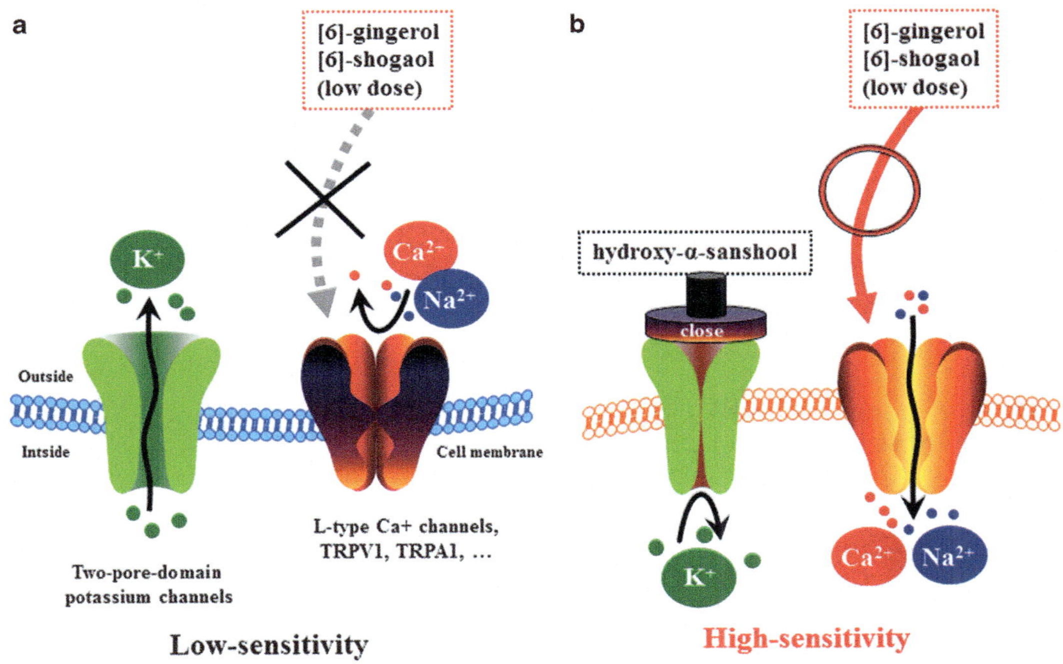

Fig. 3 Hypotheses. (**a**) Two-pore-domain potassium channels (i.e., KCNKs family channels) are expressed in many types of excitable cells throughout the body and have been implicated in various cellular functions, including the maintenance of the resting potential and regulation of excitability. Low doses of ginger ingredients cannot evoke action potentials. (**b**) One of ingredients of daikenchuto, hydroxy-α-sanshool, acts as a blocker of two-pore-domain potassium leak channels (KCNK3 and KCNK9) and alters the excitability of a cell via voltage-activated cation channels. Low doses of ginger ingredients can evoke action potentials. From Kono, T. et al (2015) (ref. 5)

suggest that DKT ingredients could induce a therapeutic effect at concentrations lower than those required for each ingredient to exert its effect by itself. Indeed, Japanese pepper and processed ginger ingredients have no or the least effect on colonic motility when administered separately, but concomitant administration generates a significant prokinetic action (Fig. 4). Likewise, at doses for which Japanese pepper and ginseng ingredients administered independently do not affect colonic blood flow, the combination significantly increases flow (Fig. 5). Unraveling the precise mechanisms underpinning these synergistic effects would be a herculean task, nevertheless, our hypothesis appears robust and credible enough that is poised on the brink of elucidation.

We believe that systems biology is particularly beneficial for the elucidation of multicomponent remedies and has the potential of producing groundbreaking results that could instigate a paradigm shift in health care.

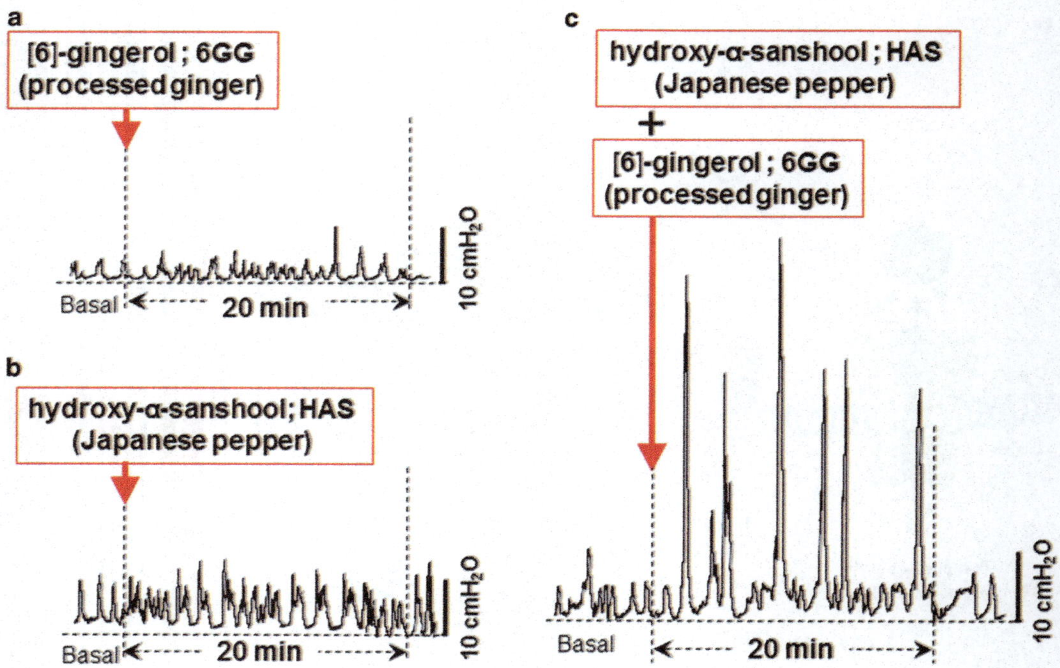

Fig. 4 Mixture of hydroxy-α-sanshool and [6]-gingerol increased colonic motility. Isolated segments of the proximal rat colons were placed in an organ bath containing aerated Kreb's solution. Motility was evaluated by monitoring the intestinal tract pressure and videography. (**a**) Bath application of [6]-gingerol (1 μM), [6]-shogaol (1 μM), or hydroxy-α-sanshool (HAS) (3 μM), from serosal side did not alter colonic motility. (**b**) A simultaneous addition of three ingredients increased colonic motility. Video imaging showed a typical squeezing

5 How to Work: Clinical Evidence of Daikenchuto

5.1 Postoperative Ileus

The objective of this section is to address the concept of appropriate use of DKT in the field of gastroenterology. In the digestive surgery area, DKT has been employed for speeding the recovery from postoperative ileus after abdominal surgery and its clinical efficacy has been reported in open label studies [43–46]. In order to clarify the clinical benefits of DKT, several double blind placebo-controlled trials on the patients with postoperative ileus (POI), CD, functional constipation, and irritable bowel syndromes are currently underway in the U.S. and Japan.

A double-blind, placebo-controlled study on healthy volunteers in the U.S., Mayo Clinic, has shown that treatment with TU-100 significantly accelerates ascending colon emptying [47].

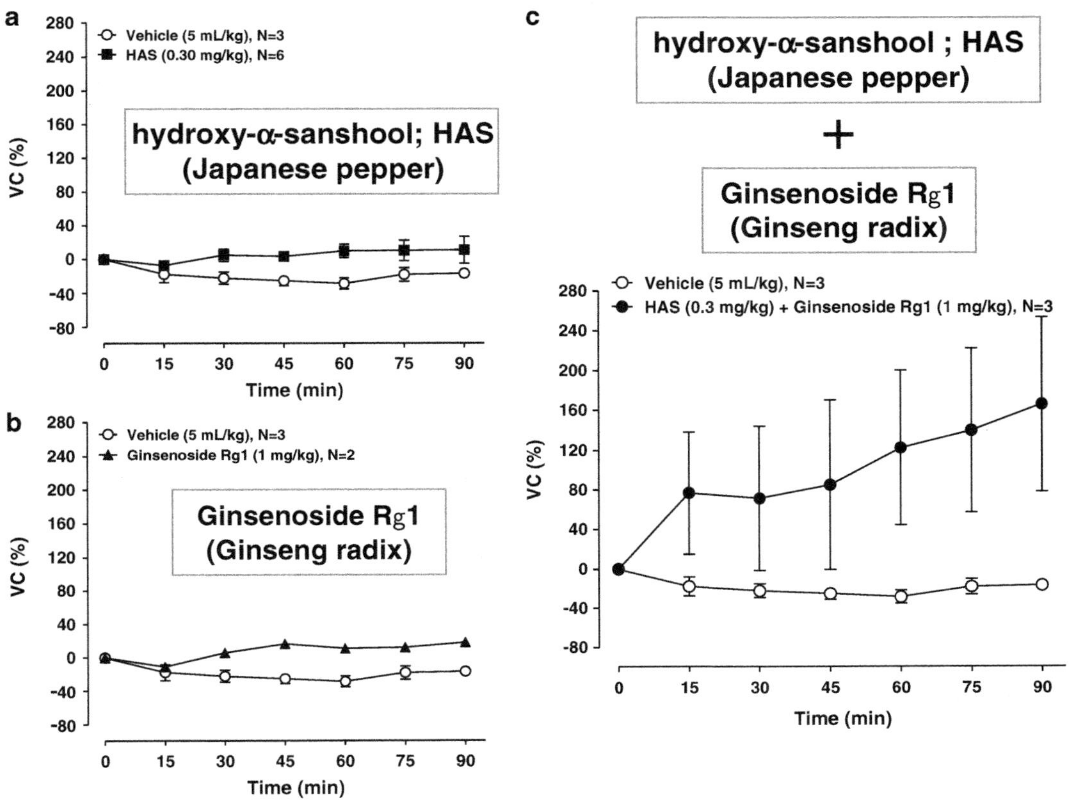

Fig. 5 Mixture of hydroxy-α-sanshool and ginsenoside Rg1 increased intestinal blood flow. Systemic mean arterial blood pressure (MAP) and heart rate (HR) were recorded. Red blood cell flux in colonic blood flow, CBF was measured using noncontact laser tissue blood flowmetry, and colonic vascular conductance (VC) was calculated as the ratio of flux to MAP. (**a**) Intracolonal administration of hydroxy-α-sanshool (0.3 mg/kg) or vehicle did not alter VC. (**b**) Intracolonal administration of ginsenoside Rg1 (1 mg/kg) or vehicle did not alter VC. (**c**) Intracolonal administration of mixture of hydroxy-α-sanshool (0.3 mg/kg) and ginsenoside Rg1 (1 mg/kg) increased VC from the first 15-min observation period (% of basal, 80 %) and kept the increase during whole experimental period (90 min, 165 %). Vehicle did not alter VC. Vehicle: Tween 80

In Japan, several multicenter, double-blind, placebo-controlled studies of DKT involving 80 % of nationwide university hospitals were launched to explicate the benefits and mechanism of action of DKT at the clinical level.

Shimada revealed that DKT administration accelerated the time of first bowel movement after hepatic resection in patients with liver cancer [48]. This multicenter, phase II trial assesses the efficacy of DKT on POI after hepatic resection.

A total of 209 patients (DKT: $n = 108$, placebo: $n = 101$), who underwent hepatic resection at 26 Japanese centers, were included in the statistical analysis. Patients were randomly assigned to receive either oral doses (15 g/day, three times a day) of DKT or placebo control from preoperative day 3 to postoperative day 10, except on the day of surgery. The median of the time from extubation until the first postoperative bowel movement was 88.2 h (95 % CI 74.0–94.1) in the DKT group and 93.1 h (95 % CI 83.3–99.4) in the placebo group, demonstrating that DKT accelerated the time to first bowel movement significantly more than placebo control. TU-100 is an effective treatment option after hepatic resection in patients with liver cancer.

Another multicenter, randomized, controlled phase II trial in patients with total gastrectomy for gastric cancer showed the efficacy of DKT on postoperative bowel motility and for prevention of POI [49]. A total of 195 patients (DKT, $n = 96$; placebo, $n = 99$) were included in the analysis. Patients received either DKT (15.0 g/d) or matching placebo from postoperative days 1–12. Median time to first bowel movement was shorter in the DKT group than in the placebo group (94.7 h vs. 113.9 h; $p = 0.051$). In patients with high medication adherence, median time to first bowel movement was significantly shorter in the DKT group than in the placebo group (93.8 h vs. 115.1 h; $p = 0.014$). Significantly fewer patients in the DKT group had ≥two symptoms of gastrointestinal dysfunction than those in the placebo group on postoperative day 12 ($p = 0.026$). A prospective randomized trial (DKT, $n = 41$, control, $n = 40$), but no placebo-controlled, also showed that DKT improved bowel movements, stool properties, and bowel gas [50]. These lines strongly suggested that DKT promoted early postoperative bowel functions after total gastrectomy.

5.2 Crohn's Disease

Adrenomedullin, which is a potent Crohn's diseasevasodilator in the microvascular system as well as having some immunoregulatory effects, may be a potential treatment approach in CD. Indeed, the anticolitis effect of ADM was demonstrated in mouse and rat models of CD [11, 12, 51] and acetic acid-induced colonic ulceration in rats [52]. In addition, several investigators have suggested that the effect of ADM might play an important role in mucosal defense as an antimicrobial peptide [53, 54]. Invasion of microbes through the mucosal barrier stimulates the host immune system and intimately correlates with development of morbidity in experimental and human inflammatory bowel disease (IBD).

Interestingly, immunoreactive ADM was shown to distribute at the apical surface of the epithelial cells of the intestinal mucosa. This observation may indicate that epithelial ADM contributes to the control of intestinal microflora. Invasion of microbes through the mucosal barrier stimulates the host immune system and intimately correlates with the development of morbidity in experimental and human IBD [55].

It has already been also verified that ADM diminishes proinflammatory cytokine production (TNFα and IFNγ). Thus, ADM may play a regulatory role in inflammatory gut diseases such as CD.

Actually, the anticolitis effect of ADM was previously demonstrated in mouse4 and rat5 models of CD. Combined results of these studies support the potential treatment of CD with ADM, as exogenous ADM administration has proven efficacy in animal models.

Other clinical and experimental studies in the field of gastrointestinal pathology support stronger associations between CGRP, ADM, and CD than previously speculated [51, 56]. Decreases in colonic flow and augmentation of the inflammation of CD appear to correlate with decreased CGRP secretion from damaged neuronal cells as a result of recurrent transmural inflammation; indeed experimental support for this concept derives from studies showing the successful treatment of CD with exogenous CGRP and ADM in experimental animal models of intestinal inflammation. Although the combined results of these studies suggest a novel approach to the treatment of CD with CGRP and ADM, exogenous administration of these peptides is clearly not practical because of the potential systemic effects of these agents as well as the metabolic clearance which makes chronic delivery of a small peptide impractical [20, 57–59]. Nevertheless, endogenous administration of CGRP and ADM in the experimental setting provides a protective effect in maintaining colonic mucosal flow and decreasing inflammation; therefore, a potential role for DKT in enhancing the local, endogenous secretion of CGRP and possibly ADM has led to the formulation of the following hypothesis: DKT may be effective in improving blood flow and reducing inflammatory changes via augmenting secretion of ADM from the intestinal mucosal epithelium, which in turn may supplement the decreased production of CGRP from damaged neuronal tissues in CD.

The inhibitory effect of ADM on TNFα production has also received considerable attention in the field of CD similar in many respects to therapeutic use of infliximab (TNFα antibody) and has advanced our treatment of CD [60]. Infliximab is a murine chimeric monoclonal antibody against TNFα, and has been known for some time to trigger the production of antibodies directed at the foreign protein in the drug, which limits its widespread use as therapeutics. Despite the introduction of the anti-TNFα agents, 20–40 % of patients fail to respond to initial induction therapy, and only 60–70 % of the initial responders will maintain a sustained response at 1 year. Based on these facts, use of DKT in conjunction with infliximab treatment (which is currently administered once every 8 weeks) may in theory lead to a decrease in the frequency and dosage of the antibody treatment.

The rapidly increasing number of patients with CD in Japan has prompted an upsurge of clinical trials with DKT. A large-scale retrospective study showed that continuous DKT therapy is a clinically useful and feasible maintenance therapy for the prevention of postoperative reoperation in patients with CD [61]. A total of 258 patients who underwent surgery for CD were identified for the study. For the prevention of postoperative recurrence, patients were stratified to receive 5-aminosalicylic acid (ASA), azathioprine or DKT, and their effects on preventing reoperation at 3 years were evaluated. Of the 258 patients, 44 required reoperation with intestinal resection within 3 years due to disease recurrence. The 3-year reoperation rate was significantly lower in the postoperative DKT group than in the non-DKT group (11.3 vs. 24.5 %, $P = 0.01$). A multivariate Cox analysis showed that postoperative DKT ($P = 0.035$) was significantly and independently associated with the rate of reoperation at 3 years in patients with CD. Although further prospective, randomized, placebo-controlled trials are needed to confirm these findings, DKT may be a viable option for the postoperative management of CD.

DKT is a classic example of the harmonization between traditional herbal medicine and modern medicine. Rigorous scientific investigations are now beginning to reveal the complex therapeutic effects mediated by DKT. The ancient adage of maximizing the temporal differences in pharmacological effects may be similar to the modern concept of a combination chemotherapy regimen, except that one Kampo prescription by itself fulfills the role of a combination regimen. We believe the worldwide availability of Kampo medicines.

References

1. Motoo Y, Seki T, Tsutani K (2011) Traditional Japanese medicine, Kampo: its history and current status. Chin J Integr Med 17:85–87
2. Kono T, Kanematsu T, Kitajima M (2009) Exodus of Kampo, traditional Japanese medicine, from the complementary and alternative medicines: is it time yet? Surgery 146:837–840
3. Terasawa K (2004) Evidence-based reconstruction of Kampo medicine: part-III-how should Kampo be evaluated? Evid Based Complement Alternat Med 1:219–222
4. Terasawa K (2004) Evidence-based reconstruction of Kampo medicine: part I-Is Kampo CAM? Evid Based Complement Alternat Med 1:11–16
5. Kono T, Shimada M, Yamamoto M et al (2015) Complementary and synergistic therapeutic effects of compounds found in Kampo medicine: analysis of daikenchuto. Front Pharmacol 6:159
6. Munekage M, Ichikawa K, Kitagawa H et al (2013) Population pharmacokinetic analysis of daikenchuto, a traditional Japanese medicine (Kampo) in Japanese and US health volunteers. Drug Metab Dispos 41:1256–1263
7. Munekage M, Kitagawa H, Ichikawa K et al (2011) Pharmacokinetics of daikenchuto, a traditional Japanese medicine (kampo) after single oral administration to healthy Japanese volunteers. Drug Metab Dispos 39:1784–1788
8. Li J, Zhong W, Wang W et al (2014) Ginsenoside metabolite compound K promotes recovery of dextran sulfate sodium-induced colitis and inhibits inflammatory responses by suppressing NF-kappaB activation. PLoS One 9: e87810
9. Zhang Z, Du GJ, Wang CZ et al (2013) Compound K, a ginsenoside metabolite, inhibits colon cancer growth via multiple pathways including p53-p21 interactions. Int J Mol Sci 14:2980–2995
10. Kaneko A, Kono T, Miura N et al (2013) Preventive effect of TU-100 on a type-2 model of colitis in mice: possible involvement of enhancing adrenomedullin in intestinal epithelial cells. Gastroenterol Res Pract 2013:384057
11. Kono T, Kaneko A, Hira Y et al (2010) Anti-colitis and -adhesion effects of daikenchuto via endogenous adrenomedullin enhancement in Crohn's disease mouse model. J Crohns Colitis 4:161–170
12. Kono T, Kaneko A, Omiya Y et al (2013) Epithelial transient receptor potential ankyrin 1

(TRPA1)-dependent adrenomedullin upregulates blood flow in rat small intestine. Am J Physiol Gastrointest Liver Physiol 304: G428–G436

13. Kono T, Koseki T, Chiba S et al (2008) Colonic vascular conductance increased by Daikenchuto via calcitonin gene-related peptide and receptor-activity modifying protein 1. J Surg Res 150:78–84
14. Kono T, Omiya Y, Hira Y et al (2011) Daikenchuto (TU-100) ameliorates colon microvascular dysfunction via endogenous adrenomedullin in Crohn's disease rat model. J Gastroenterol 46:1187–1196
15. Yeoh KG, Kang JY, Yap I et al (1995) Chili protects against aspirin-induced gastroduodenal mucosal injury in humans. Dig Dis Sci 40:580–583
16. Reinshagen M, Patel A, Sottili M et al (1994) Protective function of extrinsic sensory neurons in acute rabbit experimental colitis. Gastroenterology 106:1208–1214
17. Kinoshita Y, Inui T, Chiba T (1993) Calcitonin gene-related peptide: a neurotransmitter involved in capsaicin-sensitive afferent nerve-mediated gastric mucosal protection. J Clin Gastroenterol 17(Suppl 1):S27–S32
18. Holzer P, Livingston EH, Saria A et al (1991) Sensory neurons mediate protective vasodilatation in rat gastric mucosa. Am J Physiol 260: G363–G370
19. Holm L, Phillipson M, Perry MA (2002) NO-flurbiprofen maintains duodenal blood flow, enhances mucus secretion contributing to lower mucosal injury. Am J Physiol Gastrointest Liver Physiol 283:G1090–G1097
20. Martinez V, Tache Y (2006) Carcitonin gene-related peptide and gastrointestinal function. In: Kastin AJ (ed) Handbook of biologically active peptides. Elsvier, London, pp 1005–1011
21. Guth P, Leung F, Kauffmam G (1989) Physiology of the gastric circulation. In: Schultz S (ed) Handbook of physiology. American Physiological Society, Bethesda, pp 1371–1404
22. Timmermans JP, Scheuermann DW, Barbiers M et al (1992) Calcitonin gene-related peptide-like immunoreactivity in the human small intestine. Acta Anat (Basel) 143:48–53
23. Clague JR, Sternini C, Brecha NC (1985) Localization of calcitonin gene-related peptide-like immunoreactivity in neurons of the rat gastrointestinal tract. Neurosci Lett 56:63–68
24. Miampamba M, Sharkey KA (1998) Distribution of calcitonin gene-related peptide, somatostatin, substance P and vasoactive intestinal polypeptide in experimental colitis in rats. Neurogastroenterol Motil 10:315–329
25. Murata P, Kase Y, Ishige A et al (2002) The herbal medicine Dai-kenchu-to and one of its active components [6]-shogaol increase intestinal blood flow in rats. Life Sci 70:2061–2070
26. Foord SM, Marshall FH (1999) RAMPs: accessory proteins for seven transmembrane domain receptors. Trends Pharmacol Sci 20:184–187
27. McLatchie LM, Fraser NJ, Main MJ et al (1998) RAMPs regulate the transport and ligand specificity of the calcitonin-receptor-like receptor. Nature 393:333–339
28. Brain SD, Grant AD (2004) Vascular actions of calcitonin gene-related peptide and adrenomedullin. Physiol Rev 84:903–934
29. Kato J, Kitamura K (2015) Bench-to-bedside pharmacology of adrenomedullin. Eur J Pharmacol 764:140–148
30. Chu DQ, Choy M, Foster P et al (2000) A comparative study of the ability of calcitonin gene-related peptide and adrenomedullin (13–52) to modulate microvascular but not thermal hyperalgesia responses. Br J Pharmacol 130:1589–1596
31. Tam C, Brain SD (2004) The assessment of vasoactive properties of CGRP and adrenomedullin in the microvasculature: a study using in vivo and in vitro assays in the mouse. J Mol Neurosci 22:117–124
32. Schubert ML (2006) Adrenomedullin in gastrointestinal function. In: Kastin AJ (ed) Handbook of biologically active peptides. Elesvier, London, pp 999–1004
33. Wu R, Zhou M, Wang P (2003) Adrenomedullin and adrenomedullin binding protein-1 downregulate TNF-alpha in macrophage cell line and rat Kupffer cells. Regul Pept 112:19–26
34. Sato Y, Katagiri F, Inoue S et al (2004) Daikenchu-to raises levels of calcitonin gene-related peptide and substance P in human plasma. Biol Pharm Bull 27:1875–1877
35. Shibata C, Sasaki I, Naito H et al (1999) The herbal medicine Dai-Kenchu-Tou stimulates upper gut motility through cholinergic and 5-hydroxytryptamine 3 receptors in conscious dogs. Surgery 126:918–924
36. Tokita Y, Yuzurihara M, Sakaguchi M et al (2007) The pharmacological effects of Daikenchuto, a traditional herbal medicine, on delayed gastrointestinal transit in rat postoperative ileus. J Pharmacol Sci 104:303–310
37. Jin XL, Shibata C, Naito H et al (2001) Intraduodenal and intrajejunal administration of the herbal medicine, dai-kenchu-tou, stimulates small intestinal motility via cholinergic receptors in conscious dogs. Dig Dis Sci 46:1171–1176
38. Nagano T, Itoh H, Takeyama M (1999) Effect of Dai-kenchu-to on levels of 3 brain-gut

peptides (motilin, gastrin and somatostatin) in human plasma. Biol Pharm Bull 22:1131–1133
39. Satoh K, Hashimoto K, Hayakawa T et al (2001) Mechanism of atropine-resistant contraction induced by Dai-kenchu-to in guinea pig ileum. Jpn J Pharmacol 86:32–37
40. Endo M, Hori M, Ozaki H et al (2014) Daikenchuto, a traditional Japanese herbal medicine, ameliorates postoperative ileus by anti-inflammatory action through nicotinic acetylcholine receptors. J Gastroenterol 49:1026–1039
41. Bautista DM, Sigal YM, Milstein AD et al (2008) Pungent agents from Szechuan peppers excite sensory neurons by inhibiting two-pore potassium channels. Nat Neurosci 11:772–779
42. MacKinnon R, Cohen SL, Kuo A et al (1998) Structural conservation in prokaryotic and eukaryotic potassium channels. Science 280:106–109
43. Iwai N, Kume Y, Kimura O et al (2007) Effects of herbal medicine Dai-Kenchu-to on anorectal function in children with severe constipation. Eur J Pediatr Surg 17:115–118
44. Endo S, Nishida T, Nishikawa K et al (2006) Dai-kenchu-to, a Chinese herbal medicine, improves stasis of patients with total gastrectomy and jejunal pouch interposition. Am J Surg 192:9–13
45. Suehiro T, Matsumata T, Shikada Y et al (2005) The effect of the herbal medicines dai-kenchu-to and keishi-bukuryo-gan on bowel movement after colorectal surgery. Hepatogastroenterology 52:97–100
46. Itoh T, Yamakawa J, Mai M et al (2002) The effect of the herbal medicine dai-kenchu-to on post-operative ileus. J Int Med Res 30:428–432
47. Manabe N, Camilleri M, Rao A et al (2010) Effect of daikenchuto (TU-100) on gastrointestinal and colonic transit in humans. Am J Physiol Gastrointest Liver Physiol 298: G970–G975
48. Shimada M, Morine Y, Nagano H et al (2015) Effect of TU-100, a traditional Japanese medicine, administered after hepatic resection in patients with liver cancer: a multi-center, phase III trial (JFMC40-1001). Int J Clin Oncol 20:95–104
49. Yoshikawa K, Shimada M, Wakabayashi G et al (2015) The effect of DKT, a traditional Japanese herbal medicine, after total gastrectomy for gastric cancer: a multi-center, randomized, double-blind, placebo-controlled phase II trial (JFMC42-1002). J Am Coll Surg 221 (2):571–578
50. Akamaru Y, Takahashi T, Nishida T et al (2015) Effects of daikenchuto, a Japanese herb, on intestinal motility after total gastrectomy: a prospective randomized trial. J Gastrointest Surg 19:467–472
51. Talero E, Sanchez-Fidalgo S, de la Lastra CA et al (2008) Acute and chronic responses associated with adrenomedullin administration in experimental colitis. Peptides 29:2001–2012
52. Ashizuka S, Ishikawa N, Kato J et al (2005) Effect of adrenomedullin administration on acetic acid-induced colitis in rats. Peptides 26:2610–2615
53. Allaker RP, Kapas S (2003) Adrenomedullin and mucosal defence: interaction between host and microorganism. Regul Pept 112:147–152
54. Marutsuka K, Nawa Y, Asada Y et al (2001) Adrenomedullin and proadrenomudullin N-terminal 20 peptide (PAMP) are present in human colonic epithelia and exert an antimicrobial effect. Exp Physiol 86:543–545
55. Clavel T, Haller D (2007) Bacteria- and host-derived mechanisms to control intestinal epithelial cell homeostasis: implications for chronic inflammation. Inflamm Bowel Dis 13:1153–1164
56. Gonzalez-Rey E, Fernandez-Martin A, Chorny A et al (2006) Therapeutic effect of urocortin and adrenomedullin in a murine model of Crohn's disease. Gut 55:824–832
57. Westphal M, Booke M, Dinh-Xuan AT (2004) Adrenomedullin: a smart road from pheochromocytoma to treatment of pulmonary hypertension. Eur Respir J 24:518–520
58. Eto T, Kitamura K, Kato J (1999) Biological and clinical roles of adrenomedullin in circulation control and cardiovascular diseases. Clin Exp Pharmacol Physiol 26:371–380
59. Meeran K, O'Shea D, Upton PD et al (1997) Circulating adrenomedullin does not regulate systemic blood pressure but increases plasma prolactin after intravenous infusion in humans: a pharmacokinetic study. J Clin Endocrinol Metab 82:95–100
60. Sandborn WJ (2007) Clinical perspectives in Crohn's disease. Moving forward with anti-TNF-alpha therapy: current needs and future treatments. Rev Gastroenterol Disord 7(Suppl 2):S23–S35
61. Kanazawa A, Sako M, Takazoe M et al (2014) Daikenchuto, a traditional Japanese herbal medicine, for the maintenance of surgically induced remission in patients with Crohn's disease: a retrospective analysis of 258 patients. Surg Today 44:1506–1512

Chapter 12

Memory/Learning, Dementia, and Kampo

Kinzo Matsumoto and Hironori Fujiwara

Abstract

Impairment of cognitive function and learning/memory is a core symptom of patients with Alzheimer's disease (AD), vascular dementia (VaD), and other forms of dementia. Because the number of dementia patients is increasing explosively as the world population is growing and aging, a lot of effort have been made to develop innovative drugs to overcome dementia; however, it has not succeeded yet. On the other hand, a potential usefulness of Kampo medicines for the treatment of cognitive deficits of patients with dementia has been suggested by clinical and/or preclinical studies reported during the last two decades. Those are yokukansan (YKS), chotosan, kihi-to, and kami-kihi-to (KKT), a "kihi-to"-based formula. Pharmacological and molecular biological evidence or chemical constituents, which may account for the antidementia effects of those Kampo medicines, have also been provided by lines of studies employing animal models of dementia or in vitro neurodegeneration models of dementia pathology. In this chapter, we discuss the clinical and preclinical effects of these Kampo medicines and their putative mechanisms of actions, which have been demonstrated by our own research and other laboratories.

Key words Dementia, Animal models, Kampo therapy, Yokukansan, Chotosan, Kihi-to (kami-kihi-to), Molecular mechanism

1 Introduction

Dementia like Alzheimer's disease (AD) and vascular dementia (VaD) is one of the most problematic diseases that is characterized by neurological damages including neurodegeneration as well as by deterioration of learning/memory, cognitive and emotional functions, and ability to perform daily activities. This disease not only provides a huge impact on the person diagnosed and their family members but also becomes a rapidly increasing threat to public health because caring for people with AD or dementia needs a lot of tasks from family members and public healthcare services. Dementia is also becoming a global public health problem because the worldwide population is explosively growing and aging [1].

Akio Inui (ed.), *Herbal Medicines: New Horizons*, Methods in Pharmacology and Toxicology,
DOI 10.1007/978-1-4939-4002-8_12,

Based on these backgrounds, a number of scientists in academic institutions and pharmaceutical industries have been challenging to clarification of exact pathophysiology of dementias and exploration/development of innovative drugs effective for prevention and/or therapy of dementia. In terms of AD, more than 200 chemicals and several monoclonal antibodies targeting a β-amyloid cascade, a causal mechanism of AD [2, 3], have been developed and examined by clinical trials; however, none of them has become available for the treatment of dementia patients yet.

Lines of epidemiological studies indicate that various risk factors can lead to be AD and VaD, major causes of dementia. Those includes genetic/inherent factor and aging that cannot be controlled and the controllable and life style-related factors such as hypertension, hypercholesterolemia, diabetes (higher glucose levels), obesity, etc. [4–8]. Indeed, AD and/or VaD patients reportedly suffer from diabetes mellitus or have a higher blood glucose level and an insulin signaling deficit that may be associated with accumulation of the neurofibrillary tangles and β-amyloid plaques in AD [9, 10], suggesting a possible linkage of cerebrovascular disorder and diabetes mellitus to AD and VaD [11]. Therefore, it is very likely that the pathophysiological/pathogenic mechanism underlying dementia is more complicated than it was considered before [12]. Currently, two types of chemical drugs have been used as anti-AD and anti-VaD drugs [13–15]; one is acetylcholinesterase inhibitors such as donepezil, galantamine, and rivastigmine and the other memantine, an *N*-methyl-D-aspartate-type (NMDA) glutamate receptor antagonist. However, their clinical effects are very limited and are not curable. In some cases, the interventions with these chemicals are needed to be terminated because of their unpleasant side effects.

The limited availability of these antidementia drugs as well as of etiology and risk factors of dementia, application of traditional medicines, has been attracting a lot of interest in Kampo medicines and traditional Chinese medicines as an alternative and effective strategy for dementia therapy or prevention because of a couple of reasons. First, they consist of systematic combination of various crude drugs including multiple chemicals which may be able to interact with various factors implicated in the etiology of dementia. Second, they have been believed to exert less side effects compared to western chemicals drugs. On the basis of such anticipation, a number of researches have been focusing on exploration of interventions including traditional medicines like Kampo medicines (traditional Sino-Japanese medicines) that may be able to prevent or ameliorate AD and other dementias.

2 Kampo Medicine TreatmentKampo therapy of Dementia and Experimental Evidence for the Intervention

Several lines of clinical studies on dementia therapy with Kampo medicines (Table 1) have been conducted under protocols which were designed to provide higher levels of evidence such as randomized, double-blind, placebo-controlled clinical trials. The Kampo medicines has been shown to be beneficial mainly to behavioral and psychological symptoms of patients with dementia (BPSD) and some of them appear to be effective for cognitive function of dementia patients as well. There are also many preclinical studies elucidating potentials of Kampo medicines to ameliorate cognitive dysfunction in animal models of AD, VaD, and other cognitive/emotional dysfunction. The studies have substantiated the beneficial effects of Kampo medicines in patients with dementia and provided the underlying (putative) mechanisms of Kampo medicines as well. These clinical and preclinical studies allow us to consider a rational use of some Kampo medicines for the treatment of patients with dementia including AD and VaD. Here, we review the potential availabilities of yokukansan (YKS), chotosan (CTS), kihi-to and its conger formula, kami-kihi-to (KKT) as formulae with antidementia effects.

2.1 Yokukansan (YKS)

YKS is a Kampo medicine consisting of seven different crude herbal drugs (Table 1). In Kampo medicine or traditional Chinese medicine (TCM), YKS is generally prescribed for patients with weak physical constitution and "defect of Liver." In traditional medicine, "Liver" is believed to represent mood stabilization, autonomic nerve control, and storing of nutritious substance but is not the same as the liver meant in Western medicine. The therapeutic potential of YKS has been extensively investigated by intervention studies in which patients with AD and other types of dementia were subjected. Accumulated evidence including a meta-analysis study [16] indicates that YKS exerts beneficial effects particularly on BPSD. Readers should refer to the other article [17] and Chapter 13 in terms of YKS's alleviation of BPSD.

2.1.1 YKS-Induced Amelioration of Memory and Cognitive Dysfunction in Animal Models of Dementia

Compared with evidence for YKS amelioration of BPSD, effects of this formula on cognitive and learning/memory dysfunction, core symptoms of patients with dementia, have not been clearly reported in the clinical intervention studies. However, there are several preclinical studies demonstrating a potential of YKS to improve disturbance of learning/memory and cognitive performance in animal models of AD and other types of dementias. In the studies in which amyloid precursor protein (APP) transgenic mice expressing human form of APP685SWE were used as an animal model of AD [18, 19], the administration of YKS, at doses three to ten times

Table 1
Representative Kampo formulae candidates for antidementia therapy

	Yokukansan (YKS) (Yi-gan-san)	Chotosan (CTS) (Diaoteng San)	Kihito (Guipi tang) or Kami-kihito (KKT)[a] (Jia Wei Gupi Tang)	Hachimi-jio-gan (Ba Wei Di Huang Wan)
Pattern	Patients with weak physical constitution and "defect of Liver"	Middle-aged and elderly patients with weak physical constitution, "Blood stasis", "Qi deficiency", and "defect of Liver"	Patients with weak physical constitution, "Qi deficiency", "Blood deficiency", and cold syndrome	Patients with dry mouth or a tired feeling/edema/numbness in legs due to beriberi
Clinical effects	Improvement of insomniac and neurotic symptoms	Improvement of chronic headache, neck stiffness, dizziness, insomnia, or hypertension	Improvement of the gastric intestinal function and anemia. Improvement of falling asleep via attenuating anxiety and tension	Improvement of nephritis, diabetes, sciatic neuralgia, dysuria, pollakiuria, hypertension
Combination and ratio of crude drugs	*Atractylodis Lanceae Rhizoma* (4) *Hoelen* (4) *Uncariae Uncis cum Ramulus* (3) *Glycyrrhizae Radix* (1.5) *Cnidii Rhizoma* (3) *Angelicae Radix* (3) *Bupleuri Radix* (2)	*Ginseng Radix* (2) *Hoelen* (3) *Uncariae Uncis cum Ramulus* (3) *Glycyrrhizae Radix* (1) *Zingiberis Rhizome* (1) *Pinelliae Tuber* (3) *Ophiopogonis Tuber* (3) *Aurantii Nobilis pericarpium* (3) *Saposhnikoviae Radix* (2) *Chrysanthemi flos* (2) *Gypsum fibrosum* (5)	*Ginseng Radix* (3) *Hoelen* (3) *Atractylodis Lanceae Rhizoma* (3) *Glycyrrhizae Radix* (1) *Zingiberis Rhizome* (1.5) *Zizyphi Fructus* (2) *Zizyphi Spinosi Semen* (3) *Longanae Arillus* (3) *Polygalae Radix* (2) *Angelicae Radix* (2) *Astragali Radix* (3) *Saussureae Radix* (1) *Bupleuri Radix* (3) *Gardeniae Fructus* (2)	*Rehmanniae Radix* (steamed) (6) *Hoelen* (3) *Corni Fructus* (3) *Alismatis Rhizoma* (3) *Moutan Cortex* (2.5) *Cinnamomi Cortex* (1) *Aconiti Tuber* (processed) (0.5)

The number in each parenthesis indicates ratio of crude drug composition

[a]KKT but not kihito includes *Bupleuri Radix* and *Gardeniae Fructus* in its formula

more than the daily dose used for human therapy, for 5–10 months not only improved emotional and memory/cognitive deficits but also prevented β-amyloid accumulation. The ameliorative effects of YKS have also been observed in other animal models of dementia. Those include a mouse model of intracerebroventricular (i.c.v.) injection of β-amyloid [20], a thiamine-deficient model rat [21], and a mouse model of olfactory bulbectomy (OBX) [22].

A rat model of thiamine deficiency is known to exhibit selective neuronal loss, cholinergic dysfunction, amyloid precursor protein accumulation, and memory deficits, etc. [23]. Ikarashi et al. [21] found that the daily administration of YKS (500–1000 m/kg) attenuated memory disturbance observed in by thiamine-deficient rats. Olfactory bulbectomy is also known to cause neurodegeneration of septo-hippocampal cholinergic innervation [24], elevation of Aβ level in the brain [25], and increase in spontaneous locomotor activity susceptible to antidepressant treatment, therefore, providing an animal model of AD with depression-like emotional deficits [22, 26, 27]. Yamada et al. have demonstrated that the OBX-induced disruption of spatial (Fig. 1) and nonspatial working memory but not of the long-term fear memory was attenuated by YKS given at doses of 375–750 mg/kg which were in the range of 6–7-fold more than the daily dose for human therapy [22]. Together, these behavioral observations have led to the idea that YKS is able to exert beneficial effects on core symptoms of patients with dementia as well as on BPSD.

2.1.2 Putative Mechanisms Underlying YKS-Induced Amelioration of Cognition/Learning and Memory Deficits

Yamada et al. [22] have reported that the ameliorative effect of YKS on OBX-induced deficit in short-term memory can be reversed by scopolamine, an anticholinergic drug, suggesting possible involvement of central cholinergic mechanism(s) in the action of YKS. Their hypothesis was supported by the neurochemical findings that the administration of YKS reversed the expression levels of central cholinergic marker proteins which were down-regulated by OBX as well. Moreover, a rat model of thiamine deficiency has selective neuronal loss, cholinergic dysfunction, amyloid precursor protein accumulation, memory deficits, etc. [23]. Ikarashi et al. [21] found that the daily administration of YKS attenuated not only memory disturbance observed in thiamine-deficient rats but also degeneration of neuronal and astroglial cells caused by glutamate excitotoxicity resulting from thiamine deficiency. Based on these findings, they proposed the idea that inhibition of glutamate-mediated excitotoxicity is one of mechanisms underlying the antidementia effect of YKS.

There are several lines of in vitro studies clarifying the underlying mechanisms involved in the antidementia action of YKS. Fujiwara et al. [28] found that the extract from YKS had a potent antiaggregation effect on β-amyloid proteins and that the effect

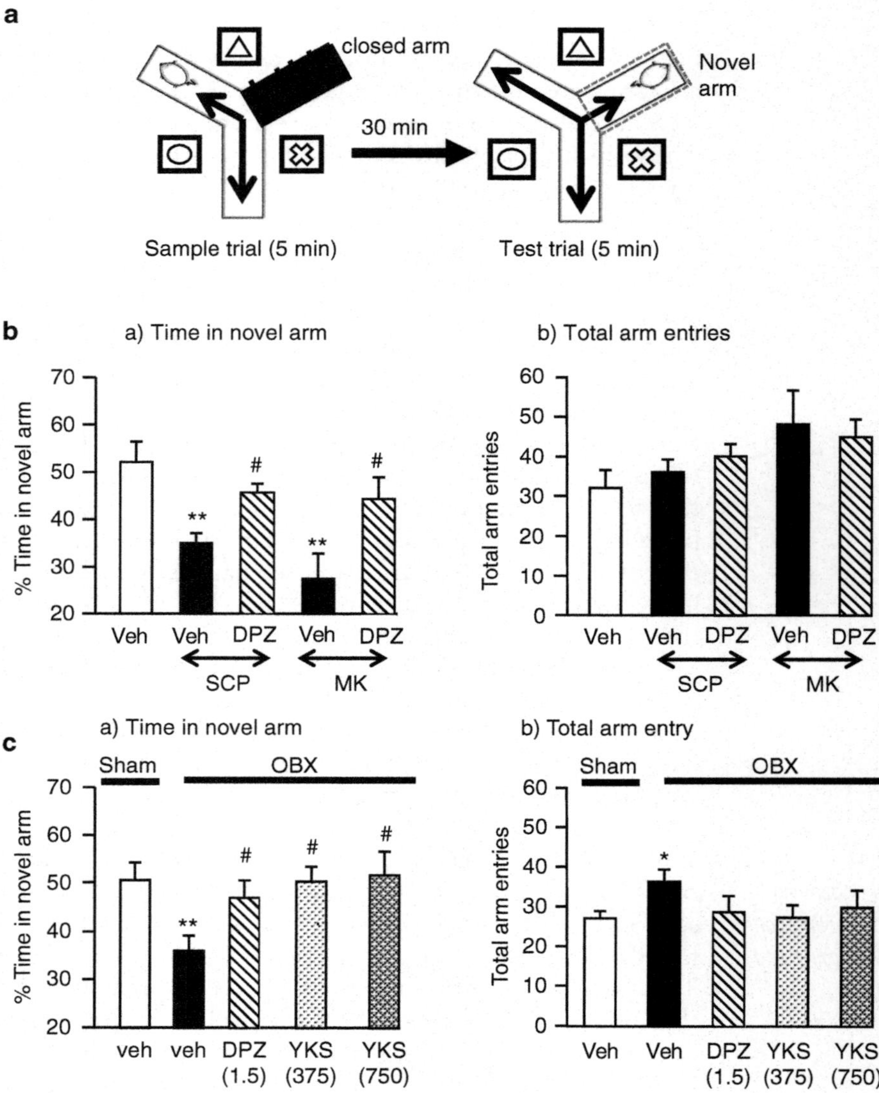

Fig. 1 OBX-induced spatial working memory deficit in the modified Y-maze test and its reversal by test drugs. (**a**) Schematic drawings of the Y-maze and the experimental procedure. The maze was surrounded by different spatial cues. The sample trial and test trials were conducted for 5 min at a 30-min interval as described in the text. (**b**) Evaluation of the modified Y-maze test using reference drugs, scopolamine (SCP), MK801 (MK), and donepezil (DPZ). Surgical operation-naïve mice were injected i.p. with vehicle (Veh) or DPZ (1.5 mg/kg) 60 min before the sample phase trial. Thirty min after DPZ, Veh, SCP (1 mg/kg, i.p.), or MK (0.2 mg/kg, i.p.) was given. The values in *parentheses* indicate the dose (mg/kg/day) of test drugs and each data column represents the mean $\pm$ S.E.M. ($n = 6$–8). **$P < 0.01$ compared with vehicle control group. #$P < 0.05$ compared with SCP or MK alone. (**c**) The effects of DPZ and YKS on OBX-induced spatial working memory deficit in the modified Y-maze test. The animals received daily administration of 375–750 mg/kg YKS from 3 days after OBX. Two weeks after the drug administration period, the modified Y-maze test was conducted as described in **a.** Each data column represents the mean $\pm$ S.E.M. ($n = 13$–17). **$P < 0.01$ compared with vehicle-treated sham group (*t*-test). #$P < 0.01$ compared with vehicle-treated OBX group (Student–Newman–Keuls test). Cited from Ref. [22] (Journal of Ethnopharmacology 135: 737–746, 2011)]

was mainly attributable to *Uncariae Uncis cum Ramulus*, an important component herb of YKS (Table 1). They suggested that YKS had a therapeutic/preventive potential for AD which might be due to *Uncariae Uncis cum Ramulus.*

YKS also appears to have a neuroprotective effect against Aβ oligomer- and glutamate-induced neurotoxicity in primary cultured rat cortical neurons [29] and PC12 cells [30, 31], respectively. According to Kannno et al. [29, 31], the effect of YKS is exhibited mainly via suppression of caspase-3 activity by *Uncariae Uncis cum Ramulus* and *Glycyrrhiza Radix* in cultured neurons, whereas, in PC12 cells, the effect is exhibited via activation of glutamate transport and cysteine/glutamate antiporter system Xc^- by *Uncaria*-derived alkaloids such as geissoschizine methyl ether and hirsuteine'. An important role of *Uncariae Uncis cum Ramulus* in the action of YKS observed in in vivo and in vitro studies is true of the effects of chotosan (CTS) [32–35], a Kampo formula including the same plant as an herbal component. The pharmacological profile of this plant is overviewed in detail in the following section of this chapter.

2.2 Chotosan (CTS)

2.2.1 Clinical Findings

CTS is a Kampo formulaChotosan (CTS), the clinical interventions of which have been conducted in patients with AD or VaD or both. This formula consists of 11 different crude drugs (Table 1) including *Uncariae Uncis cum Ramulus.* In Kampo medicine, CTS is mainly prescribed for patients with "Blood stasis," "Qi deficiency," and "defect of Liver." In the concept of Kampo medicine and TCM, "Blood" is considered to be nutritious materials composing human body as well as the blood defined in Western medicine, while "Qi" is invisible and ever-flowing energy of life [17]. The concept of "Liver" is stated in the previous section concerning YKS. In clinic, CTS is generally prescribed for middle-age and/or elderly patients with weak physical constitution and symptoms related to hypertension and chronic headache (Table 12.1).

Based on the clinical features of CTS in Kampo medicine or TCM, Terasawa et al. [36] conducted a double-blind, randomized placebo-controlled study in 1997 in which patients with VaD were subjected to daily administration of CTS (7.5 g/day) over 12 weeks. In this intervention study, CTS showed a potential to improve BPSD and impaired activities of daily living in VaD patients, suggesting usefulness of CTS in the treatment of patients with dementia, particularly BPSD.

Two other groups also independently reported the effects of CTS on the core symptoms in patients with dementia including VaD, AD, or both. In a clinical study where chronic stroke patients with mild cognitive impairments were subjected, Yamaguchi et al. [37] analyzed cognitive function of the patients by recording P3 event-related brain potentials, the mini mental state examination (MMSE)Mini mental state examination (MMSE), and verbal fluency test. They found that the administration of CTS (7.5 g/kg per day) over a 12-week period significantly improved both neuropsychological test scores and electrophysiological indices related to attention and decision making. Moreover, in a double-blind, randomized, placebo-controlled study where AD and VaD patients were subjected to CTS treatment, Suzuki et al. [38] found that cognitive functions and daily living activities are improved in the group treated with CTS, whereas no improvement was observed in the groups treated with placebo or gosya-jinki-gan (Niu-Che-Shen-Qi-Wan in TCM), a Kampo formula with different clinical indications and crude drug composition. Taken together, the available clinical data allow us to consider that CTS is useful for the treatment of core symptoms of dementia patients as well and that the ameliorative effect of CTS on cognitive function may represent one of distinctive pharmacological and clinical features of this formula [17].

2.2.2 CTS-induced Amelioration of Cognitive Dysfunction and Its Mechanism in Animal Models of Dementia

CTS is one of the Kampo formulae that have been reported to exhibit ameliorative or preventive effects on learning and memory deficits in various animal models of cognitive dysfunction. The reported findings are likely to support the clinical utilities of CTS in therapy of dementia patients.

The effects of CTS on cognitive function have been first reported by Yuzurihara et al. [39]. In their study employing mice with transient cerebral ischemia (T2VO) as a model of VaD, the postischemic treatment with CTS extract (0.5–2 g/kg per day) for 7 days improved the impaired memory performance in the passive avoidance test in a manner that was reversed by a serotonin (5-HT)$_{1A}$ receptor antagonist. Their findings suggested the involvement of serotonergic mechanism(s) in the action of CTS. On the other hand, our group reported that a single administration of CTS extract, at doses (375–750 mg/kg per day, p.o.) which were equivalent to about 10–30 times more than the daily dose for human therapy, prevented T2VO-induced spatial cognitive deficits in a manner that could be reversed by a muscarinic M_1 receptor antagonist but not by a nicotinic receptor antagonist [34]. Moreover, in a mouse model of permanent occlusion of common carotid arteries (P2VO), the daily administration of CTS (750 mg/kg per day, p.o.) post P2VO also improved spatial and nonspatial cognitive deficits (Fig. 2) caused by P2VO and the amelioration of cognitive performance was abolished by withdrawal of CTS administration as well as by treatment with a muscarinic M_1 receptor antagonist [35]. These findings suggest that the effect of CTS is reversible and is in part mediated by central cholinergic systems. Moreover, as in the case of YKS, *Uncariae Uncis cum Ramulus*, a major and distinctive herbal constituent of CTS, is likely to play a key role in the anti-dementia effect of CTS because the *Uncariae* extract but not the *Uncaria*-free CTS extract could improve cognitive dysfunction in the T2VO and P2VO animals when given at doses equivalent to the effective doses of CTS [34, 35].

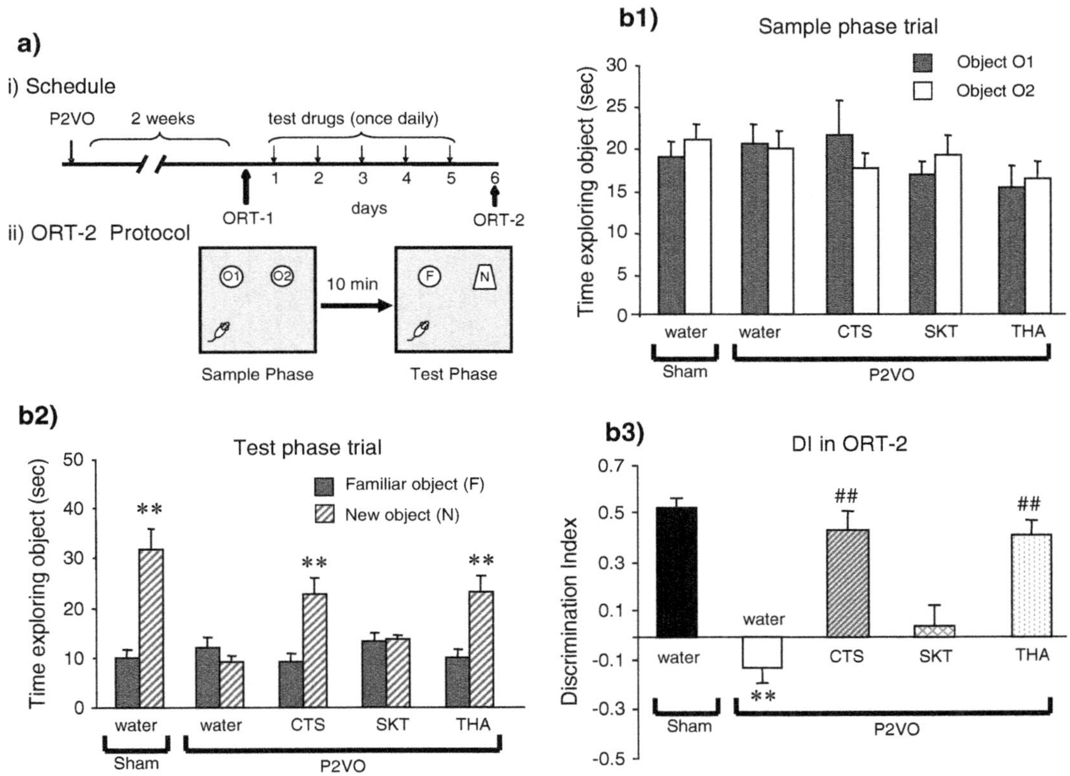

Fig. 2 Effects of CTS, SKT, and THA on P2VO-induced object recognition deficit in mice. (**a**) Experimental schedule (i) and representation of sample and test phase conditions in the second object recognition test (ORT-2) (ii). The P2VO mice were randomly divided into four groups after the ORT-1. They received water, CTS (750 mg/kg), SKT (750 mg/kg), or THA (2.5 mg/ kg) daily for 5 consecutive days. The sham-operated group was given water. The second object recognition test (ORT-2) was conducted on day 6. Each datum represents the mean ± S.E.M. (10–12 mice per group). (**b1**) Object recognition performance in the sample phase trial of the ORT-2. The animal was placed into the arena where two identical sample objects made of glass were placed in two adjacent corners of the arena and was allowed to explore for 5 min. The time animals spent exploring the objects were measured. (**b2**) Object recognition performance in the test phase trials conducted 10 min after the sample trials. The time animals spent exploring each object was measured during a 5-min observation period. $^{**}P < 0.01$ vs. the time spent exploring a familiar object. (**b3**) Discrimination index (DI) in the ORT-2. $^{**}P < 0.01$ vs. vehicle-treated sham-operated group. $^{\#\#}P < 0.01$ vs. vehicle-treated P2VO group. Cited from Ref. [46] Fig. 2, J Pharmacol Sci 103, 360–373, 2007

The antidementia effects and the underlying mechanism(s) of CTS have also been elucidated by preclinical studies in which employed animal models of aging/AD [40] and diabetes mellitus, risk factors for AD and VaD [9, 11, 41, 42]. Zhao et al. [43, 44] examined the therapeutic potentials of CTS for aging- and type 2 diabetes-induced decline of cognitive function in senescence accelerated prone mouse SAMP8 and C57BLKS/J-*db/db* mice, respectively. They demonstrated using several types of learning and memory tasks that daily administration of CTS extract (750 mg/kg per day, p.o.) for about 6–7 weeks improved spatial and nonspatial

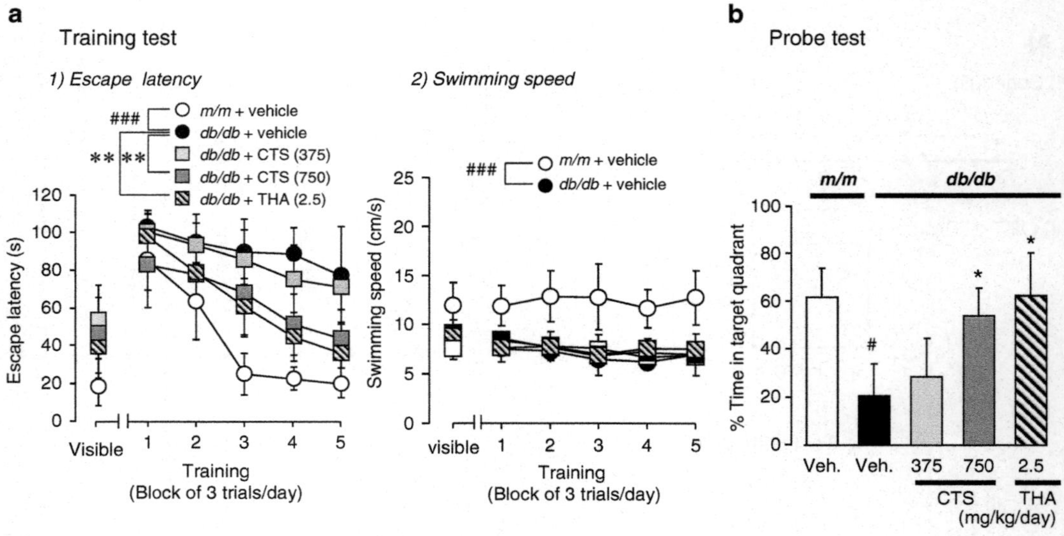

Fig. 3 Effects of CTS and THA on water maze performance of *db/db* mice. Learning performance of the animals was analyzed in the training test by latency (**a**) and swimming speed (**b**). Each data point indicates the mean ± S.D. for 6–9 animals in each group. ###$P < 0.001$ vs. vehicle-treated m/m group, and **$P < 0.01$ vs. vehicle-treated db/db group (one-way repeated measures ANOVA). Memory retrieval performance (D) elucidated in the probe test. Each datum represents the mean of time spent in the target quadrant ± S.D. ###$P < 0.001$ vs. vehicle-treated m/m group (*t*-test). *$P < 0.05$ vs. respective vehicle-treated *db/db* group (one-way repeated measure ANOVA followed by Tukey test). [Ref. [44], BMC Complement Altern Med 12: 188, 2012]

cognitive disturbance caused by aging [43] and diabetes (Fig. 3) [44]. Interestingly, they excluded the possibility that the ameliorative effect of CTS on diabetes-induced cognitive dysfunction is apparently due to the antidiabetic effect of this formula since the administration of CTS failed to reduce serum glucose levels or body weights in an animal model of type 2 diabetes [44]. This idea seemed to be applicable to a type 1 diabetes since the administration of CTS could improve cognitive deficits observed in type 1 diabetes model of streptozotocin-treated rats without affecting their serum glucose levels [45]. These preclinical studies employing animal models especially relevant to risk factors of dementia support the clinical data concerning the beneficial effects exhibited by CTS in the treatment of patients with AD or VD or both.

2.2.3 Molecular Biological Evidence for the Antidementia Effects of CTS

Several lines of neurochemical findings have provided evidence for the ameliorative effects of CTS on impaired cognitive function in animal models of dementia.

1. Cholinergic systems

   The central cholinergic system is a major mechanism responsible for cognitive function and learning and memory and deterioration of this mechanism is considered to be a major cause of the core symptom of patients with dementia. Therefore, improvement of cholinergic dysfunction has been an effective strategy for dementia therapy in not only AD but also VaD patients [15].

In animal models of VaD; i.e., T2VO and P2VO mice [34, 35], acetylcholine levels in the cerebral cortex and hippocampus were reduced compared to the sham-operated control groups and the decreased levels were attenuated in the groups treated with CTS as well as with tacrine. These neurochemical results accounted for the behavioral studies in which the anti-dementia effects of CTS were abolished by muscarinic acetylcholine receptor antagonists and suggested an involvement of central cholinergic systems in the effect of CTS. Moreover, we found that the expression levels of genes coding cholinergic marker proteins (choline acetyltransferase (ChAT) and M_3 and M_5 muscarinic receptor subtypes) in the brain were down-regulated in P2VO model mice and that these changes were prevented in the groups treated with the daily administration of CTS and tacrine [46]. These findings allowed us to infer that enhancement of cholinergic function is likely to prevent or rescue central cholinergic systems from ischemic damage. Since, in our ex vivo experiments, the daily administration of tacrine (2.5 mg/kg, i.p.) but not of CTS (750 mg/kg per day, p.o.) for 6 days significantly inhibited the activity of cholinesterase in the brain tissue; CTS may improve dysfunction of central cholinergic systems in animal models of dementia by a mechanism(s) differing from that of tacrine [46].

Dysfunction of central cholinergic systems has also been reported in animal models of diabetes [44, 47–49]. Zhao et al. found [50] that the expression levels of cholinergic marker proteins, ChAT and muscarinic receptors, in the hippocampus (Fig. 4) and the ChAT-immunopositive neurons in the medial septum and basal forebrain, nuclei origins of cholinergic systems, are decreased in 18-week-old *db/db* mice than in the age-matched nondiabetic *m/m* mice, whereas no difference in ChAT-immunopositive neurons was found at the age of 7 weeks. Their findings suggested aging-dependent occurrence of cholinergic dysfunction in the brain which may be accelerated by diabetes [44, 50]. Moreover, the down-regulation of cholinergic marker proteins expression and decrease of the septal cholinergic neurons were prevented in the *db/db* mice treated daily with CTS (375–750 mg/kg per day, p.o.) from the age of 7 weeks [44]. Therefore, CTS-induced amelioration of cognitive deficits in diabetic animals may be in part attributable to suppression of neurodegeneration of central cholinergic systems which was accelerated by diabetes.

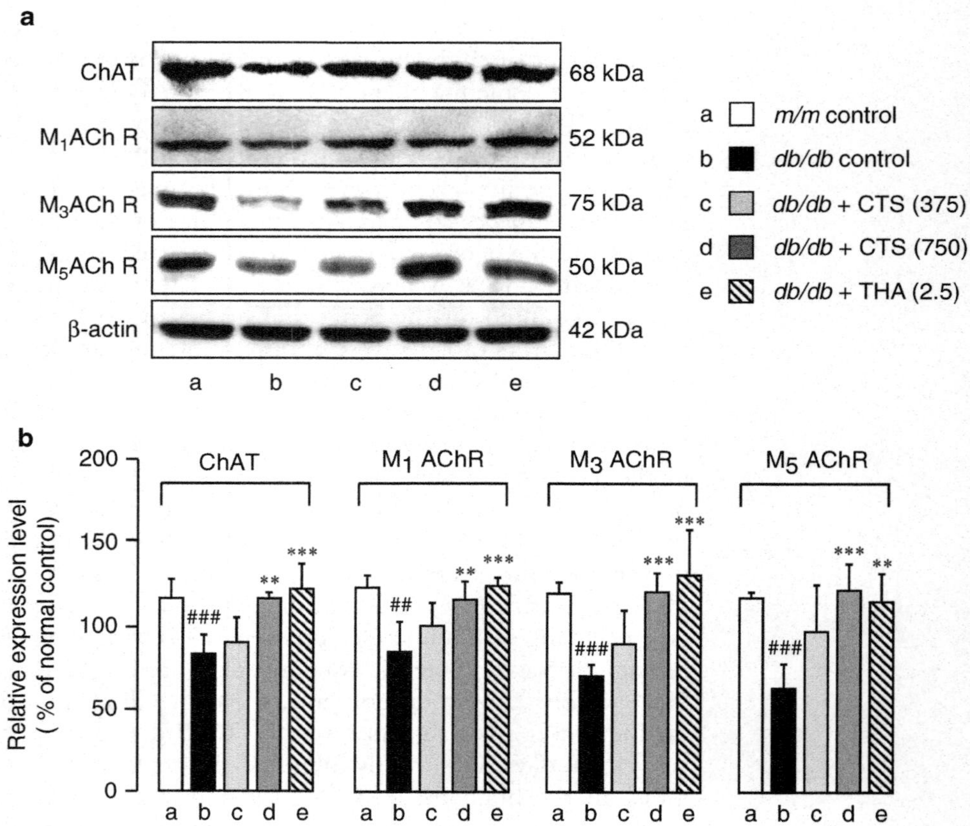

Fig. 4 Effects of CTS and THA on ChAT, M1, M3, and M5 receptor protein expression in the hippocampus of db/db mouse. (**a**)Typical photos indicating the expression levels of each factor in the hippocampus of vehicle-treated m/m (*lane a*), and vehicle (*lane b*)-, CTS (325 mg/kg per day: *lane c*; 750 mg/kg per day: *lane d*)-, and THA (2.5 mg/kg per day; *lane e*)-treated db/db mice. (**b**) Quantitative comparisons of each factor among different animal groups were conducted as described in the text. The data are expressed as the percentage of the value obtained from naïve control m/m mice. Each data column represents the mean ± S.D. obtained from 5 to 6 brain samples. ##$P < 0.01$, ###$P < 0.01$ vs. vehicle treated m/m group (Student's *t*-test). **$P < 0.01$, ***$P < 0.001$ vs. respective vehicle-treated db/db group (one-way ANOVA followed by Tukey test). [Ref. [44], BMC Complement Altern Med 12: 188, 2012]

2. Neuroplasticity-related neuronal signaling
   A glutamatergic system including *N*-methyl-D-aspartate receptor (NMDAR) function is one of the neuronal bases of learning and memory [51]. Stimulation of this system triggers neurosignaling process linked to phosphorylation of some key proteins such as NMDAR, calmodulin-dependent protein kinase II (CAMKII), and cAMP response element-binding protein (CREB) and production of brain-derived neurotrophic factor (BDNF) and thereby plays a role in neuronal plasticity, an important molecular mechanism underlying learning and memory [52–54]. Improvement of neuroplasticity-related

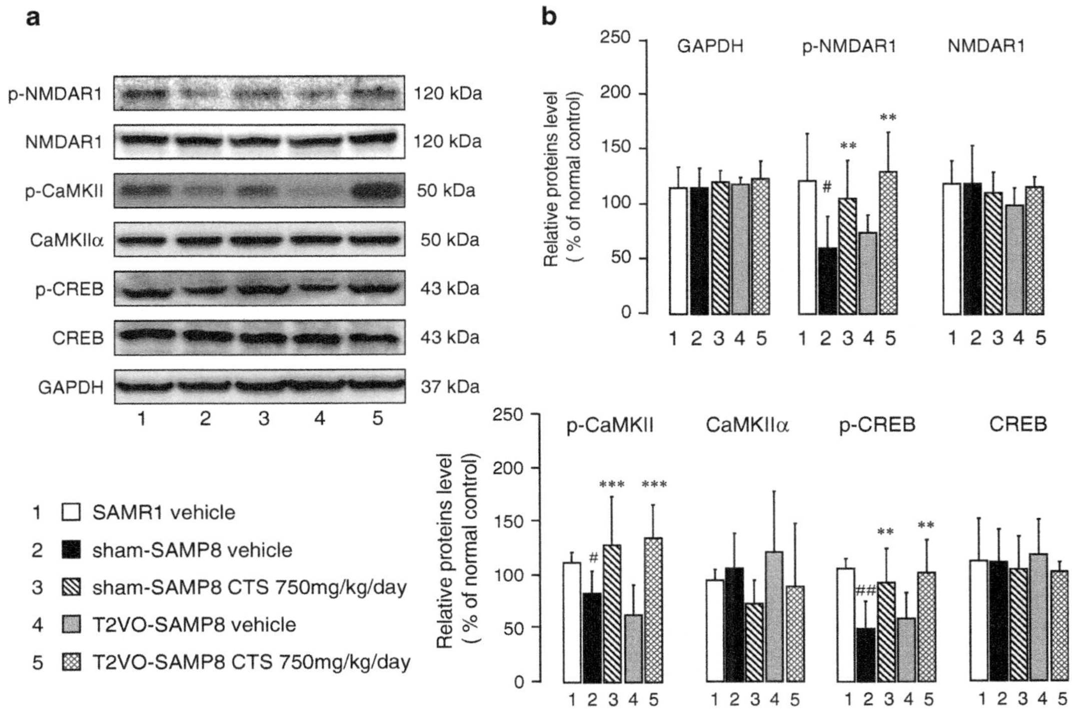

Fig. 5 Effects of CTS on expression levels of p-NMDAR1, NMDAR1, p-CaMKII, CaMKIIα, p-CREB, CREB, and GAPDH in the cerebral cortex of SAMP8 with and without ischemic insult. (**a**) Typical photos indicating the expression levels of each factor in the cerebral cortex of vehicle-treated SAMR1 control (*lane 1*), vehicle-treated sham-SAMP8 (*lane 2*), CTS (750 mg/kg/day)-treated sham-SAMP8 (*lane 3*), vehicle-treated T2VO-SAMP8 (*lane 4*), and CTS-treated T2VO-SAMP8 group (*lane 5*). After completing the behavioral studies, the animals were decapitated and proteins were extracted from the cerebral cortices in each animal group. (**b**) Quantitative comparisons of CTS-induced changes in expression levels of each parker proteins in the cerebral cortex of SAMP8 with and without are chemic insult. The data are expressed as the percentage of the value obtained from naïve control SAMR1 mice. Each data column represents the mean ± SD obtained from 4 to 5 brain samples. #$P < 0.05$ or ##$P < 0.01$ vs. compared with vehicle-treated SAMR1 group (*t*-test). ***$P < 0.001$, **$P < 0.01$ vs. respective vehicle-treated sham- or T2VO-SAMP8 group (two-way ANOVA). Cited from Ref. [43]

signaling systems by CTS has been proposed to be evidence for the ameliorative effects of this formula on cognitive dysfunction in animal models of dementia (Fig. 5). Indeed, the SAMP8 at the age of 22 weeks or older had reduced levels of p-NMDAR1, p-CaMKII, p-CREB, and BDNF in the cortex compared to the age-matched control strain SAMR1 or 8-week-old young SAMP8, suggesting that these changes contribute to aging-induced cognitive dysfunction [43, 48]. Importantly, the daily administration of CTS (750 mg/kg per day, p.o.) and tacrine reversed the reduced expression levels of these neuroplasticity-related signaling proteins in the SAMP8 group [43], providing molecular biological evidence for the potential of CTS to improve cognitive function in an animal model of dementia.

3. Vascular endothelial growth factor (VEGF)/platelet-derived growth factor (PDGF) systems
VEGF and PDGF systems are likely to be one of targets for antidementia effects of CTS [43, 44, 48]. VEGF is a hypoxia-inducible secreted signaling molecule which activates receptor tyrosine kinases such as VEGFR2 expressed on endothelial cells to promote angiogenesis, proliferation, and migration of endothelial cells [55]. The VEGF/VEGFR2 systems are expressed in neurons, astrocytes, and neural progenitor cells [56] as well and are involved in reducing neurological deficits during stroke recovery [57, 58]. VEGF reportedly elevates intracellular Ca^{2+}, activates CaMKII, and potentiates long-term potentiation [59] in the hippocampal neurons and also protects hippocampal neurons against hypoxic damage via activating the phosphatidylinositol 3-kinase (PI3-K) signaling pathway [60]. Similarly, PDGF-A and -B and their receptors (PDGFRα and PDGFRβ) play a variety of roles in the brain such as proliferation, migration, and differentiation of oligodendrocytes, neurite outgrowth [61], and neuroprotection [62]. On the basis of a beneficial effect of CTS reported in dementia patients as well as of the CTS-applicable pattern in Kampo medicine (Table 1), Zhao et al. [43, 48] elucidated the effects of CTS on the VEGF/PDGF systems in the brain. They found that the expression levels of VEGF and VEGFR2 and PDGF and PDGFRα in the brain were decreased in an aging mouse model of SAMP8 with and without transient cerebral ischemia, and that the daily administration of CTS reversed the down-regulated expression of these factors at the same doses which improved the cognitive performance of this model [43].
Susceptibility of the hippocampal VEGF/PDGF systems to CTS is also found in *db/db* mice, a type 2 diabetes model [44]. Indeed, *db/db* mice with impaired cognitive function showed down-regulated expression levels of VEGF, VEGFR2, PDGF, PDGFRα, and phosphorylated-Akt in the hippocampus compared with a nondiabetic control and these neurochemical alterations were attenuated by the daily administrations of CTS and tacrine [44]. The molecular mechanism underlying the effects of CTS and tacrine modulate is unclear. However, in an in vitro study using the organotypic hippocampal slice culture systems, we suggested that the muscarinic receptor function was partly linked to VEGF-VEGFR2 signaling involved in protection of hippocampal cells from excitotoxicity-induced damage [63, 64]. Therefore, the facilitatory effects of CTS on central cholinergic systems allow us to speculate that the linkage between cholinergic and VEGF systems in the brain may be at least responsible for the behavioral and neurochemical actions of CTS in animal models of dementia.

4. Herbal components and chemical constituents which may account for antidementia effect of CTS

   Uncaria rhynchophylla (Miq.) Jacks is one of the major herbal components of CTS that characterize the clinical effects of this formula in Kampo medicine and TCM. Indeed, CTS is termed originally from the Chinese name of this plant. Lines of pharmacological studies have demonstrated an important role of this plant in the pharmacological action of CTS including an antidementia effect. For instance, the *Uncaria* extract but not the *Uncaria*-free CTS mimicked apparently the effect of CTS on spatial cognitive dysfunction observed in animal models of VaD [34, 35]. Moreover, in vitro electrophysiological studies conducted in our laboratory [32, 33] demonstrated that rhynchophylline and isorhynchophylline, alkaloid components of *Uncaria*, can act as noncompetitive NMDA receptor antagonists and exert neuroprotective actions against oxygen and glucose deprivation-induced neuronal damage in the hippocampus. It has been confirmed by a recent metabonomic study [65] that major Uncaria alkaloid components including rhynchophylline and isorhynchophylline can be transported to the central nervous system after the systemic administration of CTS.

   This crude drug is also likely to play an important role in the antidementia effect of CTS in AD patients as well as in an animal model of AD. Fujiwara et al. [28] demonstrated that the *Uncaria* extract had a potent antiaggregation effect on β-amyloid protein in in vitro, suggesting that *Uncaria rhynchophylla* has inhibitory effects on the regulation of Aβ and is able to prevent and/or cure AD. Since this crude drug is an important herbal component in CTS and YKS, these in vitro studies suggest at least significance of this plant in the beneficial action of CTS (and probably YKS) in amelioration of cognitive and emotional dysfunction in dementia patients.

   Citrus Unshiu Peel is also an herbal component of CTS which is likely to have a potential antidementia effect in an animal model of AD. A chemical feature of this plant is to contain methoxy-flavone compounds such as nobiletin. Evidence indicates that the systemic administration of nobiletin can ameliorate deficits in learning and cognitive performance caused in a transgenic mouse model of AD [66] as well as in other AD models such as an acute intracerebroventricular (i.c.v.) injection model of Aβ [67]. In these models, nobiletin suppressed amyloidosis and reversing Aβ-induced inhibition of CREB phosphorylation and CRE-mediated transcription. Interestingly, the extract from a nobiletin-rich *Citrus Unshiu* Peel (designated N-Chinpi) reportedly facilitates CRE-mediated transcription in culture hippocampal neurons more potently than the standard *Citrus Unshiu* Peel extract [68].

5. Biomolecules susceptible to CTS treatment
   To clarify biomolecules susceptible to CTS, in in vivo, we have conducted a metabonomic analysis of CTS in *db/db* type 2 diabetic mice and *m/m* nondiabetic control mice [65]. In this study, blood and brain tissue samples were obtained from the animals which had previously received the administration of either vehicle water or the CTS extract for 20 days, and then, subjected to high performance liquid chromatography equipped with an orbitrap hybrid Fourier transform mass spectrometer. The levels of 59 chemicals in the plasma and 13 chemicals in the brain were found to be affected in only the db/db group treated with CTS. Their analysis revealed that CTS affected four major metabolic pathways in in vivo: purine, tryptophan, cysteine, and methionine, and glycerophospholipids in *db/db* mice and that glycerophosphocholine (GPC) Glycerophosphocholine (GPC) levels in the plasma and brain were significantly elevated in the CTS-treated *db/db* mice (Fig. 6) [65]. They suggested GPC as a putative biomolecule responsible for the tacrine-like antidementia effect of CTS in diabetic mice, since GPC exhibited a neuroprotective action against excitotoxicity-induced hippocampal cell damage in a manner that was reversed by a muscarinic receptor antagonist (Fig. 7) [65].

2.3 Kihi-to and Kami-kihi-to

Kihi-to and kami-kihi-to (KKT) are Kampo formulae consisting of 12 and 14 crude drugs, respectively, with a constant ratio of each herbal component (Table 1). A major difference between these two formulae is that kami-kihito contains two crude drugs, *Bupleurum falcatum* and *Gardenia jasminoides*, more than kihi-to. Based on TCM- and Kampo-based diagnosis, these formulae are generally prescribed for patients with weak constitution, deficiency of visible and ever-flowing energy of life (Qi deficiency), and insufficient nutritious material composing human body and the blood (Blood deficiency), expecting improvement of symptoms such as insomnia, anemia, amnesia, depression, and neurosis. On the basis of such clinical features in TCM and Kampo medicine, the antidementia effects of kihi-to and KKT have been investigated using several animal models of dementia.

2.3.1 Effects on Aging- and Cholinergic Dysfunction-induced Deficits in Cognitive Function and Learning/Memory

The ameliorative effects of KKT on cognitive/learning dysfunction were first reported by Nishizawa et al. [69], although the effects have not yet been confirmed by clinical intervention studies with a high evidence level. They employed SAMP8 mice as animal models of aging and SAMR1 as control normal animals and demonstrated that the repeated administration of 8 % KKT extract as diet improved learning performance of SAMP8 but not SAMR1 in the passive and conditioned avoidance tests. The ameliorative effect has

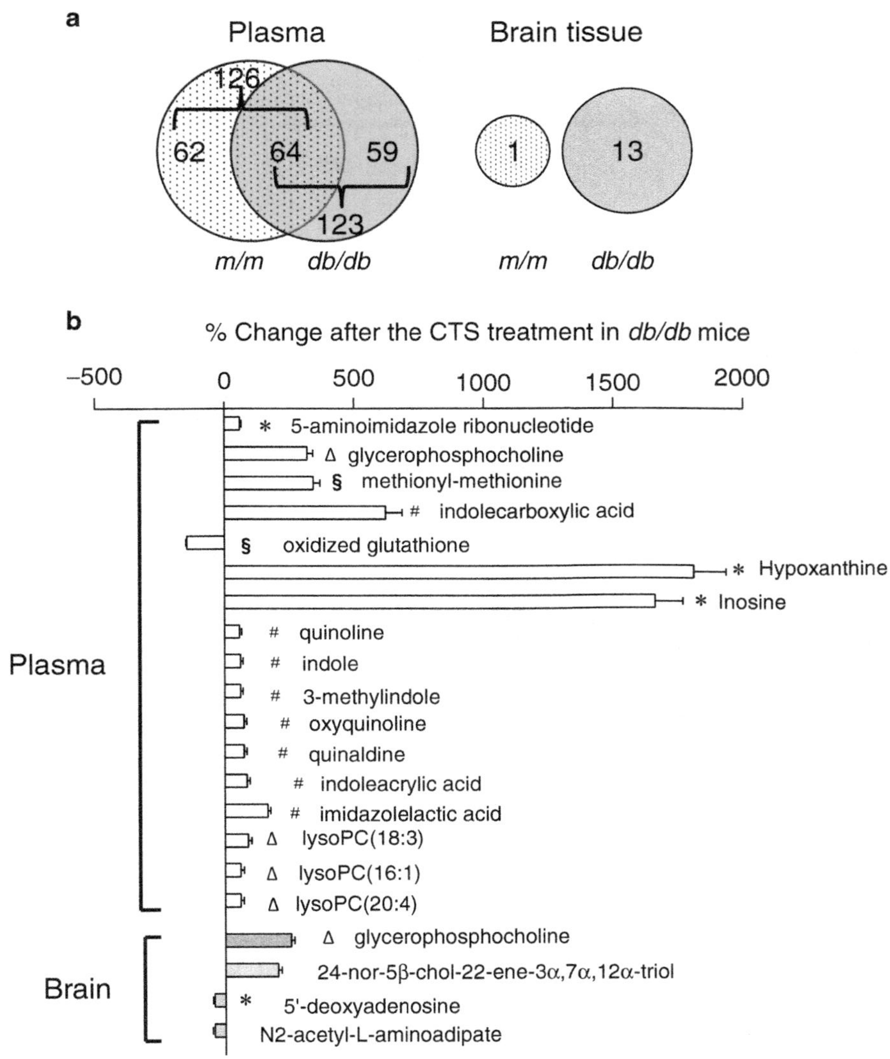

Fig. 6 Differential expression analysis of endogenous chemicals responsive to the CTS treatment in the plasma and brain tissues of m/m and *db/db* mice. (**a**) Summary of CTS-induced changes in the levels of endogenous chemicals in the plasma and brain tissue samples of *m/m* and *db/db* mice. In the plasma, 126 and 123 chemicals in the *m/m* and *db/db* groups, respectively, showed significant changes in their levels after the administration of CTS, and 64 chemicals were detected in both groups. In brain tissues, 1 and 13 chemicals showed significant changes in their or its level after the CTS treatment. (**b**) Extent of CTS-induced changes in the levels of the identified endogenous chemicals in the plasma and brain tissue samples of *db/db* mice. Each data column represents percentage changes from the levels detected in the vehicle-treated group. Asterisks: *, #, §, and Δ, represent metabolic pathways for purine, tryptophan, cysteine/methionine, and glycerophospholipids, respectively. Each data column represents the mean ± S.D. ($n = 6$). Cited from Ref. [65]

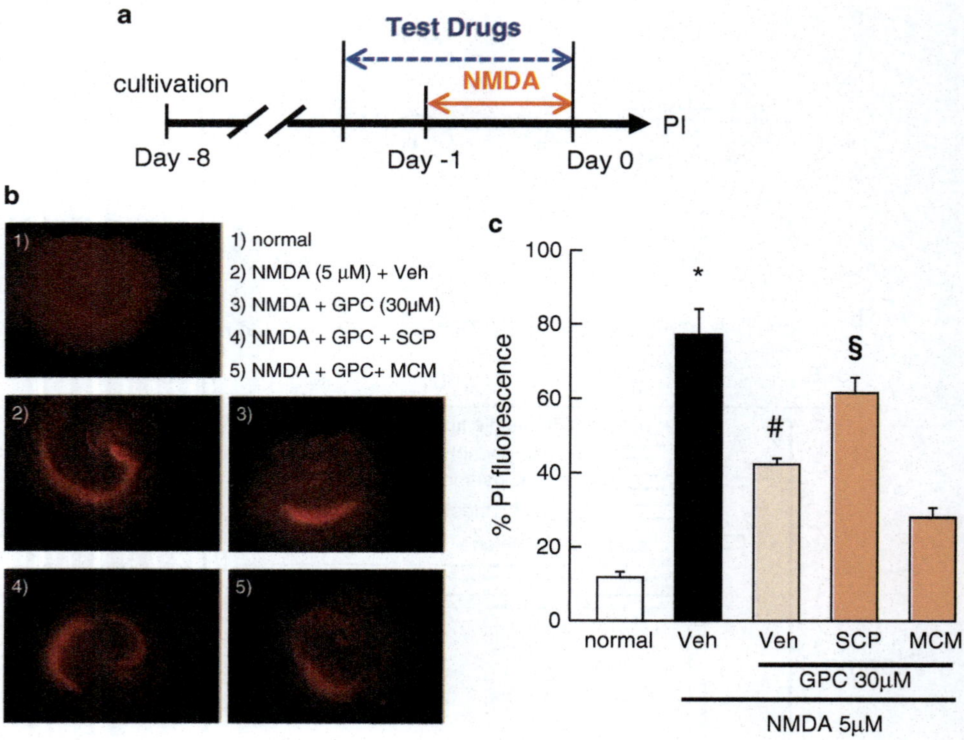

Fig. 7 Possible involvement of endogenous acetylcholine in the protective effects of glycerophosphocholine (GPC) on NMDA-induced hippocampal cell damage. (**a**) Experimental schedule. (**b**) Typical propidium iodide (PI) staining images of NMDA-induced hippocampal cell damage in OHSCs treated with the test drugs. (**c**) The effects of scopolamine and mecamylamine on the GPC-mediated suppression of 5 μM NMDA-induced cell damage. Either scopolamine (SCP: 30 μM) or mecamylamine (MCM: 30 μM) was added together with 30 μM GPC 30 min before the 5 μM NMDA treatment. Each data column represents the mean ± S.E.M. ($n = 4$). $^{*}P < 0.05$ compared with normal slice preparations. $\#P < 0.05$ compared with NMDA alone. Cited from Ref. [65]

been confirmed by other studies in which aged rats or a scopolamine model of memory deficits was employed as an animal model of dementia [70, 71]. In these studies, KKT ameliorated not only cognitive/learning performance impaired by scopolamine but also the dysfunction of central cholinergic systems caused by aging, suggesting that KKT is useful for the treatment of senile dementia.

2.3.2 Animal Models of AD

The antidementia effects of KKT and kihi-to, a basic formula of KKT (Table 1), have also been elucidated using an acute Aβ toxicity model mouse or a transgenic mouse model of AD mouse. In the study where reported by Tohda C and her colleagues [72], mice were subjected to the i.c.v. injection of $A\beta_{2-35}$ and then administered kihi-to extract daily at a dose of 100 mg/kg (p.o.) for

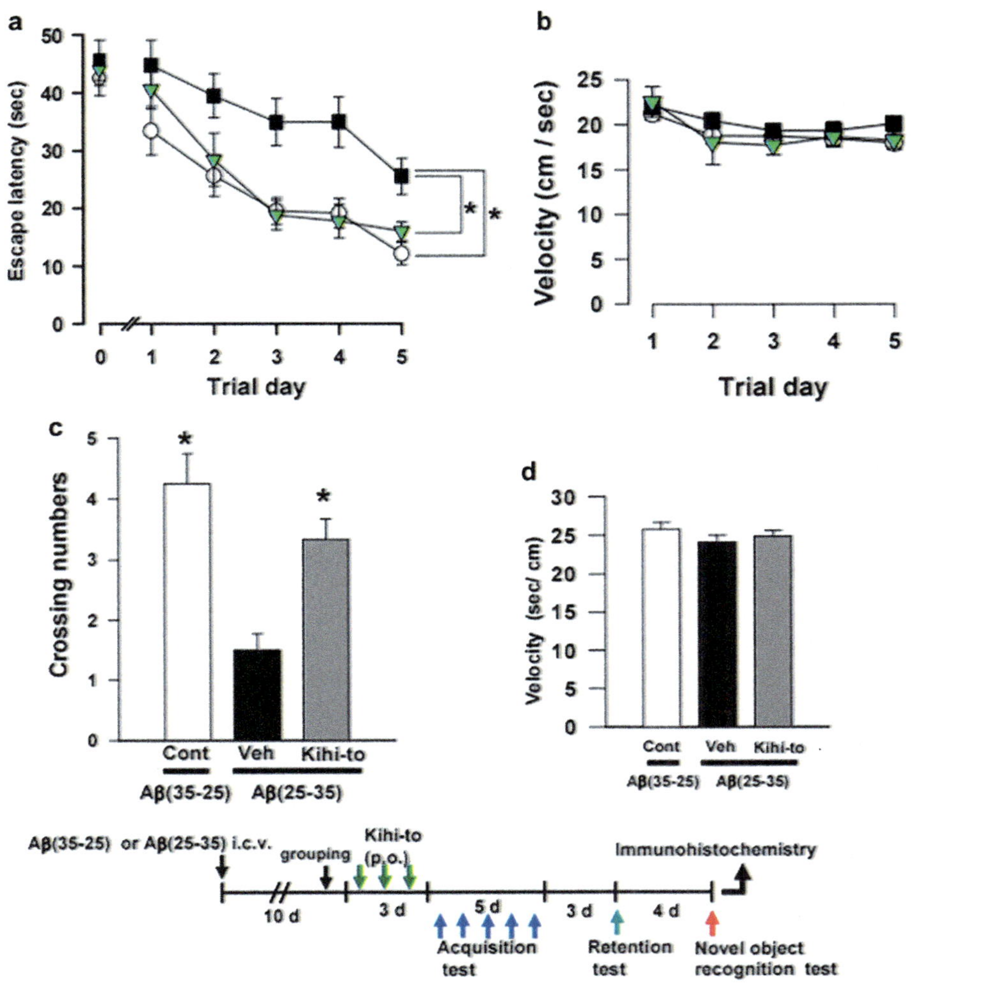

Fig. 8 Effects of Kihi-to on Aβ(25–35)-induced spatial memory deficits. Aβ(25–35) (25 nmol) was injected into the right lateral ventricle of mice. From ten days after the injection, mice were administered vehicle (Veh, water by p.o.; DMSO by i.v., $n = 10$; *squares*) or Kihi-to (100 mg/kg B.W., p.o., $n = 9$; *triangles*) for 3 days. The control mice (Cont, $n = 8$; *circles*) were injected with a reverse peptide, Aβ(35–25), and then administered vehicle. After that, memory acquisition tests were continued for 5 days in a Morris water maze (**a**). Escape latencies to a hidden platform were measured. Three days after the last trial of the memory acquisition test, the memory retention test was performed (**c**). The number of crossings over the position at which the platform had been located was measured for 60 s. Swimming velocities of mice in the memory acquisition test (**b**) and the retention test (**d**) are shown. $^*p < 0.05$ vs. Veh. (**a** Repeated measures two-way ANOVA followed by Holm-Sidak post hoc test, **c** one-way ANOVA followed by Holm-Sidak post hoc test). Cited from Ref. [72]

consecutive 3 days before the behavioral and neurochemical experiments. According to their results, the administration of kihi-to significantly attenuated $A\beta_{2-35}$-induced cognitive dysfunction (Fig. 8) as well as $A\beta_{2-35}$-induced loss of neurites and synapses in the brain even 2 weeks after the administration was discontinued.

The antidementia effect of KKT has also been confirmed by Tohda's group using a transgenic AD model of 5XFAD mice. They found that the administration of KKT at a daily dose of 200 mg/kg/day [73] or 500 mg/kg/day (p.o.) [74] for 15 days also improved memory deficits in the transgenic AD mice and restore degenerated axons and synapses in the brain. Moreover, in their in vitro study using primary neuronal cell cultures, KKT reversed Aβ-induced progression of tau phosphorylation and axon atrophy [74]. These findings, therefore, raise the possibility that kihi-to and kihi-to-based formula, KKT, can exert an ameliorative effect on cognitive and neurological dysfunction in patents with AD. However, it is still unclear about which chemical constituents in kihi-to or KKT are responsible for their antidementia effects. Moreover, it remains to be clarified whether central cholinergic systems are involved in the effects of these formulae in the animal models of AD because recently it was reported that the cholinergic systems play an important role in regulation of Aβ biosynthesis as well as of Aβ-induced neurodegeneration [75, 76]. Nevertheless, kihi-to and KKT are very likely to be beneficial for the treatment of aging-related dementia, particularly AD. Clinical studies with high levels of evidence are required to translate these preclinical findings to clinic application for patients with dementia.

3 Conclusion

In this chapter, we reviewed about several Kampo medicines with a potential to ameliorate cognitive dysfunction in patients with dementia and their neuromolecular mechanism(s) or evidence proposed from animal models of dementia on the basis of clinical and preclinical studies conducted during the last two decades. The findings surveyed offer new insights into the potential usefulness of Kampo medicines as an alternative and effective strategy for intervention of cognitive dysfunction and emotional symptoms in patients with dementia, including AD and VaD. However, less progress has been made on studies on identification, pharmacokinetics, and biotransformation of active ingredients of plant origin. It is also true that little information is available on target biological molecules for the mechanisms underlying the pharmacological and clinical action of the formulae. Therefore, studies aiming to solve these issues are required not only to obtain a better understanding of the mechanistic basis by which the Kampo formulae improve cognitive dysfunction but also to promote scientific evidence-based application of the formulae to therapy of dementia patients. Such studies may also allow us to identify new seed compounds and/or new target molecules useful for the development of potential therapeutic drugs for dementia.

Acknowledgments

This work was supported in part by a Grant-in-Aid for the 2012 and 2013 Cooperative Research Project I from the Institute of Natural Medicine, University of Toyama and a Grant-in-Aid for Young Scientists (B), #25860075 (to H.F.) for Scientific Research from the Ministry of Education, Culture, Sports, Science and Technology, Japan.

References

1. Wortmann M (2012) Dementia: a global health priority - highlights from an ADI and World Health Organization report. Alzheimers Res Ther 4:40
2. Roher AE, Maarouf CL, Kokjohn TA, Whiteside CM, Kalback WM, Serrano G, Belden C, Liebsack C, Jacobson SA, Sabbagh MN, Beach TG (2014) Neuropathological and biochemical assessments of an Alzheimer's disease patient treated with the gamma-secretase inhibitor semagacestat. Am J Neurodegener Dis 3:115–133
3. Arrighi HM, Barakos J, Barkhof F, Tampieri D, Jack C Jr, Melancon D, Morris K, Ketter N, Liu E, Brashear HR (2016) Amyloid-related imaging abnormalities-haemosiderin (ARIA-H) in patients with Alzheimer's disease treated with bapineuzumab: a historical, prospective secondary analysis. J Neurol Neurosurg Psychiatry 87:106–112
4. Bekris LM, Yu CE, Bird TD, Tsuang DW (2010) Genetics of Alzheimer disease. J Geriatr Psychiatry Neurol 23:213–227
5. Kivipelto M, Helkala EL, Hanninen T, Laakso MP, Hallikainen M, Alhainen K, Soininen H, Tuomilehto J, Nissinen A (2001) Midlife vascular risk factors and late-life mild cognitive impairment: a population-based study. Neurology 56:1683–1689
6. Biessels GJ, Staekenborg S, Brunner E, Brayne C, Scheltens P (2006) Risk of dementia in diabetes mellitus: a systematic review. Lancet Neurol 5:64–74
7. Crane PK, Walker R, Hubbard RA, Li G, Nathan DM, Zheng H, Haneuse S, Craft S, Montine TJ, Kahn SE, McCormick W, McCurry SM, Bowen JD, Larson EB (2013) Glucose levels and risk of dementia. N Engl J Med 369:540–548
8. Larson EB, Yaffe K, Langa KM (2013) New insights into the dementia epidemic. N Engl J Med 369:2275–2277
9. Janson J, Laedtke T, Parisi JE, O'Brien P, Petersen RC, Butler PC (2004) Increased risk of type 2 diabetes in Alzheimer disease. Diabetes 53:474–481
10. Matsuzaki T, Sasaki K, Tanizaki Y, Hata J, Fujimi K, Matsui Y, Sekita A, Suzuki SO, Kanba S, Kiyohara Y, Iwaki T (2010) Insulin resistance is associated with the pathology of Alzheimer disease: the Hisayama study. Neurology 75:764–770
11. de la Torre JC (2008) Pathophysiology of neuronal energy crisis in Alzheimer's disease. Neurodegener Dis 5:126–132
12. Humpel C (2011) Chronic mild cerebrovascular dysfunction as a cause for Alzheimer's disease? Exp Gerontol 46:225–232
13. Erkinjuntti T, Kurz A, Gauthier S, Bullock R, Lilienfeld S, Damaraju CV (2002) Efficacy of galantamine in probable vascular dementia and Alzheimer's disease combined with cerebrovascular disease: a randomised trial. Lancet 359:1283–1290
14. Wilkinson D, Doody R, Helme R, Taubman K, Mintzer J, Kertesz A, Pratt RD, Donepezil 308 Study G (2003) Donepezil in vascular dementia: a randomized, placebo-controlled study. Neurology 61:479–486
15. Roman GC, Salloway S, Black SE, Royall DR, Decarli C, Weiner MW, Moline M, Kumar D, Schindler R, Posner H (2010) Randomized, placebo-controlled, clinical trial of donepezil in vascular dementia: differential effects by hippocampal size. Stroke 41:1213–1221
16. Matsuda Y, Kishi T, Shibayama H, Iwata N (2013) Yokukansan in the treatment of behavioral and psychological symptoms of dementia: a systematic review and meta-analysis of randomized controlled trials. Hum Psychopharmacol 28:80–86
17. Matsumoto K, Zhao Q, Niu Y, Fujiwara H, Tanaka K, Sasaki-Hamada S, Oka J (2013) Kampo formulations, chotosan, and yokukansan, for dementia therapy: existing clinical and preclinical evidence. J Pharmacol Sci 122:257–269

18. Tabuchi M, Yamaguchi T, Iizuka S, Imamura S, Ikarashi Y, Kase Y (2009) Ameliorative effects of yokukansan, a traditional Japanese medicine, on learning and non-cognitive disturbances in the Tg2576 mouse model of Alzheimer's disease. J Ethnopharmacol 122:157–162
19. Fujiwara H, Takayama S, Iwasaki K, Tabuchi M, Yamaguchi T, Sekiguchi K, Ikarashi Y, Kudo Y, Kase Y, Arai H, Yaegashi N (2011) Yokukansan, a traditional Japanese medicine, ameliorates memory disturbance and abnormal social interaction with anti-aggregation effect of cerebral amyloid β proteins in amyloid precursor protein transgenic mice. Neuroscience 180:305–313
20. Sekiguchi K, Imamura S, Yamaguchi T, Tabuchi M, Kanno H, Terawaki K, Kase Y, Ikarashi Y (2011) Effects of yokukansan and donepezil on learning disturbance and aggressiveness induced by intracerebroventricular injection of amyloid beta protein in mice. Phytother Res 25:501–507
21. Ikarashi Y, Iizuka S, Imamura S, Yamaguchi T, Sekiguchi K, Kanno H, Kawakami Z, Yuzurihara M, Kase Y, Takeda S (2009) Effects of yokukansan, a traditional Japanese medicine, on memory disturbance and behavioral and psychological symptoms of dementia in thiamine-deficient rats. Biol Pharm Bull 32:1701–1709
22. Yamada M, Hayashida M, Zhao Q, Shibahara N, Tanaka K, Miyata T, Matsumoto K (2011) Ameliorative effects of yokukansan on learning and memory deficits in olfactory bulbectomized mice. J Ethnopharmacol 135:737–746
23. Calingasan NY, Gandy SE, Baker H, Sheu KF, Kim KS, Wisniewski HM, Gibson GE (1995) Accumulation of amyloid precursor protein-like immunoreactivity in rat brain in response to thiamine deficiency. Brain Res 677:50–60
24. Hozumi S, Nakagawasai O, Tan-No K, Niijima F, Yamadera F, Murata A, Arai Y, Yasuhara H, Tadano T (2003) Characteristics of changes in cholinergic function and impairment of learning and memory-related behavior induced by olfactory bulbectomy. Behav Brain Res 138:9–15
25. Aleksandrova IY, Kuvichkin VV, Kashparov IA, Medvinskaya NI, Nesterova IV, Lunin SM, Samokhin AN, Bobkova NV (2004) Increased level of beta-amyloid in the brain of bulbectomized mice. Biochemistry (Mosc) 69:176–180
26. Cryan JF, Mombereau C (2004) In search of a depressed mouse: utility of models for studying depression-related behavior in genetically modified mice. Mol Psychiatry 9:326–357
27. Mizuki D, Matsumoto K, Tanaka K, Le Thi X, Fujiwara H, Ishikawa T, Higuchi Y (2014) Antidepressant-like effect of Butea superba in mice exposed to chronic mild stress and its possible mechanism of action. J Ethnopharmacol 156:16–25
28. Fujiwara H, Iwasaki K, Furukawa K, Seki T, He M, Maruyama M, Tomita N, Kudo Y, Higuchi M, Saido TC, Maeda S, Takashima A, Hara M, Ohizumi Y, Arai H (2006) *Uncaria rhynchophylla*, a Chinese medicinal herb, has potent antiaggregation effects on Alzheimer's β-amyloid proteins. J Neurosci Res 84:427–433
29. Kanno H, Kawakami Z, Iizuka S, Tabuchi M, Mizoguchi K, Ikarashi Y, Kase Y (2013) Glycyrrhiza and Uncaria Hook contribute to protective effect of traditional Japanese medicine yokukansan against amyloid beta oligomer-induced neuronal death. J Ethnopharmacol 149:360–370
30. Kawakami Z, Kanno H, Ueki T, Terawaki K, Tabuchi M, Ikarashi Y, Kase Y (2009) Neuroprotective effects of yokukansan, a traditional Japanese medicine, on glutamate-mediated excitotoxicity in cultured cells. Neuroscience 159:1397–1407
31. Kanno H, Kawakami Z, Mizoguchi K, Ikarashi Y, Kase Y (2014) Yokukansan, a kampo medicine, protects PC12 cells from glutamate-induced death by augmenting gene expression of cystine/glutamate antiporter system Xc. PLoS One 9:e116275
32. Kang TH, Murakami Y, Matsumoto K, Takayama H, Kitajima M, Aimi N, Watanabe H (2002) Rhynchophylline and isorhynchophylline inhibit NMDA receptors expressed in *Xenopus oocytes*. Eur J Pharmacol 455:27–34
33. Kang TH, Murakami Y, Takayama H, Kitajima M, Aimi N, Watanabe H, Matsumoto K (2004) Protective effect of rhynchophylline and isorhynchophylline on in vitro ischemia-induced neuronal damage in the hippocampus: putative neurotransmitter receptors involved in their action. Life Sci 76:331–343
34. Zhao Q, Murakami Y, Tohda M, Watanabe H, Matsumoto K (2005) Preventive effect of chotosan, a Kampo medicine, on transient ischemia-induced learning deficit is mediated by stimulation of muscarinic M_1 but not nicotinic receptor. Biol Pharm Bull 28:1873–1878
35. Murakami Y, Zhao Q, Harada K, Tohda M, Watanabe H, Matsumoto K (2005) Chotosan, a Kampo formula, improves chronic cerebral hypoperfusion-induced spatial learning deficit via stimulation of muscarinic M_1 receptor. Pharmacol Biochem Behav 81:616–625
36. Terasawa K, Shimada Y, Kita T, Yamamoto T, Tosa H, Tanaka N, Saito E, Kanaki E, Goto S, Mizushima N, Fujioka M, Takase S, Seki H, Kimura I, Ogata T, Nakamura S, Araki G,

Maruyama I, Maruyama Y, Takaori S (1997) Choto-san in the treatment of vascular dementia: a double-blind, placebo-controlled study. Phytomedicine 4:15–22

37. Yamaguchi S, Matsubara M, Kobayashi S (2004) Event-related brain potential changes after Choto-san administration in stroke patients with mild cognitive impairments. Psychopharmacology (Berl) 171:241–249
38. Suzuki T, Futami S, Igari Y, Matsumura N, Watanabe K, Nakano H, Oba K, Murata Y, Koibuchi H, Kigawa Y (2005) A Chinese herbal medicine, choto-san, improves cognitive function and activities of daily living of patients with dementia: a double-blind, randomized, placebo-controlled study. J Am Geriatr Soc 53:2238–2240
39. Yuzurihara M, Goto K, Sugimoto A, Ishige A, Komatsu Y, Shimada Y, Terasawa K (1999) Effect of Choto-san, a kampo medicine, on impairment of passive avoidance performance in mice. Phytother Res 13:233–235
40. Morley JE, Farr SA, Kumar VB, Armbrecht HJ (2012) The SAMP8 mouse: a model to develop therapeutic interventions for Alzheimer's disease. Curr Pharm Des 18:1123–1130
41. Zhao WQ, Townsend M (1792) Insulin resistance and amyloidogenesis as common molecular foundation for type 2 diabetes and Alzheimer's disease. Biochim Biophys Acta 2009:482–496
42. Whitmer RA, Karter AJ, Yaffe K, Quesenberry CP, Selby JV (2009) Hypoglycemic episodes and risk of dementia in older patients with type 2 diabetes mellitus. JAMA 301:1565–1572
43. Zhao Q, Yokozawa T, Tsuneyama K, Tanaka K, Miyata T, Shibahara N, Matsumoto K (2011) Chotosan (Diaoteng San)-induced improvement of cognitive deficits in senescence-accelerated mouse (SAMP8) involves the amelioration of angiogenic/neurotrophic factors and neuroplasticity systems in the brain. Chin Med 6:33
44. Zhao Q, Niu Y, Matsumoto K, Tsuneyama K, Tanaka K, Miyata T, Yokozawa T (2012) Chotosan ameliorates cognitive and emotional deficits in an animal model of type 2 diabetes: possible involvement of cholinergic and VEGF/PDGF mechanisms in the brain. BMC Complement Altern Med 12:188
45. Sasaki-Hamada S, Tamaki K, Otsuka H, Ueno T, Sacai H, Niu Y, Matsumoto K, Oka J (2014) Chotosan, a Kampo formula, ameliorates hippocampal LTD and cognitive deficits in juvenile-onset diabetes rats. J Pharmacol Sci 124:192–200
46. Zhao Q, Murakami Y, Tohda M, Obi R, Shimada Y, Matsumoto K (2007) Chotosan, a kampo formula, ameliorates chronic cerebral hypoperfusion-induced deficits in object recognition behaviors and central cholinergic systems in mice. J Pharmacol Sci 103:360–373
47. Sherin A, Peeyush KT, Naijil G, Nandhu MS, Jayanarayanan S, Jes P, Paulose CS (2011) The effects of abnormalities of glucose homeostasis on the expression and binding of muscarinic receptors in cerebral cortex of rats. Eur J Pharmacol 651:128–136
48. Zhao Q, Yokozawa T, Yamabe N, Tsuneyama K, Li X, Matsumoto K (2010) Kangen-karyu improves memory deficit caused by aging through normalization of neuroplasticity-related signaling system and VEGF system in the brain. J Ethnopharmacol 131:377–385
49. Rocco ML, Pristera A, Pistillo L, Aloe L, Canu N, Manni L (2013) Brain cholinergic markers and Tau phosphorylation are altered in experimental type 1 diabetes: normalization by electroacupuncture. J Alzheimers Dis 33:767–773
50. Zhao Q, Matsumoto K, Tsuneyama K, Tanaka K, Li F, Shibahara N, Miyata T, Yokozawa T (2011) Diabetes-induced central cholinergic neuronal loss and cognitive deficit are attenuated by tacrine and a Chinese herbal prescription, kangen-karyu: elucidation in type 2 diabetes *db/db* mice. J Pharmacol Sci 117:230–242
51. Lau GC, Saha S, Faris R, Russek SJ (2004) Up-regulation of NMDAR1 subunit gene expression in cortical neurons via a PKA-dependent pathway. J Neurochem 88:564–575
52. Zhao H-F, Li Q, Zhang Z-F, Pei X-R, Wang J, Li Y (2009) Long-term ginsenoside consumption prevents memory loss in aged SAMP8 mice by decreasing oxidative stress and up-regulating the plasticity-related proteins in hippocampus. Brain Res 1256:111–122
53. Vaynman S, Ying Z, Pinilla FG (2007) The select action of hippocampal calcium calmodulin protein kinase II in mediating exercise-enhanced cognitive function. Neuroscience 144:825–833
54. Lamprecht R (1999) CREB: a message to remember. Cell Mol Life Sci 55:554–563
55. Lay I-S, Ciu J-H, Shiao M-S, Lui W-Y, Wu C-W (2003) Crude extract of Salvia miltiorrhiza and salvianolic acid B enhance in vitro angiogenesis in murine SVR endothelial cell line. Planta Med 69:26–32
56. Gong Y, Liu L, Xie B, Liao Y-C, Yang E, Sun Z (2008) Ameliorative effects of lotus seedpod

proanthocyanidins on cognitive deficits and oxidative damage in senescence-accelerated mice. Behav Brain Res 194:100–107

57. Wada T, Haigh JJ, Ema M, Hitoshi S, Chaddah R, Rossant J, Nagy A, van der Kooy D (2006) Vascular endothelial growth factor directly inhibits primitive neural stem cell survival but promotes definitive neural stem cell survival. J Neurosci 26:6803–6812
58. Udo H, Yoshida Y, Kino T, Ohnuki K, Mizunoya W, Mukuda T, Sugiyama H (2008) Enhanced adult neurogenesis and angiogenesis and altered affective behaviors in mice overexpressing vascular endothelial growth factor 120. J Neurosci 28:14522–14536
59. Kim BW, Choi M, Kim YS, Park H, Lee HR, Yun CO, Kim EJ, Choi JS, Kim S, Rhim H, Kaang BK, Son H (2008) Vascular endothelial growth factor (VEGF) signaling regulates hippocampal neurons by elevation of intracellular calcium and activation of calcium/calmodulin protein kinase II and mammalian target of rapamycin. Cell Signal 20:714–725
60. Wu KW, Yang P, Li SS, Liu CW, Sun FY (2015) VEGF attenuated increase of outward delayed-rectifier potassium currents in hippocampal neurons induced by focal ischemia via PI3-K pathway. Neuroscience 298:94–101
61. Matsui T, Sano K, Tsukamoto T, Ito M, Takaishi T, Nakata H, Nakamura H, Chihara K (1993) Human neuroblastoma cells express α and β platelet-derived growth factor receptors coupling with neurotrophic and chemotactic signaling. J Clin Invest 92:1153–1160
62. Zheng L, Ishii Y, Tokunaga A, Hamashima T, Shen J, Zhao Q-L, Ishizawa S, Fujimori T, Nabeshima Y-I, Mori H, Kondo T, Sasahara M (2010) Neuroprotective effects of PDGF against oxidative stress and the signaling pathway involved. J Neurosci Res 88:1273–1284
63. Inada C, Niu Y, Matsumoto K, Le XT, Fujiwara H (2014) Possible involvement of VEGF signaling system in rescuing effect of endogenous acetylcholine on NMDA-induced long-lasting hippocampal cell damage in organotypic hippocampal slice cultures. Neurochem Int 75:39–47
64. Inada C, Le Thi X, Tsuneyama K, Fujiwara H, Miyata T, Matsumoto K (2013) Endogenous acetylcholine rescues NMDA-induced long-lasting hippocampal cell damage via stimulation of muscarinic M(1) receptors: Elucidation using organic hippocampal slice cultures. Eur J Pharmacol 699:150–159
65. Niu Y, Li F, Inada C, Tanaka K, Watanabe S, Fujiwara H, Sasaki-Hamada S, Oka J, Matsumoto K (2015) Chemical profiling with HPLC-FTMS of exogenous and endogenous chemicals susceptible to the administration of chotosan in an animal model of type 2 diabetes-induced dementia. J Pharm Biomed Anal 104:21–30
66. Onozuka H, Nakajima A, Matsuzaki K, Shin RW, Ogino K, Saigusa D, Tetsu N, Yokosuka A, Sashida Y, Mimaki Y, Yamakuni T, Ohizumi Y (2008) Nobiletin, a citrus flavonoid, improves memory impairment and Abeta pathology in a transgenic mouse model of Alzheimer's disease. J Pharmacol Exp Ther 326:739–744
67. Nakajima A, Yamakuni T, Matsuzaki K, Nakata N, Onozuka H, Yokosuka A, Sashida Y, Mimaki Y, Ohizumi Y (2007) Nobiletin, a citrus flavonoid, reverses learning impairment associated with N-methyl-D-aspartate receptor antagonism by activation of extracellular signal-regulated kinase signaling. J Pharmacol Exp Ther 321:784–790
68. Kawahata I, Yoshida M, Sun W, Nakajima A, Lai Y, Osaka N, Matsuzaki K, Yokosuka A, Mimaki Y, Naganuma A, Tomioka Y, Yamakuni T (2013) Potent activity of nobiletin-rich citrus reticulata peel extract to facilitate cAMP/PKA/ERK/CREB signaling associated with learning and memory in cultured hippocampal neurons: identification of the substances responsible for the pharmacological action. J Neural Transm 120:1397–1409
69. Nishizawa K, Saito H, Nishiyama N (1990) Effects of Kamikihi-To, a traditional Chinese medicine, on passive and conditioned avoidance performance impairment in senescence accelerated mouse (SAM). Jpn J Pharmacol 54:375–382
70. Egashira N, Manome N, Kurauchi K, Matsumoto Y, Iwasaki K, Mishima K, Shoyama Y, Fujiwara M (2007) Kamikihi-to, a Kampo medicine, ameliorates impairment of spatial memory in rats. Phytother Res 21:126–129
71. Egashira N, Sudo S, Murayama F, Kohno S, Kudo Y, Goto S, Takayama F, Yamanaka Y (1991) Effects of kamikihi-to, a Chinese traditional medicine, on various cholinergic biochemical markers in the brains of aged rats. Folia Pharmacol Japon 98:273–281
72. Tohda C, Naito R, Joyashiki E (2008) Kihi-to, a herbal traditional medicine, improves Abeta (25–35)-induced memory impairment and losses of neurites and synapses. BMC Complement Altern Med 8:49
73. Tohda C, Nakada R, Urano T, Okonogi A, Kuboyama T (2011) Kamikihi-to (KKT) rescues axonal and synaptic degeneration

associated with memory impairment in a mouse model of Alzheimer's disease, 5XFAD. Int J Neurosci 121:641–648

74. Watari H, Shimada Y, Tohda C (2014) New treatment for Alzheimer's disease, Kamikihito reverses amyloid-beta-induced progression of tau phosphorylation and axonal atrophy. Evid Based Complement Alternat Med 2014:706487
75. Welt T, Kulic L, Hoey SE, McAfoose J, Spani C, Chadha AS, Fisher A, Nitsch RM (2015) Acute effects of muscarinic M1 receptor modulation on AβPP metabolism and amyloid-β levels in vivo: a microdialysis study. J Alzheimers Dis 46:971–982. doi:10.3233/JAD-150152
76. Del Pino J, Zeballos G, Anadon MJ, Moyano P, Diaz MJ, Garcia JM, Frejo MT (2016) Cadmium-induced cell death of basal forebrain cholinergic neurons mediated by muscarinic M1 receptor blockade, increase in GSK-3β enzyme, β-amyloid and tau protein levels. Arch Toxicol 90:1081–1092. doi:10.1007/s00204-015-1540-7

Chapter 13

Inchinkoto and Jaundice

Junichi Shoda, Eiji Warabi, Kosuke Okada, and Masahiro Yamamoto

Abstract

Patients suffering from cholestasis and jaundice are frequently encountered in daily clinical practice. Cholestasis is a pathological condition characterized by impaired bile formation and secretion in livers. The accompanying oxidative stress may damage hepatocytes and thereby result in severe jaundice (hyperbilirubinemia), leading to liver fibrosis. Kampo formulation inchinkoto (IKCT) has been recognized as a "magic bullet" for the treatment of jaundice. Although the potent hepatoprotective and choleretic actions and main active ingredients of IKCT have long been known, the recent advances in research of bile formation and hepatic transporters have opened a road to the understanding of the action mechanism. In this chapter, the molecular mechanism of the clinically useful actions induced by ICKT is described in detail.

Key words Jaundice, Cholestasis, Bilirubin, Inchikoto, Genipin, Abcc2 (Mrp2), Nrf2

1 Bile Formation and Secretion

In the liver, bile is produced at a volume of about 600–800 mL daily and is secreted into the bile canaliculi, where the biliary tract begins. Bile in the bile canaliculi flows from the center of hepatic lobules to the portal region. Bile enters the cholangioles, which are located in the portal regions, and flows toward the interlobular bile ducts. The biliary tract is a major pathway for detoxification and excretion of foreign bodies and wastes in the living body. Foreign bodies and wastes are carried by bile flow into the duodenum and are eventually excreted in the feces. Thus, the formation and secretion of bile in liver cells play an important role in the maintenance of homeostasis in the living body.

The hepatocyte membranes, which serve as the canalicular membranes, form the lumen of the bile canaliculi (0.5–2.5 μm in diameter), and the initial form of bile is secreted from hepatocytes. The canalicular membranes are known to hold transporter proteins involved in bile formation and secretion (Fig. 1). The co-operative role of the ATP-dependent transporters present in the hepatic sinusoidal membranes and bile canalicular membranes are

Akio Inui (ed.), *Herbal Medicines: New Horizons*, Methods in Pharmacology and Toxicology, DOI 10.1007/978-1-4939-4002-8_13,

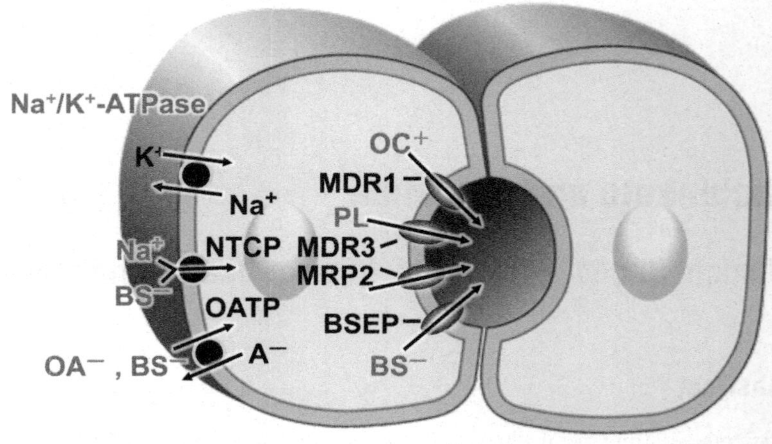

Fig. 1 Sinusoidal and canalicular membrane transporters in rat hepatocytes. Na^+-dependent bile acid (BA) uptake at a sinusoidal membrane is mediated by NTCP and is driven by the electrochemical Na^+ gradient generated and maintained by the Na^+/K^+-ATPase. The Na^+-independent hepatic uptake of organic anions (OA^-) and BA is mediated by members of the OATP family. Canalicular excretion of BA is mediated by another ABC transporter, BSEP. Excretion of non-BA OA^-, such as bilirubin diglucuronides, as well as sulfated and glucuronidated BA, is mediated by MRP2. Transport across the canalicular membrane represents the rate-limiting step in the overall blood-to-bile transfer of most endogenous bile constituents and xenobiotics. It is driven mainly by ATP-dependent export pumps, which belong to the superfamily of the ATP-binding cassette (ABC) transporters

important for secretion of bile acid and reduced glutathione into the bile from hepatocytes. Abcc2 (Mrp2), a protein associated with multidrug resistance, functions as a transporter for bilirubin conjugate and reduced glutathione Inchinkoto (ICKT)on the canalicular membrane. Abcb4 (Bsep), a bile acid transporter, plays an essential role in bile acid-dependent bile secretion [1]. The formation and secretion of bile in hepatocytes (choleresis) involves both bile acid-dependent and -independent mechanisms. Both ends of the bile canaliculi are closed by the bound complex, and microvilli are present in the lumen of this structure. Bile flow is then produced by contraction of the actin-myosin filaments around the lumen.

2 Cholestasis and Altered Expression of Hepatic Transporters

Cholestasis is encountered frequently during clinical practice and is defined as a condition involving disruption of initial bile formation and secretion in hepatocytes. Cholestasis (bile stasis-induced hepatic dysfunction) is a disease accompanying viral hepatitis or drug-induced liver injuries or developing in cases of obstructive cholangitis secondary to bile duct stone incarceration or malignant hepatobiliary tumor and in cases after extensive hepatectomies or liver transplantation. In some cases of cholestasis, the accompanying oxidative stress causes severe jaundice (hyperbilirubinemia) and prolonged persistence of hepatic dysfunction. Persistence of cholestasis induces compromised liver cell function, reduced hepatic tissue blood flow, and morphological changes. In cases where cholestasis is difficult to cure, these symptoms become irreversible, leading to biliary liver cirrhosis.

In the presence of cholestasis, hepatocytes are severely affected by disturbed bile flow due to bile duct obstruction, increased inflammatory cytokines due to cholangitis etc., and oxidative stress associated with bile retention, and so on. Under such conditions, hepatocytes show reduced intercellular communication because of malfunction of the hepatocyte cytoskeleton (particularly in gap junctions and tight junctions), disturbed vesicular transport of endogenous substances needed for bile secretion, and abnormal rhythmical contraction of the canalicular membranes due to disorders of the action-myosin complex around the bile canaliculi [2]. These cytoskeletal changes also cause abnormalities in the expression of transporters on the sinusoidal membranes and the bile canalicular membranes and disrupt smooth intake and secretion of bile acid or organic ions, leading to disturbances in both bile acid-dependent and -independent bile secretion. Importantly, since the transport function of the bile canalicular membrane transporters are thought to have about one-tenth the function of the sinusoidal membrane transporters, the functional activity of the canalicular membrane transporters serve as a more important factor associated with pathophysiology in cases of cholestasis.

The association of Mrp2 expression with bile secretion has been analyzed in patients with obstructive cholestasis who have undergone biliary drainage. In this study, Mrp2 expression levels were analyzed in patients who showed good excretion of bilirubin into bile (i.e., the well-excreted group) and in patients who showed poor excretion of bilirubin into bile (i.e., the poorly excreted group). In analysis of Mrp2 transcription and protein levels, the expression of Mrp2 was shown to remain almost unchanged in the well-excreted group as compared with that in the control group, while the expression of Mrp2 was shown to be markedly reduced in the poorly excreted group (Fig. 2) [3]. From immunohistochemical analysis of Mrp2 expression, the results demonstrated that intense accumulation of Mrp2 was observed in the canalicular membranes in the control group, while markedly reduced accumulation was observed in the poorly excreted group. Furthermore, canalicular membrane transporters have incorporated into the cytoplasm. In contrast, in the well-excreted group, accumulation of Mrp2 was similar to that observed in the control group, with Mrp2 mostly localized in the canalicular membranes and minimally

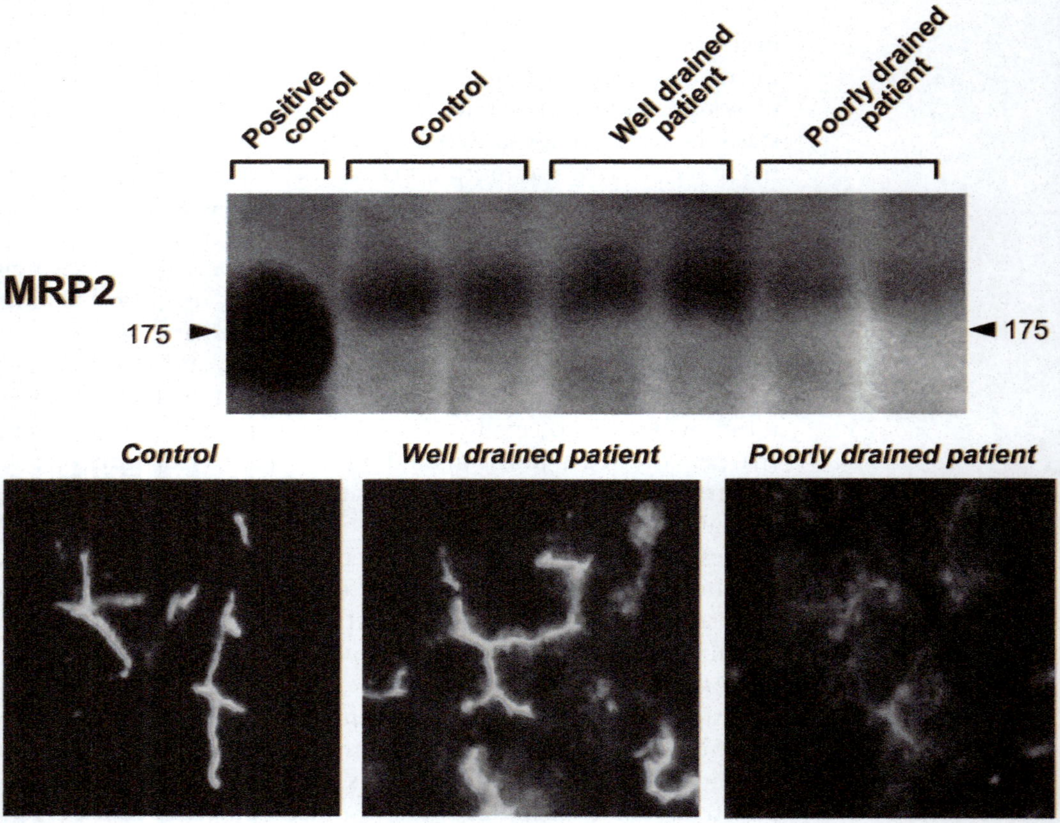

Fig. 2 (**a**) Immunoblot analysis of MRP2 in the crude plasma membrane fractions isolated from liver tissue specimens of control subjects, cholestatic patients well drained by percutaneous transhepatic biliary drainage (PTBD), and patients poorly drained. *Lane* P, positive control; *Lanes* 1 and 2, control subjects; *Lanes* 3 and 4, patients well drained; *Lanes* 5 and 6, patients poorly drained. (**b**) Immunofluorescence localization of MRP2 in liver tissue sections. Liver specimens were obtained from a control subject, a cholestatic patient well drained by PTBD, and a patient poorly drained. The immunofluorescence stainings of MRP2 outlined the canalicular membrane domain of the liver sections from the control subject and the well-drained patient. However, in the section from the poorly drained patient, the stainings disrupted a linear and intense localization in the canalicular membrane domain and appeared fuzzy. The magnitude of the alterations was greater in the patients poorly drained than those well drained

incorporated into the cytoplasm (Fig. 2) [3]. These findings revealed that the expression levels of Mrp2 affects bile secretion and serves as an important factor mediating the pathogenesis of cholestasis. Steroid hormones, phenobarbital, cholestyramine, etc. are conventionally used for empirically treating cholestasis; however, the efficacies of these treatments are inconsistent and have not been clearly established.

3 Preparation of Inchinkoto (ICKT)

ICKT, a pharmaceutical-grade traditional Japanese (kampo) medicine, has been widely used for the treatment of various liver disorders including jaundice and chleostasis. The drug has been approved as a prescription drug by the Ministry of Health, Labor and Welfare of Japan and fully integrated into the modern medical care system in Japan. ICKT is typically prepared as follows: A mixture of 5.0 g of the spike of *Artemisia capillaris* Thunberg, 4.0 g of the fruit of *Gardenia jasminoides* Ellis, and 1.0 g of the rhizome of certain Rheum species (*Rheum palmatum* Linne, *Rheum tanguticum* Maximowicz, *Rheum officinale* Baillon, or *Rheum coreanum* Nakai) in ten times its weight of water is boiled for 60 min and filtered. The liquid extract is then spray- or freeze-dried to obtain the extracted powder. Kampo medicines such as ICKT are presently manufactured according to the Ethical Kampo Medicine Drug GMP regulation and the self-imposed regulations of the Japan Kampo-Medicine Manufacturers Association.

ICKT contains a large number of constituents derived from various classes of compounds. All manufacturers of Kampo medicines as ethical drugs in Japan ensure that their extracts contain two or more of the major compounds characterizing the particular medicine group. Chemical analyses of the constituent compounds in Kampo medicines including ICKT and its constituent herbs, have generally been performed by HPLC combined with photodiode array (PDA) and evaporative light scattering (ELS) detection to obtain an overall view of as many compounds in the Kampo formulation as possible at a glance. The representative Kampo medicine supplier Tsumura & Co. (Tokyo, Japan) has been constructing a database that includes retention times and ultraviolet-visible light profiles of approximately 1000 compounds purified from various herbs, and more than 100 fingerprint patterns of Kampo medicines and constituent herbs made by 3-dimensional HPLC analysis. Such a database will enable us to provide a convenient method of assigning constituent compounds contained in herbs and Kampo medicines. It will also provide the means to control extract quality from a more comprehensive and global viewpoint, by providing the "fingerprint" for each medicine and herb. A number of routine quality controls have been carried out: these include quality inspection for residual agrichemicals, heavy metals, mycotoxins and microorganisms, determination of uniformity of content and disintegration time, accelerated and long-term stability studies, stability tests of active ingredients, and other characteristic ingredients. In all cases, high batch-to-batch reproducibility is obtained.

4 Pharmacological Actions

ICKT is composed of Artemisia Capillaris Flower (inchinko), Gardenia Fruit (sanshishi), and Rhubarb (daio). This mix has been used to treat jaundice for centuries, with its efficacy attributed to the choleretic effect of geniposide (contained in sanshishi) or 6,7-dimethylescultin (contained in inchinko). The choleretic effect of geniposide is thought to be manifested through increasing bile acid-independent bile secretion (particularly through potentiation of Mrp family function) by its active form, genipin. However, the specific molecular mechanism involved in this process had been unclear.

In the intestine, geniposide is hydrolyzed by enterobacteria to yield its active form genipin through loss of the glucose moiety (Fig. 3) [4]. Genipin is transported by the portal blood to the liver, where it exerts choleretic effect and subsequently undergoes addition of glucuronide to its 1-poisition, followed by excretion into the bile in the form of 1β-O-glucuronide [4].

We intravenously injected genipin or bile acid (ursodeoxycholic acid [UDCA]) into rats via the carotid vein and evaluated the choleretic effect of these substances in SD rats harboring Mrp2 and in Mrp2-deficient EHBR rats. In SD rats, both genipin and

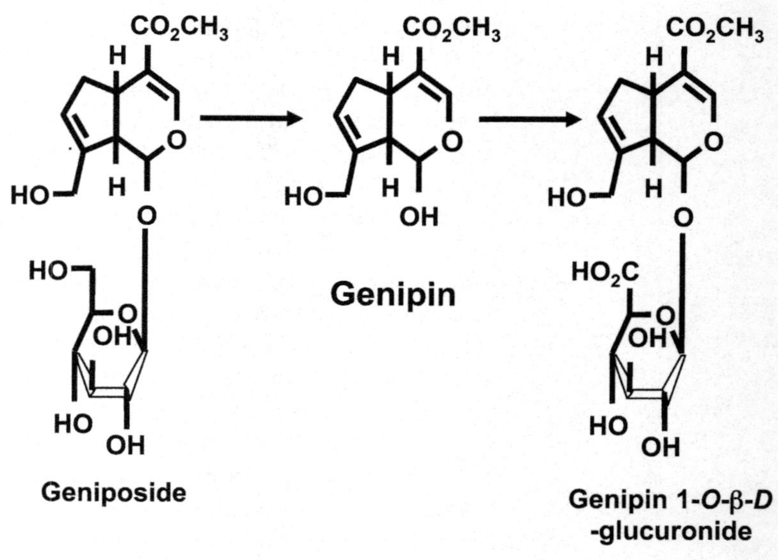

Fig. 3 Structures of geniposide (*left*), genipin (*middle*), and genipin 1-*O*-β-D-glucuronide (*right*). A major ingredient of Inchinkoto (ICKT), geniposide, is converted to an active metabolite, genipin, by intestinal bacteria. Genipin is then transported to the liver via portal circulation and subject to conjugation (mainly with glucuronide). About 20 % of infused genipin was secreted into the bile as the main metabolite 1-*O*-β-D-glucuronide

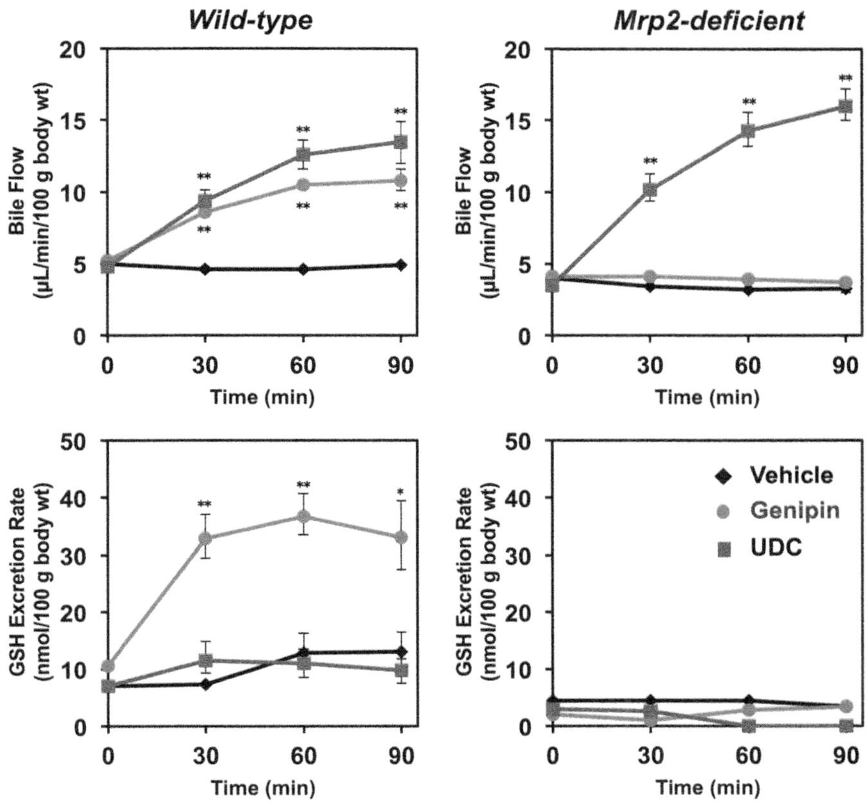

Fig. 4 Bile flow and rate of biliary secretion of GSH after bolus infusion of genipin. The bile was collected over a 30-min period before infusion in SDRs and Mrp2-defective EHBRs, and the initial values of bile flow and rate of GSH secretion were calculated. The rats were continuously infused with a vehicle (*open circle*), genipin (*filled circle*) or UDC (*open square*). The choleretic activity and rate of GSH secretion were measured at 30-min intervals over a 90-min period. Date are given as means $\pm$ SEM ($n = 6$). $^{**}P < 0.01$, significantly different from the vehicle-treated group

UDCA caused increased bile flow volume after intravenous injection. In Mrp2-deficient EHBR rats, only UDCA caused increased bile flow, and genipin failed to exert choleretic effect (Fig. 4) [5]. Monitoring of glutathione, a substance driving bile acid-independent bile secretion, revealed that genipin caused increased excretion of glutathione only in SD rats expressing Mrp2 (Fig. 4). These results suggest that Mrp2 mediates the choleretic effect of genipin. Analysis of the volume of bile acid excreted into the bile revealed that intravenous genipin treatment did not increase the volume of bile acid excreted, but did cause a significant increase in conjugate bilirubin excretion (Table 1) [5].

Genipin, UDCA, or physiological saline was injected intravenously to SD rats, followed by preparation of a canalicular membrane vesicle (CMV) fraction from the liver of each rat. ATP-dependent intake of Mrp2 substrates (i.e., E217βG, LTC4, MTX,

Table 1
Biliary bile acid secretion rates and concentrations of total bilirubin after bolus infusion of genipin

Time	0 min	30 min	60 min	90 min
Bile acid secretion rate (nmol/min/100 g/BW)				
Vehicle	262.8 ± 42.2	166.8 ± 13.6	144.2 ± 7.5	137.1 ± 6.5
Genipin	318.2 ± 28.7	166.8 ± 8.5	120.3 ± 6.6	116.8 ± 8.8
UDC	265.2 ± 18.3	461.0 ± 41.7‡	591.7 ± 34.4‡	566.8 ± 19.2‡
Total bilirubin (mg/dl)				
Vehicle	2.4 ± 0.2	1.8 ± 0.2	1.7 ± 0.2	1.7 ± 0.2
Genipin	3.2 ± 0.6	6.3 ± 2.0	9.1 ± 3.4	12.3 ± 3.2‡
UDC	2.8 ± 0.4	1.8 ± 0.1	1.0 ± 0.1	1.0 ± 0.1

Data are mean ± SEM ($n = 10$)
†$P < 0.05$, ‡$P < 0.01$: significantly different from the vehicle-treated group

and TLC-3S) by the CMV was then analyzed. ATP-dependent intake of each substrate for Mrp2 was found to be significantly increased in CMVs prepared from the livers of genipin-treated rats [5], indicating that genipin activates the transport function of Mrp2. When CMVs were prepared in the same way from Mrp2-deficient EHBR rats following genipin treatment, analysis of ATP-dependent E217βG intake revealed no increase in E217βG intake following genipin treatment. When the pharmacokinetic parameters of Km (affinity for the substrate) and Vmax (maximum initial velocity of reaction) were calculated using CMVs treated with each drug, the Km in the genipin treatment group was found to be similar to that from the other groups, indicating that genipin did not affect substrate affinity. However, Vmax rose markedly in CMVs after genipin treatment, suggesting that genipin induced an increase in Mrp2 protein levels in CMVs.

Western blotting of CMVs prepared from the livers of rats treated with each drug revealed a significant increase in Mrp2 protein levels following genipin treatment (Fig. 5) [5]. Because analysis of the crude membrane fraction revealed no changes in Mrp2 protein levels for samples of the entire liver, these data suggested that the increase in Mrp2 protein levels in the canalicular membrane may reflect genipin-induced Mrp2 protein redistribution.

Immunostaining for Mrp2 revealed a significant increase in Mrp2 density along the canalicular membrane following genipin treatment as compared with the other two groups (Fig. 5) [5]. Moreover, calculation of the membrane density with a densitometer in 800–1000 liver cells showed that the membrane density

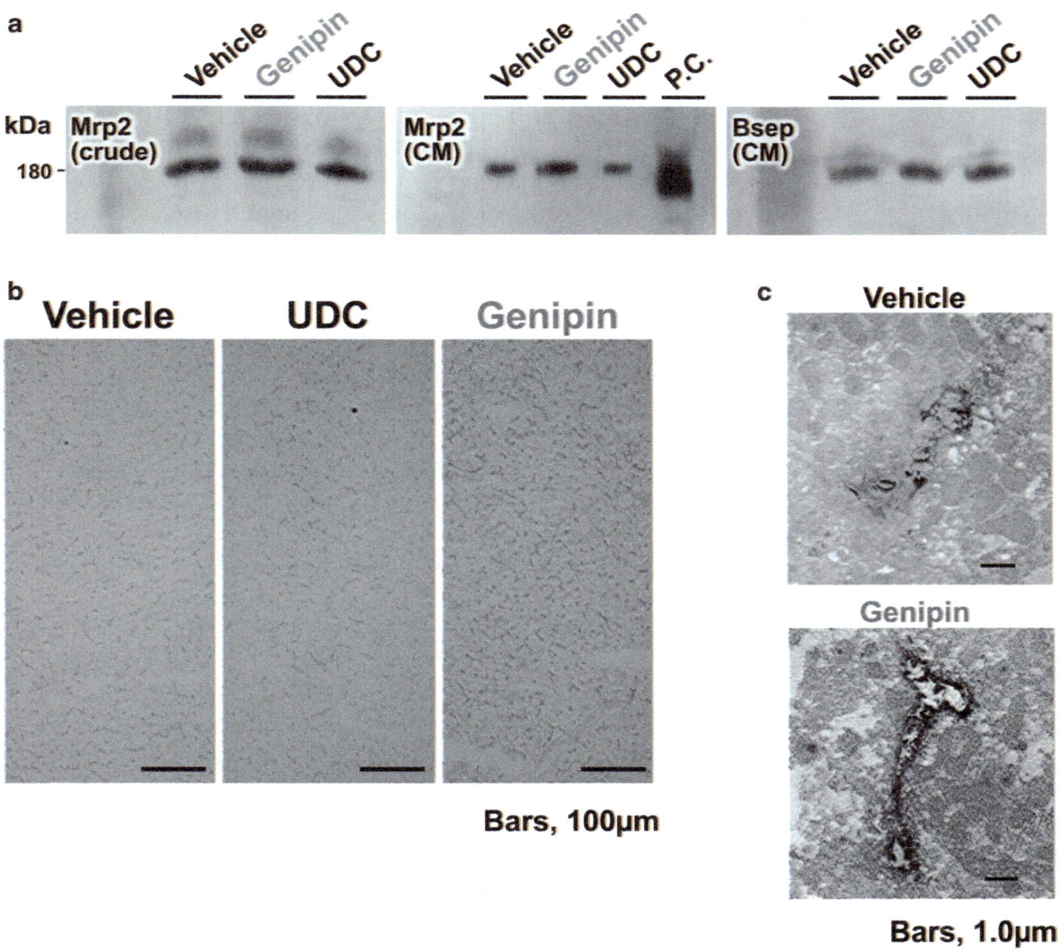

Fig. 5 (**a**) Immunoblot analysis of Mrp2 in crude plasma membrane (crude) fractions and canalicular membrane (CM) fractions isolated from livers of vehicle-, genipin-, and UDC-treated SDRs. Membrane-enriched fractions were prepared from rat livers 30 min after intravenous administration of vehicle, UDC or genipin. *P* positive control. The membrane vesicles from LLC-PK1 cells transfected with rat Mrp2 cDNA were used as a positive control for Mrp2. (**b**) Immunohistochemical localizations of Mrp2 in the livers (light-microscopic view). Liver sections were prepared from SDR livers 30 min after intravenous administration of vehicle, UDC or genipin. Mrp2 immunostaining shows a diffuse and linear pattern outlining the canalicular membrane domain of each liver section from vehicle-, UDC-, and genipin-treated rats. Bars, 100 μm. (**c**) Immunohistochemical localizations of Mrp2 in the SDR livers (electron-microscopic view). Liver sections were prepared from rat livers 30 min after intravenous administration of vehicle or genipin. The Mrp2 protein was localized mostly in canalicular microvilli in vehicle-treated livers, whereas, the localization was predominant in both microvilli and canalicular membrane in genipin-treated livers. Bars, 1.0 μm

increased close to two-fold following genipin treatment (Fig. 5) [5]. Subsequent immunoelectron microscopy analysis of Mrp2 expression demonstrated that Mrp2 distribution was restricted to part of the microvilli in the bile canaliculus lumen in rats treated with physiological saline, while intense accumulation of Mrp2 along the canalicular membrane was observed in the livers of rats following intravenous genipin treatment (Fig. 5) [5]. The number of microvilli containing Mrp2 was also larger in rats treated with genipin. Of about 300 microvilli, approximately 80–90 % became enriched in Mrp2 following genipin treatment in the liver [5]. On the other hand, no changes in the expression of Bsep, a bile acid transporter, were observed following genipin treatment.

The genipin-induced change in Mrp2 expression appeared to be a post-translation change (an early event) because it occurred 30 min after genipin treatment. Such post-translational changes are generally thought to be attributable to classical second messengers, such as cAMP, MAP kinases, and PKC [6]. In the literature, PKC has been reported to be activated by increased cAMP levels [7], and Mrp2 sorting occurs as a result of PKC isoform translocation [8]. In the present study, no significant changes in cAMP levels of PKC isoform translocation were noted in the liver or in liver cells following genipin treatment.

To evaluate the usefulness of genipin in clinical medicine, rats were treated with ICKT, geniposide, or genipin for 1 week. Oral administration of ICKT, geniposide or genipin to rats for 7 days increased bile flow and biliary excretion of bilirubin conjugates (Table 2) [5]. Biliary excretion of reduced GSH was similarly increased in the rats (Table 2) [5]. Moreover, the glutathione level, which is important for liver function, was significantly elevated in each drug treatment group compared with that in the control group (Table 2) [5].

Table 2
Comparison of the choleretic activities of ICKT, geniposide, and genipin in vivo

	Bile		Liver	Serum
Group	File flow (μl/min/100 g•BW)	GSH secretion rate (nmol/min/100 g•BW)	GSH concentration (μmol/g•liver)	GSH concentration (μmol/ml)
H_2O	5.4 ± 0.2	12.6 ± 0.9	5.5 ± 0.1	4.1 ± 0.0
ICKT (2 g/kg)	7.4 ± 0.3‡	25.1 ± 1.4‡	7.1 ± 0.1‡	4.0 ± 0.1
Geniposide (150 mg/kg)	6.8 ± 0.3†	23.3 ± 1.4‡	6.8 ± 0.2‡	4.0 ± 0.1
Genipin (100 mg/kg)	7.6 ± 0.4‡	27.5 ± 2.9‡	6.9 ± 0.3‡	3.9 ± 0.1

Each value represents the mean ± SEM ($n = 10$)
†$P < 0.05$, ‡$P < 0.01$: significantly different from the vehicle-treated group

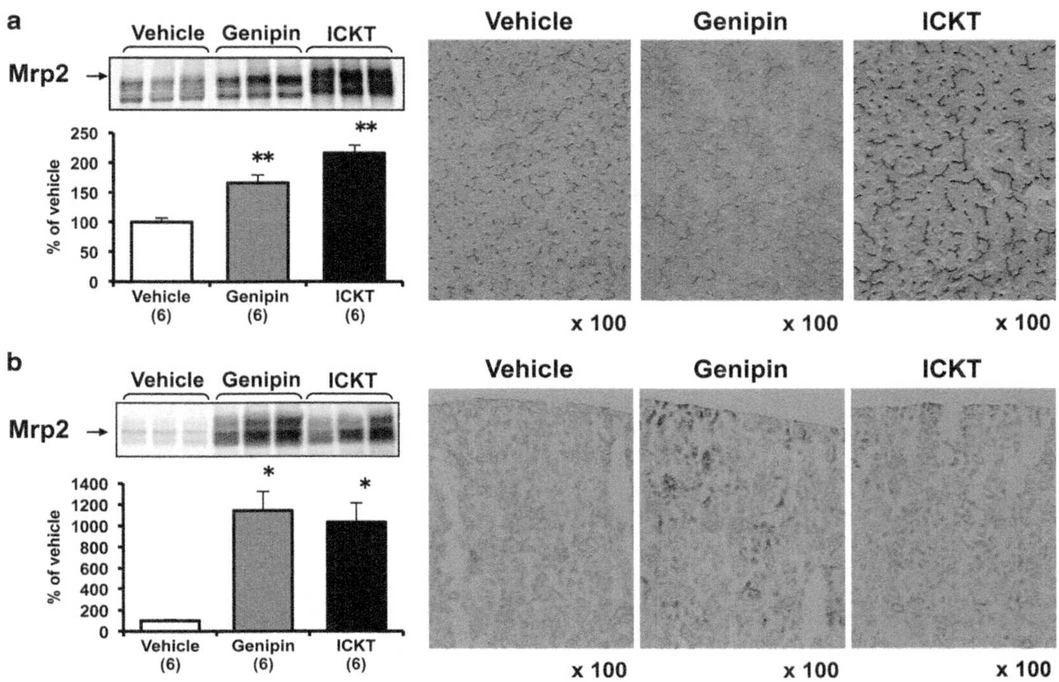

Fig. 6 Immunoblot analysis of Mrp2 in crude plasma membrane fractions isolated from livers (**a**) and kidneys (**b**) of vehicle-, genipin-, and ICKT-treated rats, and immunohistochemical localizations of MRP in their livers (**c**) and kidneys (**d**)

For the 1-week administration, Mrp2 protein and mRNA levels and Mrp2 membrane densities in the bile canaliculi and renal proximal tubules were significantly increased in ICKT- or genipin-treated rat livers (Fig. 6) [9] and kidneys (Fig. 6) [9]. ICKT and genipin, thereby, accelerated the disposal of intravenously infused bilirubin [9]. The treatment also increased hepatic levels of heme oxygenase-1 and GSH by a nuclear factor-E2-related factor (Nrf2)-dependent mechanism. Similar effects of ICKT on MRP2 expression levels were observed in humanized livers of chimeric mice (Fig. 7) [9]. These findings provide the rationale for therapeutic options of ICKT and its ingredients that should potentiate bilirubin disposal in vivo by enhancing Mrp2/MRP2-mediated secretory capacities in both livers and kidneys as well as Nrf2-mediated anti-oxidative actions in the treatment of cholestatic liver diseases associated with jaundice (Fig. 8).

Besides geniposide or genipin, 6, 7-dimethylesculetin was reported to exert a choleretic action [10]. The mechanism of action of this ingredient has been elucidated in recent studies by Huang et al. [11] using Yin Zhi Huang, a Chinese herbal drug closely related to ICKT. Yin Zhi Huang contains extracts from four different plants: *A. capillaris, G. jasminoides* Ellis, *R. officinale* Baillon,

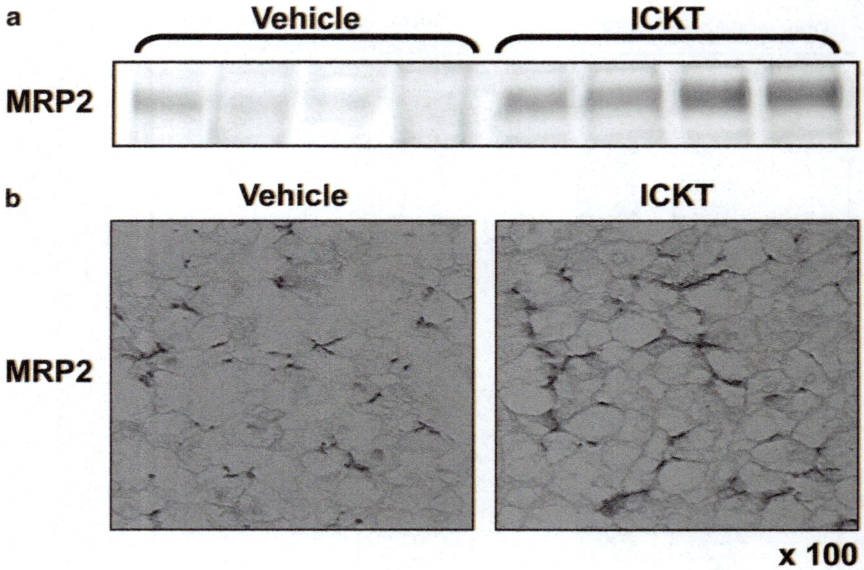

Fig. 7 Effects of ICKT and its ingredients on expression levels of MRP2 in humanized livers of chimeric mice. (**a**) Immunoblot analysis of human MRP2 in crude plasma membrane fractions isolated from livers of vehicle-, geniposide-, and ICKT-treated chimeric mice. (**b**) Immunohistochemical localizations of MRP2 in human livers of chimeric mice

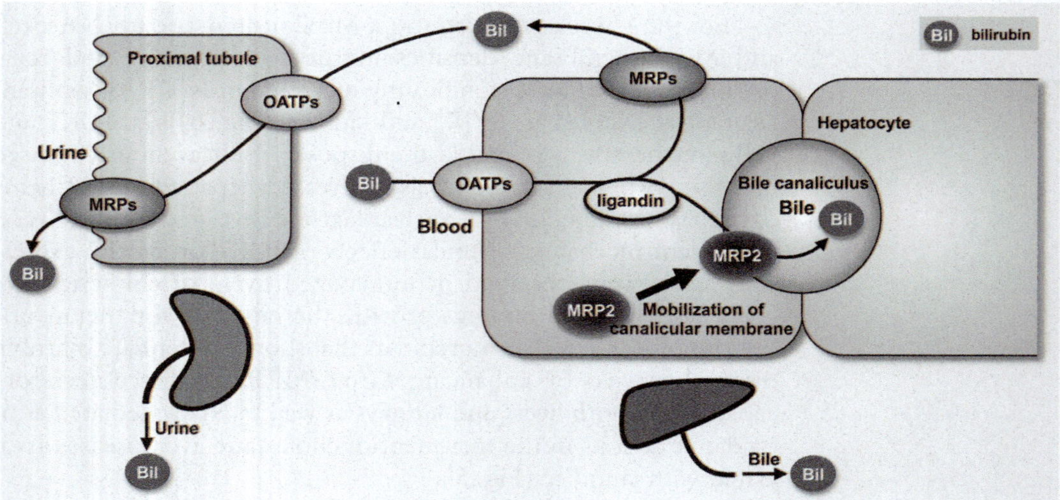

Fig. 8 Schematic summary of the stimulatory effects of ICKT on bilirubin and organic anion transport systems in rat liver and kidneys. ICKT upregulates major basolateral uptake, canalicular export, alternative export into the systemic circulation, and bilirubin conjugation in livers as well as apical export and alternative export into the systemic circulation in kidneys. *BA* bile acid, *GSH* glutathione, *OA*$^-$ organic anions, *Bili-Glc* glucuronidated bilirubin (Bili)

and *Scutellaria baicalensis* Georgi. Three of these four constituent herbs are also present in ICKT. Yin Zhi Huang, the decoction of *A. capillaris* and 6, 7-dimethylesculetin, accelerated the clearance of exogenously injected bilirubin. It was likely that the effect of these agents is mediated by the constitutive androstane receptor (CAR), a key regulator of bilirubin clearance in the liver, because the effect was completely abrogated in CAR knockout mice. In primary hepatocytes from both wild-type mice and mice expressing only human CAR, 6, 7-dimethylesculetin activated CAR and also accelerated bilirubin clearance in vivo. These effects were accompanied by an increase in the transcription of various components involved in bilirubin metabolic pathways: a sinusoidal organic anion transporter (OATP2), ligandin carrier proteins (glutathione *S*-transferase A1 and/or A2), the conjugating enzyme UDP-glucuronosyltransferase 1A1 (UGT1A1) and Mrp2. While the possible stimulatory effect of ICKT on CAR has not been studied directly, the well-known contribution of 6, 7- dimethylesculetin to the beneficial effect of ICKT suggests the drug has a similar action.

Capillarisin, isolated from *A. capillaris*, has been described as a more potent choleretic agent than 6, 7- dimethylesculetin [12]. However, the content of capillarisin in ICKT is rather small [13–16], and for this reason, a possible contribution of capillarisin to the choleretic effect of ICKT remains to be determined [17]. The detailed mechanism by which capillarisin exerts choleretic effects also remains to be clarified. There are preliminary reports of choleretic activity of compounds such as *p*-hydrocyacetophenone, capillartemisin A, B, and B1, artepillin A and C, scopoletin, isoscopoletin, and capillene from *A. capillaris* [18, 19], but further investigations have not been carried out.

In terms of the mechanism through which ICKT exerts its choleretic activity, the herbal component genipin was thought to stimulate accumulation of Mrp2, a liver transport protein serving as the molecular target of genipin and 6, 7-dimethylesculetin, in the liver cell canalicular membrane, resulting in increased bile acid-independent bile secretion. Thus, ICKT may be useful as a means of treating cholestatic liver disease, even in children.

In an experimental study [20], the effects of ICKT were studied in the rat mode of sepsis-induced intrahepatic cholestasis. Available information on the effects of ICKT on experimental cholestasis was scare, and therefore, the effects were examined in the rats administered LPS in terms of bile flow, glutathione secretion (but not bile acid secretion), and hepatobiliary transporter expression levels. Supplementation of ICKT restored LPS-induced decreases in the bile flow, glutathione secretion, bile acid secretion, and Mrp expression levels. ICKT has beneficial effects on the LPS-induced cholestasis and the ability to increase the bile acid-independent bile flow. In relation to the inhibitory effects of LPS-induced cholestasis, it was also reported that ICKT inhibits the activation of NF-kB that is involved in the process of bacterial translocation under cholestatic conditions [21].

These results of this study may encourage us to conduct clinical trials to evaluate the therapeutic efficacy of ICKT on hepatobiliary diseases associated with cholestasis.

5 Clinical Studies

Much of the published work reporting the beneficial effects of ICKT for the treatment of acute liver failure, viral hepatitis, jaundice, cholestasis, postoperative liver injury, primary biliary cirrhosis, primary sclerosing cholangitis, and biliary atresia has been written in Japanese. For English papers, a number of case reports from Japan reported the clinical effectiveness of ICKT for the treatment of severe acute hepatitis with prolonged jaundice [22, 23] and prolonged intrahepatic cholestasis associated with the drug use [24].

Moreover, Onji et al. [25] reported that the combined use of ursodeoxycholic acid and ICKT in three jaundiced patients with primary biliary cirrhosis resulted in clinical and biochemical improvement, including a decrease in bilirubin levels in all patients. Kobayashi et al. [26] reported a beneficial effect for ICKT in postoperative biliary artesia patients. Eighteen such patients aged 3–23 years, with elevated ALT and γ-glutamyltranspeptidase (γ-GT) but normal serum total bilirubin levels, were treated with ICKT for 2 years. All patients had been receiving ursodeoxycholic acid for at least 1 year without improvement before ICKT treatment. All subjects tolerated the drugs well and completed the study without difficulty. Measurements were made before and after treatment of AST, ALT, γ-GT, total bile acid and serum total bilirubin as markers of liver failure, and of hyaluronic acid, procollagen type III, and type IV collagen as liver fibrosis markers. The percentage of subjects who improved (defined by a > 25 % decrease in the parameter for each patient) after treatment was 72 % for ALT, γ-GT, and total bile acid and 67 % for hyaluronic acid. The mean values for all serum markers significantly decreased after ICKT treatment.

In addition, the effectiveness on postoperative hyperbilirubinemia after hepatic resection was also reported in the fields of gastrointestinal surgery [27]. The patient group given ICKT pre- and post-operative periods showed a significant decrease in the serum bilirubin levels compared with the control patient group. Bile acid-independent bile secretion exerts its action mainly in zone III. Many ischemic changes associated with major hepatectomy injure zone III, the most vulnerable region in ischemic attack, which in turn leads to a reduction in the bile acid independent bile secretion.

ICKT may be useful for postoperative management of liver resection by its potent Mrp2-mediated choleretic action.

Thus, although a considerable number of clinical reports have been published and the pharmacological effects of ICKT become recognized in clinical practice, the use of ICKT has failed to become widespread because of emphasis on evidence-based medicine and the lack of molecular mechanisms underlying these beneficial effects. Unfortunately, large-scale well-controlled clinical studies have not yet been conducted.

Therefore, we designed a randomized controlled study to determine the choleretic effects of ICKT on the livers of patients with biliary obstruction due to bile duct carcinoma, which subsequently underwent biliary drainage and major hepatectomy, to study if ICKT exerts choleretic effects on the cholestatic livers of the patients through an increase in biliary secretion of bilirubin and bile acid. Under these circumstances, the results of clinical trials on the usefulness of ICKT administration before hepatectomy for the treatment of biliary tract cancer have been reported recently [28]. Biliary tract cancer is often accompanied by obstructive jaundice due to bile duct obstruction. Prolongation of obstructive jaundice leads to decreased liver function. In the study, the hepatectomized patients with biliary tract cancer requiring preoperative biliary drainage for obstructive jaundice were randomly assigned to receive or not to receive ICKT to compare the clinical efficacy of ICKT. Patients receiving ICKT showed marked pre- to posttreatment increases in bile flow, total bilirubin concentration in bile, and total bile acid concentration in bile (Fig. 9) [28]. This was explained by the significant increase in the expression of Mrp2, a liver transporter protein for organic anions including bilirubin, located on the hepatocyte bile canalicular membrane (Fig. 9) [28]. The Western blotting method using liver homogenate also confirmed the significant increase in Mrp2 protein expression (Fig. 9) [28]. It has been suggested that preoperative administration of ICKT increases Mrp2 expression in the liver and Mrp2 localization on the bile canalicular lateral membrane to promote excretion of bilirubin and bile acid in bile, thereby relieving preoperative liver dysfunction and reducing the operative risk of hepatectomy. This study demonstrated choleretic effect of ICKT, a herbal medicine, in the patients with biliary obstruction due to biliary tract carcinoma. This effect was associated with an increased expression of MRP2 in the cholestatic livers, which was previously shown in animal models but has never been shown in human subjects. It is believed that ICKT has a therapeutic potential in the treatment of obstructive cholestasis associated with biliary tract carcinoma through a stimulation and restoration of both defective Mrp2/MRP2 expression and function in the livers. Thus, these findings have provided evidence for the clinical usefulness of ICKT in the fields of hepatobiliary surgery.

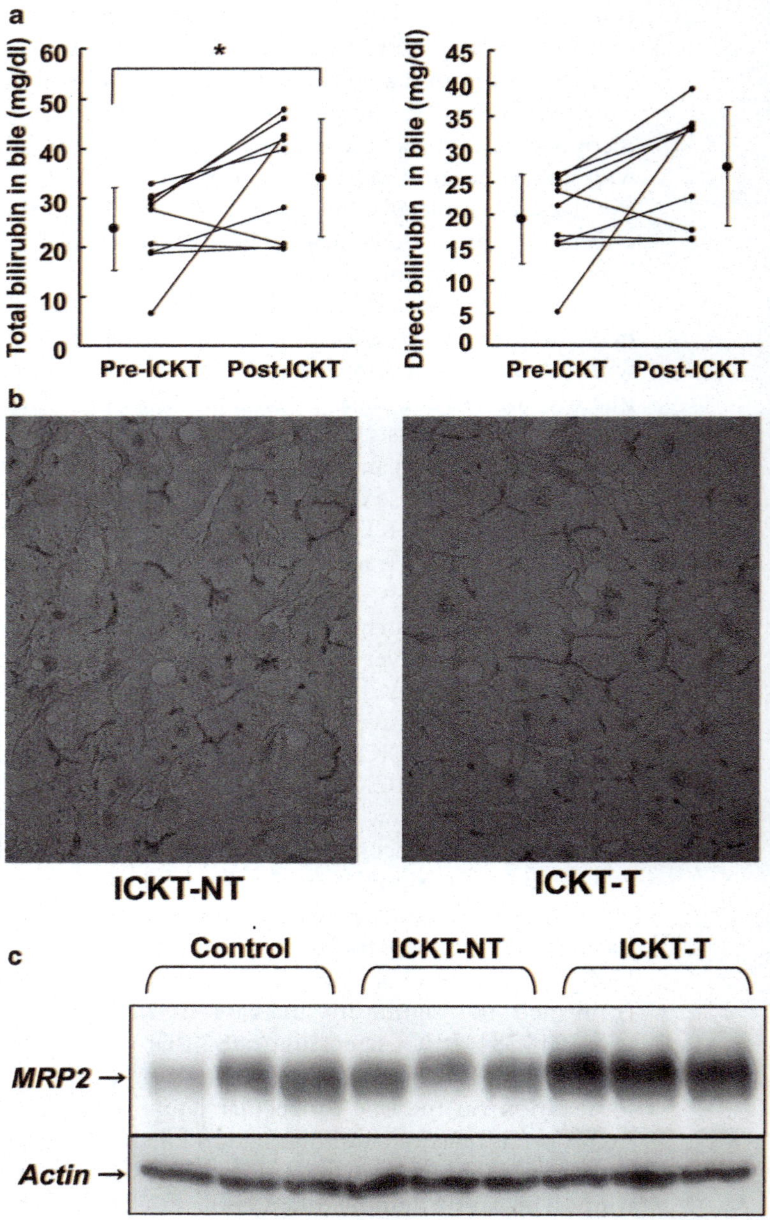

Fig. 9 (**a**) Changes of total bilirubin and direct bilirubin concentrations in bile samples obtained from nine patients before (pre-ICKT) and 2 days after (post-ICKT) oral administration of inchinkoto (ICKT). *$P < 0.05$ by paired *t*-test. Immunohistochemical localization of MRP2 in liver tissue taken before hepatectomy. (**b**) Representative staining of inchinkoto-non-treated (ICKT-NT) group (*left*) and ICKT-treated (ICKT-T) group (*right*). (**c**) Immunoblot analysis of MRP2 in crude plasma membrane fractions isolated from livers of normal (control), inchinkoto-non-treated (ICKT-NT) and ICKT-treated (ICKT-T) groups

References

1. Kullak-Ublick GA, Beuers U, Paumgartner G (2000) Hepatobiliary transport. J Hepatol 32:3–18
2. Trauner M, Meier PJ, Boyer JL (1998) Molecular pathogenesis of cholestasis. N Engl J Med 339:1217–1227
3. Shoda J, Kano M, Oda K et al (2001) The expression levels of plasma membrane transporters in the cholestatic liver of patients undergoing biliary drainage and their association with the impairment of biliary secretory function. Am J Gastroenterol 96:3368–3378
4. Aburada M, Sasaki H, Harada M (1976) Pharmacological studies of gardeniae fructus. II. Contribution of the constituent crude drugs to choleretic activity of Inchin-ko-to in rats [English abstract]. Yakugaku Zasshi 96:147–153
5. Shoda J, Miura T, Yamamoto M et al (2004) Genipin, an active metabplite of a herbalmedicine Inchinko-To, enhances multidrug resistance-associated protein 2-mediated bile formation in rats. Hepatology 39:167–178
6. Anwer MS (2004) Cellular regulation of hepatic bile acid transport in health and cholestasis. Hepatology 39:581–590
7. Beuers U, Bilzer M, Chittattu A et al (2001) Tauroursodeoxycholic acid inserts the apical conjugate export pump, Mrp2, into canalicular membranes and stimulates organic anion secretion by protein kinase C-dependent mechanisms in cholestatic liver. Hepatology 33:1206–1216
8. Roelofsen H, Soroka CJ, Keppler D et al (1998) Cyclic AMP stimulates sorting of the canalicular organic anion transporter (Mrp2/cMOAT) to the apical domain in hepatocyte couplets. J Cell Sci 111:1137–1145
9. Okada K, Shoda J, Kano M et al (2007) Inchinkoto, a herbal medicine, and its ingredients dually exert Mrp2/MRP2-mediated choleresis and Nrf2-mediated antioxidative action in rat livers. Am J Physiol 292:G1450–G1463
10. Takeda S, Endo T, Aburada M (1981) Pharmacological studies on iridoid compounds. III. The choleretic mechanism of iridoid compounds. J Pharmacobiodyn 4:612–623
11. Huang W, Zhang J, Moore DD (2004) A traditional herbal medicine enhances bilirubin clearance by activating the nuclear receptor CAR. J Clin Invest 113:137–143
12. Komiya T, Tsukui M, Oshio H (1976) Studies on "Inchinko". I. Capillarisin, a new choleretic substance [abstract in English]. Yakugaku Zasshi 96:841–854
13. Kagawa K, Okuno I, Noro Y (1984) Colorimetric determination of capillarisin. Shoyakugaku Zasshi 38:133–137
14. Okuno I, Kagawa K, Noro Y et al (1983) Pharmacological studies on the crude drug "Inchinko" in Japan (VI). Seasonal variation in chemical constituents of Artemisia capillaris THUNB. Shoyakugaku Zasshi 37:199–203
15. Akahori A, Kagawa K, Okuno I (1978) Determination of scoparone, capillarin and capllin in the crude drug "Inchinko" [abstract in English]. Shoyakugaku Zasshi 32:177–184
16. Wang X, Saito K, Kano Y et al (1993) On the evaluation of the prepa- ration of Chinese medicinal prescriptions (VII). HPLC analysis of the components in "Inchinko-to" and "Inchin-gorei-san". Shoyakugaku Zasshi 47:243–248
17. Yamahara J, Matsuda H, Sawada T et al (1982) Biologically active principles of crude drugs. Pharmacological evaluation of Artemisiae capillaris FLOS [abstract in English]. Yakugaku Zasshi 102:285–291
18. Okuno I, Uchida K, Nakamura M et al (1988) Studies on choleretic constituents in Artemisia capillaris THUNB. Chem Pharm Bull (Tokyo) 36:769–775
19. Kitagawa I, Fukuda Y, Yoshihara M et al (1983) Capillartemisin A and B, two new choleretic prin- ciples from Artemisiae capillaris herba. Chem Pharm Bull (Tokyo) 31:352–355
20. Arab JP, Ramiez C, Munoz P et al (2009) Effects of Japanese herbal medicine Inchin-ko-to on endotoxin-induced cholestasis in the rat. Ann Hepatol 8:228–233
21. Weber-Mzell D, Zaupa P, Petnehazy T et al (2006) The role of nuclear factor-kappa B in bacterial translocation in cholestatic rats. Pediatr Surg Int 22:43–49
22. Arai M, Yokosuka O, Fukai K et al (2004) A case of severe acute hepatitis of unknown etiology treated with the Chinese herbal medicine Inchinko-to. Hepatol Res 28:161–165
23. Ohwada S, Kobayashi I, Harasawa N et al (2009) Severe acute cholestatic hepatitis of unknown etiology successfully treated with the Chinese herbal medicine Inchinko-to (TJ-135). W J Gastroenterol 15:2927–2929
24. Ichikawa T, Sato H, Kaira K et al (2008) Prolonged intrahepatic cholestasis after exposure to loxoprofen. Clin Ther 30:2402–2406
25. Onji M, Kikuchi T, Michikata K et al (1990) Combined use of ursodeoxycholic acid and Inchin-ko-to in jaundiced patients with

primary biliary cirrhosis. J Med Pharm Soc Wakan-Yaku 7:161–167

26. Kobayashi H, Horikoshi K, Yamataka A et al (2001) Beneficial effect of a traditional herbal medicine (Inchin-ko-to) in postoperative biliary atresia patients. Pediatr Surg Int 17:386–389
27. Kaiho T, Tsuchiya S, Yanagisawa S et al (2008) Effect of the herbal medicine Inchin-Ko-To for serum bilirubin in hepatectomized patients. Hepatogastroenterology 55:150–154
28. Watanabe S, Yokoyama Y, Oda K et al (2009) Choleretic effect of Inchinkoto, a herbal medicine, on the livers of patients with biliary obstruction due to bile duct carcinoma: a randomized controlled study. Hepatol Res 39:247–255

Chapter 14

Chinese Herbal Medicine: Perspectives

Juei-Tang Cheng

Abstract

Traditional Chinese medicine (TCM), or Chinese traditional medicine (CTM), is widely applied as a complementary and alternative medicine (CAM) to improve the health. In this chapter, the basis of Chinese herbal medicine is examined from the ancient view to the modern idea. The chapter is divided into the following sections. An introductory section links the basic view of Chinese herbal medicine against the background of TCM. From the idea of four "Qi" (or "Chi") and/or five tastes ("Wu Wei") to the diagnosis of syndromes in TCM, four main methods are included: "inspection (observation)," "auscultation and olfaction (listening and smelling)," "interrogation (inquiry or questioning)," and "palpation (pulse examination)." The second section introduces the application of "four properties" (hot, warm, cold, and cool) using recently published views. In the third section, five tastes and other specificities of TCM are mentioned. The modern tools of Chinmedomics for herbs and/or herbal mixtures are reviewed in the fourth section. In the fifth section, clinical trials in TCM are conducted. In the sixth section, the network tools in herbal medication are discussed. The perspective of setting up an official name for each formula used in TCM is suggested in the seventh section. The same formula in Japan is generally pronounced in Japanese, which is quite different from that pronounced in China and/or other countries. Taken together, this chapter is going to make it easier for the reader to quickly understand CCTM.

Key words Traditional Chinese medicine (TCM), Chinese herbal medicine (CHM), Yin–Yang theory, Chinmedomics, Network pharmacology, Clinical trials

1 Introduction

Traditional Chinese medicine (TCM) or Chinese traditional medicine (CTM) has been widely applied in the treatment and/or prevention of diseases for a long time in China. Recently, TCM has also been introduced as a complementary and alternative medicine (CAM) around the world. Different than modern medicine, TCM is established from ancient ideas including the Yin–Yang or five routes (Wu Shin) theory, and the human body's meridian system, in addition to the Zang Fu theory [1, 2]. Essentially, TCM is applied to reverse the Yin–Yang imbalance in the human body and it is useful in improving disorders [3]. According to the Yin–Yang theory, the human body is regulated through the

Akio Inui (ed.), *Herbal Medicines: New Horizons*, Methods in Pharmacology and Toxicology,
DOI 10.1007/978-1-4939-4002-8_14, © Springer Science+Business Media New York 2016

integration of five routes (wood, fire, earth, metal, and water). Additionally, a disorder is mainly from the result of the abnormal integrations of five routes in five organs [3]. Therefore, disease is facilitated once the Yin–Yang balance is not normally regulated.

Disorders in the five organs, either one or more, may be expressed in some parts of the human body and/or in the whole body. To identify the syndromes, TCM experts in ancient times applied four diagnostic methods, including "inspection (observation)," "auscultation and olfaction (listening and smelling)," "interrogation (inquiry or questioning)," and "palpation (pulse examination)." Basically, the inspection is aimed at the visible signs and/or external condition of the patients, such as vitality, color, appearance, secretions, and excretions. Auscultation and olfaction are performed by the auditory and olfactory senses to identify signs in patients, such as in the voice, breathing, coughing, and odor. Interrogation means asking about the patient's recent history, major complaints, standard of living, diets, sleeping habits, and other physical conditions. Palpation is diagnosed using three fingers to touch on the three special sites located on the radial artery in the patient's hand. Generally, the diagnostic methods need mature skills and it will take time to train from scratch to become an expert. However, the four diagnostic methods are widely used to direct the choice of treatment in TCM, both acupuncture and/or herbal medication. In particular, four diagnostic methods may indicate two important cues, symptoms and signs, in a syndrome. Symptoms are change in function, sensations, and cognition in each patient. Additionally, signs are related to the abnormal and are indicative of disease, as identified by experts in TCM [4]. Furthermore, the diagnosis used in TCM includes another factor known as the ZHENG classification, which is similar to the classification of the syndromes. This idea is quite different than the diagnosis used in modern medicine.

Basically, syndromes should be diagnosed in TCM, according to the symptoms and/or signs, to administer suitable medication to treat patients. In general, disease indicates pathological changes in the human body and the syndrome only shows the disorder at a certain stage. Therefore, syndromes indicate several symptoms and signs, but not a simple reflex of symptoms or signs only. In TCM clinics, symptoms are identified via a detailed diagnosis using four diagnostic methods. However, some syndromes show a marked change, which makes them suitable for characterization without diagnostic criteria. Furthermore, a patient may suffer several diseases at the same time or one disorder may show several syndromes. Therefore, one syndrome may be changed during treatment to show a dynamic difference in the syndrome. The relationship between diagnosis and diseases in TCM has thus been documented as being multidimensional [5]. However, some challenges remain. In TCM, diagnosis is mainly performed by experts from personal experience. The inconsistency of the diagnostic results among TCM experts is the main challenge. Therefore, it is essential to establish (a) reliable standard(s) for diagnosis in TCM, as described previously [6].

The crude herbs used in TCM are mostly natural products. Some of the herbs are obtained from endangered species, meaning that the supply is limited. In general, the application of powder preparation is useful. The powder product can conserve the herb compared with decoction. This was discovered by the use of 28 herbal products to compare powder and decoction preparations from the Song to the Qing Dynasty (1644–1911 AD) and the results showed that doses of powder preparation are markedly smaller than those in decoction [7]. Therefore, the ratio of doses for powder and decoction is about 1:5–2:5. The powder preparation is thus more popularly applied in TCM. Additionally, the herbal products, according to the recommendation of Zhang Zhongjing, mainly include oral and/or external applications [8]. Each formula used in TCM consists in one or more herbs to form a mixture. Oral products include blended and decocted types, and the externally used product is mainly associated with topical preparations and suppositories. Basically, the herbal powder is usually mixed with fluids to assist oral administration. The fluids from Zhang's recommendation include water, fermented vegetable infusion, wine, porridge, chicken egg yolk, medicated infusion, etc. In clinics, the powder preparation can be therapeutically effective at a lower dose than decoction. Also, the powder product induces clinical effects better than decoction via two potential mechanisms [9]. First, during the preparation of decoction, each component may react with another to form the new product(s), whereas this does not occur with a powder preparation. Second, the powder preparation usually contains nonvolatile and/or nonpolar substances that were not included in decoction. The nonpolar substances are not easily extracted by water and the volatile components easily disappear through evaporation during decoction. Therefore, neither was included in decoction or was suitable to add to a powder preparation. The standardization of manufacturing and quality control and/or the rationalization of prescriptions for herbal medication in CTM are required extremely far in advance.

2 The Four Properties Applied to Chinese Medicinal Herbs

According to TCM, the Chinese medicinal herbs used include the basic properties of four "Qi" (or "Chi") and five tastes (Wu Wei). The "Qi" is related to four sensations – hot, warm, cold, and cool – depending on the integration of herbs within the human body. Therefore, the herbs effective at relieving "cold" symptoms are "hot" in "Qi" categories. In general, herbs that are shown to be "cold" and "cool" belong to "Yin" and those inducing "warm" and "hot" sensations are close to "Yang." The four feelings of "Qi" are also termed "four properties" or "four natures" in TCM.

However, it is not easy to understand the main meaning of the "Qi" theory, which is derived from ancient Chinese philosophy. It is established through the accumulation of experiences and subjective opinions in TCM. Therefore, there is no scientific background and a lack of reliable references to demonstrate the effectiveness and/or safety of herbs. From studies in rats, it has been documented that herbs belonging to "cold" can inhibit the central nervous system and/or sympathetic tone, reduce endocrine and enzyme activities, whereas "hot" herbs with produced the opposite effect, indicating that the cold and/or hot properties in herbs are associated with the excitation and/or inhibition of physiological functions [10, 11]. Moreover, the quantification of four properties has recently been proposed [12]. It was suggested that "Qi," the basic substance that constitutes in the human body a means of maintaining life activities, might be a type of energy particularly found in the form of electromagnetic radiation. This can be focused on the ultra-weak light emission originating spontaneously from the living systems ranging in intensity from a few to approximately 10^2 photons/(s $\times$ cm^2), with a spectral range of 400–720 nm. Using the biophoton analysis system, the four natures and meridian tropism of each property of herbs has been quantitatively obtained. However, it still does not apply to all cases and more data are needed to screen the herbs used in TCM in advance.

3 The Five Tastes and Other Specificities in Chinese Medicinal Herbs

The "five tastes (Wu Wei)" include five flavors of herbal medicines, including acrid, sweet, sour, bitter, and salty [13]. These seem to be associated with the "five routes or five elements (Wu Shin)" in the Yin–Yang theory. Additionally, they may relate to "five colors (Wu Sir)" in parallel to "five organs (Wu Zhan)." According to TCM theory, as shown in Table 1, one taste is believed to enter into one specific organ as indicated. For example, the herb with a bitter taste and/or that is red enters the heart more easily, whereas the herb

Table 1
Association of five tastes with others

Tastes	Acrid	Sweet	Sour	Bitter	Salty
Colors	Green	Yellow	White	Red	Black
Organs	Liver	Spleen	Lung	Heart	Kidney

with an acrid taste and/or that is green reaches the liver more directly. However, it should be remembered that each organ in TCM includes not only the organ itself, but the organ system too; for example, the heart is not the only aspect of cardiac function, because this includes the brain (mind) according to TCM theory. Therefore, it is quite different from the modern view. However, this view is mainly derived from the ancient Chinese philosophy and the scientific confirmation of this view is still not established.

A parallel view is that the main target is from up to down for each taste. For example: herbs with a sweet taste and/or that are yellow reach the spleen more easily.

Furthermore, show the direction of herbal action(s), "four functions" are proposed for herbal medications [14]. The four functions are ascending (*sheng*), descending (*jiang*), floating (*fu*), and sinking (*chen*). In TCM, for the best use of herbs to eliminate pathogenic factor(s), each herb is employed to improve the Qi flow in the Zang-Fu organs to reverse the function back to normal. Therefore, the location of the disorder is mainly introduced to produce an effect on the upper or lower, exterior, or interior sites of the human body. The pathogenesis then progresses to ascending or descending the human body. The herbal medication is mainly focused on two pairs of opposing actions. Therefore, a herb with an ascending action is employed to treat the disorder produced on the downward action. Also, a herb with a descending action is widely applied to relieve vomiting and/or hiccups owing to the abnormal ascent of Qi into the stomach. Otherwise, a herb with a floating action can easily drive out the pathogenic factor(s) from the surface of the human body and relieve the exterior syndrome. A herb applied to treat a disorder on the interior of the human body is associated with a sinking action, including purgatives and diuretics. In general, herbs with acrid and sweet, warm and hot sensations induce to ascending and floating actions. Herbs with bitter, sour and salty, cool and cold mostly have sinking and descending actions. Additionally, herbs with a light weight, including the leaf and the flower, are mostly ascending and floating, whereas the heavier herbs, including seeds and minerals, have a mainly sinking and descending application. However, this view is still not supported by the scientific evidence.

The idea of attributive meridians (Gui Jiing) for herbal medications derives the herbal actions through the theories of organs and meridians (Zhang-Fu). According to this view, the herb produces a major effect on a specific related organ. For example, in clinics, a cough, chest pain, and a sore throat represent disorders in the Lung Meridian. Thus, herb(s) belonging to the Lung Meridian, including Radix Platycodi or Semen Armeniacae Amarum, will be suitable for treating it. Moreover, the Zhang-Fu organs and the meridians are interrelated. This does not mean that the disease of a given meridian should be treated by herbs only from that meridian, as described previously [14]. The complicated interactions also limit application in modern medicine.

4 Development of Chinmedomics in TCM

In addition to the analysis and identification of biomarkers, metabolomics contributed a better understanding of pathological changes, metabolic pathways, and drug targets. Recently, the application of metabolome in TCM has been suggested to be valuable for evidence-based TCM and it has been defined as "Chinmedomics" [15], which is a combination of Chinese medicine and "omics." Omics is known as the "high throughput technologies used to analyze various kinds of macromolecules, simultaneously; such as, transcriptomics measures many transcripts, proteomics can identify many proteins and metabolomics determines the metabolites." Through the development of information-rich techniques, including genomics, proteomics, and transcriptomics, in addition to the various profiling approaches, such as metabolomics (a nontargeted analytical approach, mostly focusing on low-weight molecules) and metabonomics (a similar approach in addition to studying the effects through a system), it has been useful to find out the simultaneous molecular effects for a mixture of chemical agents [16] and, through the bioinformatics, to propose such effects with speculation with regard to the biological system influenced. The factorial analysis models are known to decode raw information in large quantities using omic techniques, and may sometimes link the relationship between multiple components that are contained in herbs to produce biological effects [17]. Additionally, high-throughput and information-rich assays may be applied to fingerprint the herbs and herbal extracts [18]. Studies addressing quality control and sample variability are useful for identifying the reproducibility and standardization of bioactivities for herbal products. Recently, the holistic systems biology approach has shown a new perspective of pharmacological sciences and embraces the entire equilibrium for a biological system through the simultaneous analysis of primary and/or secondary multiple targets [19]. This approach seems more useful in understanding the combinations in Chinese herbal medicine [20]. Such assays with advanced bioinformatics may be an opportunity to improve experimental levels. Omics are generally applied in an identical manner, in vitro, in vivo, or in clinical research. The systems biology approach may increase the system complexity at the molecular, cellular, organ, and whole organism levels. Therefore, the application of omics in experimental models is required to include the in vitro, in vivo, and the clinical applications combined. Omics are useful in all contexts, and researchers are able to share and transfer the information within the research community and to the clinics. The term "holistic" is widely used to show the application of omic technologies, whereas the information from omics is obviously at the level of physical matter to consider many compounds and effects together. It seems useful in Chinese herbal medicine research, but should be applied cautiously. It has been demonstrated that no linear path can be traced using the evolution of omics for TCM [21]. Therefore, the development of new omic strategies, including metabonomics, seems to be more achievable.

A previous report claimed that there are two main problems [21]. First, there is an significant problem in replicating the human disease in animal or cellular models and many animal or disease models have still not been established. Therefore, the standardization of animal models for the application of omics in the study of TCM is essential. Second, omics is also liable to variability. However, the presence of variability is widely observed in Chinese herbal medicine. Therefore, it is essential to establish the reliable control of each herbal preparation. Apart from the two problems mentioned above, omics research in TCM is suggested to be unsuitable, as described previously [21].

5 Clinical Trials Applied in TCM

Evidence-based medicine (EBM) is generally defined as the judicious use of recent best evidence to make decisions on patient care. Thus, the practice of EBM means integrating personal expertise with the best external evidence from the systematic research carried out in clinics [22]. EBM has recently become the standard in medical practice, elevating it to a higher level, with greater accuracy, efficacy, and safety.

Chinese herbal medicine is popularly practiced in Asian areas, including China, Hong Kong, Taiwan, Singapore, Japan, and Korea. Non-Asian countries have also recognized the therapeutic potential of TCM. However, the link between TCM and modern medicine for healthcare has still not been established, probably because of the lack of evidence from EBM perspectives. Therefore, it is essential for TCM to show efficacy and safety through evidence that is equal to the evaluation of modern medicine, particularly EBM. In the EBM system, randomized controlled trials (RCTs) or meta-analyses of RCTs for systematic reviews are the popular standard, showing the highest level of evidence, followed by other types of evidence, including cohort studies, case–control studies, case series, case reports, animal studies, and expert opinions [23]. However, application of the EBM model in TCM has still not developed in a good way.

Many challenges are indicated for the application of EBM in TCM, but these can be overcome through various approaches, as described in a previous report [23]. Bad quality control in the manufacturing of TCM products is one of the factors to be considered when integrating TCM into modern medicine. Moreover, methodological shortcomings and clinical heterogeneity also limit the application of Chinese herbal medicine in clinical trials [24]. In general, the conduction of clinical studies is suggested to follow the international guidelines, including ethical considerations, the correct sampling selection of controls/placebos, and randomizing procedures (including blinding) [25]. However, the clinical trial publications for TCM are variable and should be challenged, particularly the systematic reviews, where it is criticized as being inconclusive with a lower quality of reporting or methodology. This seems unfair, because TCM as an ancient science is believed to be helpful for greater merit in human health. The basis of TCM is quite different than that of modern medicine. In addition to the ideas on TCM mentioned above in this chapter, biochemical markers are not involved in TCM. Therefore, it is not easy to perform clinical trials in TCM from the modern point of view. Experts in TCM understand that clinical trials must be carried out, but they do not know how to perform the clinical trials as with modern medicine. Good practice in clinical trials from other countries that focus on TCM supply the details and assist TCM to integrate with modern medicine. Additionally, communications between the two modalities needs to be dynamic to facilitate the optimal health care for the individual, as described previously [25]. Therefore, the development of clinical trials in TCM is very important.

6 Development of Network Pharmacology in CTM

Many ingredients are known to be contained in herbs and/or herbal mixtures and many changes are involved in TCM syndromes. Therefore, the multiple rules and/or roles of herbal mixtures in complicated diseases should be elucidated. Owing to the progress of bioinformatics, network-based drug discovery is suggested to be a reliable approach toward drug development [26]. Basically, pharmacological approach of the TCM network possessed two main merits: it is predictable and systematic. This approach is varied with the traditional method using "trial and error" and may assist drug discovery to be predictable. Through computer analysis, this approach is also able to manage a large amount of data. Meanwhile, it is useful for making the systematic study of herbal mixtures achievable.

To estimate the synergistic effects of drugs in a dose–response manner, the model for quantitatively analyzing drug combinations is applied by simulating the kinetics of key elements (the biochemical pathway or signals) in the network target [27]. For example, a model of the TNF–NFkB pathway, using the dose–response data for treated agents targeting proteins in the pathway, identified the synergistic combinations between certain agents, such as the IKK inhibitor (PS-1145) and the HSP90 inhibitor (geldanamycin). Basically, the formula–syndrome relationship may include the "same treatment for different diseases" and/or the "same disease by different treatments" in TCM. Network analysis methods are available to clarify the potential mechanism(s) and/or biomarkers for the formula–syndrome relationship and to find out the mechanistic integrations of herbal combinations with syndromes in TCM. In the analysis of one formula, named Liu-Wei-Di-Huang (LWDH), diseases improved by this product have been documented to share a common network target associated with the neuroendocrine–immune (NEI) pathways, in addition to the imbalance of the human body [28]. It has also been indicated that the key genes regulated by the LWDH formula are enriched in NEI pathways, and are also markedly close to the genes associated with cancer, diabetes, and hypertension in the network target [28]. Therefore, LWDH-treated diseases share an overlapping molecular basis with a high phenotypic similarity. This view has been discussed in special issues of journals [29] and documented [30]. Moreover, using the established theories, TCM researchers have more facilities for the discovery of medical insights from the complicated phenotype network in clinics. However, reliable data for clinical phenotypes, symptoms and signs, and socio-environmental factors, are still not well established. Moreover, the correlation and regularity between clinical phenotypes and the underlying molecular phenotypes should be addressed using the integrated analysis of large-scale clinical and genomics data. Therefore, this tool is still challenged in the application of TCM [31]. The development of network pharmacology to apply in TCM is vital.

7 Conclusion and Perspectives

Traditional medicine is mostly focused on personalized medicine, which is not far from the modern approach in tailor-made, human genetics-based pharmacotherapy. Standardization of TCM syndromes is very helpful in assisting the molecular network for disease types to define the potential mechanism(s) of herbal medications. Moreover, disease-oriented studies using the approach of multi-indexed high-throughput technologies and functional "omics" to elucidate the action mechanisms of herbs may assist the identification of potential biomarkers to be linked with the modern point of view. Otherwise, as alternative medicine, many TCM and herbal/natural products are bought over-the-counter (OTC) and considered to be nonpharmaceutical medicines. Adverse effects, including herb–drug interactions, were ignored and this shall be considered carefully.

Chinese herbal medicine is widely practiced in Asian populations such as Japan and Korea in addition to China, including Hong Kong, Taiwan, and Singapore. However, the names of the herbal formulas generally vary according to each local language and are not the same. For example, Kampo originated from TCM and was greatly developed in Japan especially during the Edo era (1603–1868 AD). A systemic review of Kampo has been recently documented [32]. The formula named "Dai-sai-ko-to" in Japanese is the same as "Ta-Tsai-Fu-Tang" in TCM. However, it is hard to understand by the non-Asian scientist(s) and two different products are considered. Therefore, how to make a common name for each formula in TCM around the world is currently an important issue. I suggest giving each formula a representative number, for example, like the official names of enzymes. However, this should be carried out by an official Chinese institute and/or scientific society, inviting experts in TCM from Japan, Korea, and other countries to work together. The final representative name for each formula and/or herb can then be defined and applied by all scientist(s) majoring in TCM and by the scientific journals. Therefore, the difficulties caused by having various names for the same formula and/or TCM herb will be removed in the near future; this is the main perspective of this chapter.

Overall, this chapter collected many basic views of TCM from previous reports. Some sentences are cited directly from the original report(s) without modifications. The author appreciated the scientists who described useful views in the previous report(s) that were cited in this chapter.

In conclusion, this chapter reviewed the herbal medications used in TCM from ancient views to modern ideas. Perspective(s) were shown in each section for improvement of the weaknesses of TCM. Owing to variations in the basic viewpoints of TCM and modern medicine, it is not currently easy to integrate the two modalities. However, it is essential to develop a way of improving our understanding of TCM from a modern viewpoint.

References

1. Lukman S, He Y, Hui S-C (2007) Computational methods for traditional Chinese medicine: a survey. Comput Methods Prog Biomed 88(3):283–294
2. Maciocia G (1989) The foundations of Chinese medicine. Churchill Livingstone, Edinburgh
3. Lu AP, Li S (2010) Principle and application of Chinese medicine syndrome differentiation and disease classification. Zhongguo Zhong Xi Yi Jie He Za Zhi 30:84–86.
4. Dodd M, Janson S, Facione N et al (2001) Advancing the science of symptom management. J Adv Nurs 33(5):668–676
5. Jiang M, Lu C, Zhang C et al (2012) Syndrome differentiation in modern research of traditional Chinese medicine. J Ethnopharmacol 140:634–642
6. Zhao C, Li G-Z, Wang C, Niu J (2015) Advances in patient classification for traditional Chinese medicine: a machine learning perspective. Evid Based Complement Alternat Med 2015:376716
7. Cai GX, Liu BY (2004) Research on the dosage of 28 Chinese herbal pieces with traditional decoction and its powder. Zhong Guo Shi Yan Fang Ji Xue Za Zhi 10:63–64

8. Li YQ (2009) The application of powder in the treatise on cold pathogenic and miscellaneous diseases. Shanxi Zhong Yi 30:760–761
9. Wang JN, Zhang GD, Yu RH et al (2010) Thinking of the profound meaning of the dosage form by the Traditional Chinese Medicine clinical effects difference. Zhong Guo Shi Yan Fang Ji Xue Za Zhi 16:185–187
10. Liang YH, Ren H (1991) Urine catecholamines and 5-hydroxytryptamine changes of the central, viscera in the cold and heat syndrome. J Tradit Chin Med 32:38–40
11. Xu HY, Tang SH, Chen JX et al (2011) Research ideas and strategies of Chinese medicine "group activity relationship" based on the metabolomics. World Sci Technol/Modern Trad Chin Med Mater Med 13:3–35
12. Fu JL, Pang JX, Zhao XL, Han JX (2015) The quantitative ideas and methods in assessment of four properties of Chinese medicinal herbs. Cell Biochem Biophys 71:1307–1312
13. Gao XM (2007) Chinese materia medica, 2nd edn. China Press of Traditional Chinese Medicine, Beijing, p 42
14. Li JS (1999) Authentication of Chinese medicines. Scientific and Technical Publishers, Shanghai, pp 594–595
15. Zhang AH, Sun H, Yan GL, Wang P, Han Y, Wang XJ (2015) Chinmedomics: a new strategy for research of traditional Chinese medicine. Zhongguo Zhong Yao Za Zhi 40:569–576
16. Ulrich-Merzenich G, Zeitler H, Jobst D, Panek D, Vetter H, Wagner H (2007) Application of the '-Omic-' technologies in phytomedicine. Phytomedicine 14:70–82
17. Wang P, Sun H, Lu H, Sun W, Yuan Y, Han Y, Wang D, Zhang A, Wang X (2010) Thyroxine and reserpine-induced changes in metabolic profiles of rat urine and the therapeutic effect of Liu Wei Di Huang Wan detected by UPLCHDMS. J Pharm Biomed Anal 53:631–645
18. Heubl G (2010) New aspects of DNA-based authentication of Chinese medicinal plants by molecular biological techniques. Planta Med 76:1963–1974
19. Auffray C, Chen Z, Hood L (2009) System medicine: the future of medical genomics and healthcare. Genome Med 2:1–11
20. Cooper EL (2009) eCam: integrative genomics and fecundity. Evid Based Complement Alternat Med 6:129–131
21. Buriania A, Garcia-Bermejod ML, Bosisiof E et al (2012) Omic techniques in systems biology approaches to traditional Chinese medicine research: present and future. J Ethnopharmacol 140:535–544
22. Sackett DL, Rosenberg WMC, Gray JAM, Haynes RB, Richardson WS (1996) Evidence based medicine: what it is and what it isn't. Br Med J 312(7023):71–72
23. Fung FY, Linn YC (2015) Developing traditional Chinese medicine in the era of evidence-based medicine: current evidences and challenges. Evid Based Complement Alternat Med 2015:425037
24. Chung VCH, Ho RST, Wu XY et al (2015) Are meta-analyses of Chinese herbal medicine trials trustworthy and clinically applicable? A cross-sectional study. J Ethnopharmacol 162:47–54
25. Flower A, Witt C, Liu JP, Ulrich-Merzenich G, Yu H, Lewith G (2012) Guidelines for randomised controlled trials investigating Chinese herbal medicine. J Ethnopharmacol 140:550–554
26. Jia J, Zhu F, Ma X et al (2009) Mechanisms of drug combinations: interaction and network perspectives. Nat Rev Drug Discov 8:111–128
27. Yan H, Zhang B, Li S et al (2010) A formal model for analyzing drug combination effects and its application in TNF-alpha-induced NFkappaB pathway. BMC Syst Biol 4:50
28. Li S, Zhang B, Jiang D et al (2010) Herb network construction and co-module analysis for uncovering the combination rule of traditional Chinese herbal formulae. BMC Bioinformatics 11:S6
29. Jiang M, Lu C, Chen G et al (2012) Understanding the molecular mechanism of interventions in treating rheumatoid arthritis patients with corresponding traditional Chinese medicine patterns based on bioinformatics approach. Evid Based Complement Alternat Med, ID 129452.
30. Li S, Zhang B (2013) Traditional Chinese medicine network pharmacology: theory, methodology and application. Chin J Nat Med 11:110–120
31. Zhou XZ, Li YB, Peng YH et al (2014) Clinical phenotype network: the underlying mechanism for personalized diagnosis and treatment of traditional Chinese medicine. Front Med 8:337–346
32. Motoo Y, Arai I, Tsutani K (2014) Use of Kampo diagnosis in randomized controlled trials of Kampo products in Japan: a systematic review. PLoS One 9:e104422

Chapter 15

Japanese Kampo Medicine: Perspectives

Hajime Suzuki and Akio Inui

Abstract

Japanese Kampo medicine is based on traditional Chinese medicine but is adapted to the Japanese culture and bloomed in the eighteenth century when Japan closed itself off from contact with most foreign countries. Modern translational research on Kampo extending to basic science and clinical studies should be conducted for further development of complementary and alternative medicine and drug discovery for patients with many intractable diseases. Further studies, particularly double-blind studies, are needed to confirm the efficacy of Kampo and to obtain the evidence to support the use of Kampo.

Key words Kampo, Complementary and alternative medicine, Cancer anorexia–cachexia, Herbal medicine, Translational research

1 Introduction

Traditional Chinese medicine (TCM) is a complete system of healing that developed in China about 3000 years ago and reached a coherent, codified form about 2000 years ago [1]. Outside China, in other Asian countries including South Korea, Malaysia, and Vietnam, traditional medicine has formed its own distinct culture [2]. In the sixth century, TCM also spread to Japan and started to develop independently [3]. In Japan, the traditional medicine is commonly called Kampo [2]. Kampo is based on TCM but is adapted to the Japanese culture [1]. Kampo medicine shares many similarities with TCM: they both support the concept of a gradual improvement in the body's condition using natural agents, and diagnosis is made using a pattern of symptoms [3]. But over centuries of independent development, the two systems have diverged in character and practice [3]. Kampo medicine bloomed in the eighteenth century when Japan closed itself off from contact with most foreign countries [3]. A Japanese surgeon, Seishu Hanaoka (1760–1835), made one of the most memorable achievements in surgery and anesthesiology [4]. The first successful surgery for breast cancer under general anesthesia with "Tsusensan"

Akio Inui (ed.), *Herbal Medicines: New Horizons*, Methods in Pharmacology and Toxicology,
DOI 10.1007/978-1-4939-4002-8_15,

(or "Mafutsu-To") was performed on October 13, 1804 [4]. This preceded by 38 years C W Long's clinical use of ether anesthesia in 1842 [4].

In TCM, the treatment is based on the differential diagnosis, whereas Kampo uses a treatment "formulation corresponding to Sho" (the patient's symptoms at a given moment) [1]. When treating a patient, Japanese practitioners recognize the Kampo diagnosis (Sho) and choose the most suitable formula [1]. The relationship between these steps is analogous to a lock and key [1]; each pathological condition is thus related to its prescription [1]. Japanese Kampo practitioners generally tend to check the symptoms by using the traditional four diagnostic methods of observation (hearing and smelling, inquiry and palpation, and name of the disease) and then choose Kampo drugs [1].

In China, TCM practitioners prepare their own mixtures tailored to each patient (although principal ingredients may be standardized) and can choose whether to train in modern medicine or TCM [3]. In Japan, by contrast, Kampo formulas are manufactured according to rules issued by the health ministry in 1987 to ensure consistent preparations [3]. It makes Kampo many advantages over TCM treatment. In Japan, a number of Kampo formulas are manufactured on a modern industrial scale in which the quality and quantity of ingredients are standardized under strict, scientific quality controls [5]. The isolation, identification, and analysis of the active compounds in Kampo formulas are not only important for investigating candidates for new drug development from an extraordinarily rich source but also necessary for quality control and for the elucidation of the pharmacological mechanisms of actions of the drugs now in use [5]. To obtain an overall perspective of as many compounds in a Kampo formula as possible at once, three-dimensional high-performance liquid chromatography (3D HPLC) analysis is useful because Kampo medicines and herbs contain many classes of compounds with different physicochemical properties [5]. Fingerprint patterns provided by 3D HPLC analysis make it possible to identify the overall composition of Kampo drugs [5].

Kampo in palliative treatment of cancer is a fast-emerging area. Palliative care in cancer treatment aims not only for disease control but also for addressing the patient's physical and psychosocial symptoms and improving the quality of life. Recently, the results of a randomized, controlled trial of early palliative care for patients with metastatic non-small-cell lung cancer has been shown that palliative care is appropriate and potentially beneficial when it is introduced at the time of diagnosis of a serious or life-limiting illness—at the same time as all other appropriate and beneficial medical therapies are initiated [6]. Accumulating evidence from clinical studies has shown that Kampo has a significant effect on reducing cancer-related fatigue and pain; improving respiratory tract infections and gastrointestinal side effects including diarrhea, nausea, and vomiting; protecting liver function; and even ameliorating the symptoms of cachexia [7] (details are described in the later section). Kampo will take on an added significance in palliative care for cancer treatment.

At present, Kampo has become a substance of interest for scientific research. The process of acquiring quantifiable clinical trial evidence on Kampo is now clearly underway. Notwithstanding the fact that the molecular mechanisms have yet to be elucidated, the concept of personalized medicine has similarities with the individualized diagnostic and treatment methods of Kampo [8]. Recently, it has been reported that PHY906, a four-herb formulation, reduced the gastrointestinal toxicity of CPT-11 through multiple mechanisms of action that included the inhibition of multiple steps of inflammation and the promotion of intestinal progenitor cell repopulation [9]. Furthermore, recent studies have shown that the herbal medicines such as rikkunshito improve nausea, appetite loss, and cachexia associated with cancer or cancer chemotherapy which worsens QOL and life expectancy of the patients [10]. The mechanism involves an enhancement of signaling by ghrelin which was discovered in 1999 as an appetite-stimulating peptide from the stomach [11, 12]. It has a rivaling action to leptin, an afferent signal from fat tissue which informs the brain the size of body adiposity. Currently, ghrelin agonists and antagonists are being developed and tested for treatment of anorexia–cachexia and obesity, respectively (details are also described in the later section).

2 Herbal Medicine for Cancer Treatment

There are a number of identified published cases of cancer patients treated with Kampo and that reportedly experienced significant clinical benefits [13]. Since many Japanese Kampo have undergone little or no research, often there is little objective information about the potential risks and benefits of their use [13]. Unconventional therapies, such as herbs and minerals, used in ancient medical traditions have led to the identification of active anticancer agents [13]. Mechanisms to support prospective research with such approaches are discussed [13].

2.1 Bakumondoto

Coughing is a common complication in patients with non-small-cell lung cancer after undergoing surgery and chronic obstructive pulmonary disease (COPD) [14]. Bakumondoto has been used as an antitussive agent in China for centuries and is prescribed in Japan for the treatment of bronchitis and pharyngitis accompanying severe dry cough [14]. There are a couple of studies that suggest the mechanisms of bakumondoto to serve as an antitussive agent [14]. Bakumondoto had an effect to reduce cough sensitivity [15], and the antitussive effect of bakumondoto might be mediated by the inhibition of synthesis or release of NO [16]. Other studies demonstrated that bakumondoto inhibited airway hyperresponsiveness induced by ozone in guinea pigs through inhibiting the release of acetylcholine from vagal nerve terminals [17, 18]. Based on these suggested mechanisms for cough, bakumondoto can be regarded as a peripherally acting antitussive drug [14]. Centrally acting drugs, such as codeine and dextromethorphan, are currently the most used antitussives; however, they are often associated with unpleasant or intolerable side effects, including sedation, nausea, and constipation [14]. To avoid these side effects of centrally acting drugs, bakumondoto may be a more suitable antitussive drug for cough in patients with lung cancer surgery and COPD [14]. In addition, through animal or in vitro experiments, bakumondoto had various pharmacological actions, such as anti-inflammatory, anti-allergic, immunomodulatory, secretory-modulating, and metabolic regulatory effects [19, 20]. Moreover, the clinical study also showed that bakumondoto is effective in improving not only prolonged cough after lung cancer surgery but also mental health components in QOL, when compared with dextromethorphan hydrobromide hydrate or dimemorfan phosphate [21].

2.2 Juzentaihoto

Juzentaihoto is a traditional Japanese herbal medicine formula which is composed of 10 different herbs, and the content of this preparation is tightly regulated [22]. It is used in medical practice in Japan for treatment of patients with chronic disease [23]. Interestingly, several recent studies have shown that juzentaihoto has an antitumor effect in animal models [24–26]. Although the active ingredients of this traditional herbal medicines have not been determined and the mechanisms of their protective action remain obscure, some constituents of juzentaihoto have been shown to possess antioxidant activities [27, 28] and act as immunomodulators [29, 30]. Hepatocellular carcinoma (HCC) is one of the world's most common cancers, and it is commonly associated with liver cirrhosis due to alcohol and chronic viral infection (hepatitis virus B and C), aflatoxin B1 exposure, and a variety of metabolic liver diseases [31, 32]. Chronic inflammation is thought to be tightly linked to the mechanisms of HCC through increased production of free radicals from macrophages and neutrophils at the site of inflammation [33, 34]. Because a strong correlation exists between inflammatory cells in the liver, chronic inflammation is considered to be one of the prime targets for therapeutic intervention to prevent both progression of chronic liver disease into cancer and relapse of HCC [23]. The study presents new important information on the anticancer effect of juzentaihoto in humans and provides mechanistic evidence that the protective effects are, at least in part, due to the reduction in oxidant and cytokine production by Kupffer cells [23]. In view of the fact that oxidative stress in the liver infected with HCV is associated with shortened intrahepatic recurrence-free survival of patients with HCC after primary tumor removal, combating oxidative stress and intrahepatic inflammation with juzentaihoto, or other remedies that are well tolerated and easy to use, may prove to be beneficial in management of postoperative patients and improve their quality of life [23].

2.3 Goshajinkigan

In recent years, the standard chemotherapy for advanced/recurrent colorectal cancer is a continuous intravenous infusion of 5-fluorouracil (5-FU) combined with either oxaliplatin (FOLFOX, FOLFOX4 or modified FOLFOX6) or irinotecan (FOLFIRI) [35, 36]. Acute and persistent peripheral neuropathy is the characteristic of oxaliplatin therapy [37], and the oxaliplatin dose must be limited to avoid toxicity [38]. The prevalence of peripheral neurotoxicity increases with the total accumulated dose of oxaliplatin and often interferes with the continuation of FOLFOX therapy [39]. Goshajinkigan is an extracted traditional Japanese herbal medicine that is mainly used for the improvement of symptoms like numbness, cold sensation, and limb pain associated with diabetic neuropathy [40–43]. Recently goshajinkigan was shown to be effective in protecting against the peripheral neurotoxicity due to oxaliplatin in patients with advanced colorectal cancer that were receiving FOLFOX therapy [44, 45]. Two mechanisms have been suggested by which goshajinkigan may alleviate peripheral neurotoxicity [46–48]. The first is that goshajinkigan promotes the release of dynorphin and thus improves numbness/pallesthesia via the opiate system [46–48]. The second is that goshajinkigan promotes nitric oxide production and thus improves the circulation and the blood supply to the nerves [46–48]. Concomitant administration of goshajinkigan reduced the neurotoxicity of oxaliplatin in patients that received chemotherapy for colorectal cancer [38, 46–48].

2.4 Shakuyakukanzoto

Shakuyakukanzoto, a herbal medicine with anticholinergic and prostaglandin-production-inhibiting actions [49], has been reported to be effective in reducing muscle pain, muscle spasms, joint pain, and numbness [50–52]. Shakuyakukanzoto is an extract of a powder mixture of Shakuyaku and Kanzo [53]. It was reported that shakuyakukanzoto inhibits acetylcholine-induced neurogenic contraction on ileum smooth muscle of the guinea pig by the synergistic effects of Kanzo and Shakuyaku [54]. The concentrations of paeoniflorin (main ingredient of Shakuyaku) and glycyrrhizin (main ingredient of Kanzo) that were ineffective when applied individually were able to block neuromuscular synapses when applied in combination [55]. Shakuyakukanzoto also reduced paclitaxel-induced painful peripheral neuropathy, and those effects were based on synergy between Shakuyaku and Kanzo [53]. Paclitaxel is widely used in cancer chemotherapy for the treatment of solid tumors such as breast, ovarian, and lung cancer [53]. However, it sometimes induces moderate to severe muscle pain and impairs the patients' quality of life [53]. An appropriate method for relieving this pain is not well established [53]. The efficacy of the herbal medicine shakuyakukanzoto is expected [53].

2.5 Daikenchuto

Postoperative ileus (POI) is a transient bowel dysmotility after surgery [56]. The pathogenesis of POI is multifactorial and mainly thought to be neural reflex and inflammatory responses [57–59]. POI causes abdominal discomfort, nausea, and vomiting [56]. Delayed return of gastrointestinal (GI) function and resumption of oral intake are major causes for prolonged hospitalization [58]. Daikenchuto is an herbal medicine and has been used for treating adhesive bowel obstruction in Japan [60–62]. It has been suggested that the stimulatory effect of daikenchuto on GI motility is mediated via cholinergic pathways [63]. Moreover, daikenchuto-induced intestinal contractions are mediated via the release of acetylcholine from the myenteric plexus [64, 65]. Abdominal surgery may trigger inhibition of cholinergic transmission via alpha-2-adrenoceptors, resulting in delayed GI transit [56]. It is conceivable that daikenchuto may stimulate vagal activity and facilitate cholinergic transmission of the myenteric plexus in POI [56]. Daikenchuto may be useful for the patients with POI [56].

2.6 Hangeshasinto

Irinotecan hydrochloride (CPT-11) is a potent anticancer agent by inhibiting topoisomerase 1 [66] and is effective for treating colonic cancer and non-small-cell lung cancer that are resistant to many conventional chemotherapeutic drugs [67–70]. The clinical administration of CPT-11 is attended with myelosuppression and gastrointestinal toxicity that lead to severe acute diarrhea and delayed diarrhea that occur soon and 2–3 days after CPT-11 administration, respectively [71]. Delayed diarrhea induced by CPT-11 has been a knotty problem clinically due to a lack of effective treatment and/or prevention strategy available to date even though attempts have been made to control these severe side effects of CPT-11 by using some conventional antidiarrheal drugs such as loperamide [72, 73]. Hangeshasinto, a Japanese traditional medicine, is composed of seven medicinal herbs [71]. This drug is used to treat gastrointestinal disorders such as acute and chronic gastrointestinal catarrh, fermentative diarrhea, and acute gastroenteritis [71]. Hangeshasinto is effective for castor oil-induced diarrhea, but it does not affect intestinal motility [74]. Recent studies have revealed that hangeshasinto suppresses the elevation in colonic prostaglandin E2 (PGE2) level, closely associated with diarrhea, and enhances colonic water absorption [71]. It is well known that PGE2 induces diarrhea and reduces water absorption by the digestive tract [71]. PGE2 is therefore one of the major factors involved in diarrhea [75–77]. The increase in colonic PGE2 and tissue injury accompanied by significantly impaired water absorption of the descending colon has been observed in chronic diarrheal symptoms in rats treated with CPT-11 [71].

Moreover, the clinical study in the topical application of hangeshasinto for patients afflicted with chemotherapy-induced oral mucositis (COM) showed improvements in the severity of its symptoms [78]. Oral mucositis is a common toxicity associated with cytotoxic chemotherapy used for cancer treatment and results in severe discomfort and impairs patients' ability to eat, swallow, and talk [78]. One of the factors associated with COM exacerbation is the activation of cyclooxygenase pathway that mediates ulcer and pain through the upregulation of proinflammatory prostaglandins [79]. Chemotherapy-induced myelosuppression places patients at significant risk of bacteremia and sepsis from oral microorganisms resulting in increased COM [80–83]. However, the optimal treatment of chemotherapy-induced oral mucositis has not been well established [78]. A study showed that topical application of hangeshasinto may have therapeutic effects in patients with chemotherapy-induced oral mucositis via downregulation of proinflammatory prostaglandins [78].

2.7 Hochuekkito

Fatigue is regarded as a common and unavoidable side effect experienced during the course of cancer and its treatment [84]. Cancer-related fatigue is thought to be a multifactorial condition attributed to cancer itself, side effects of therapy, diminished activity, poor nutrition, depression, and intercurrent illness [84]. Cancer-related fatigue interferes with daily activities of cancer patients and affects various aspects of life, including physiological, social, and psychological level [85]. Hochuekkito, originally meaning "Tonify the Middle and Augment the Qi Decoction," has been widely used in traditional medicine in China, Japan, and Korea [84]. This herbal prescription has been identified as an effective medication to improve the function of digestive systems and treat conditions such as general fatigue, poor appetite, spontaneous sweating, and intermittent fever and as an adjunct to treating debilitating condition resulting from chronic diseases [86, 87]. Some clinical studies have been performed regarding the effect of hochuekkito on fatigue, such as a double-blind, placebo-controlled study [88] which suggested that the use of hochuekkito may be helpful for chronic fatigue syndrome [84, 88]. Animal studies also showed positive results in a murine model of chronic fatigue syndrome [89].

The effect of hochuekkito administration was attributed to the mechanism of activating the immune system through significantly increasing lymphocyte cell-surface antigens, CD3-positive cells, and CD3/CD4 double-positive cells in the treatment group [90]. Hochuekkito treats chronic fatigue by inhibiting TNF-α, IL-6, IL-10, TGF-β1, and INF-γ production in chronic fatigue syndrome patients [91]. Hochuekkito also improves systemic inflammation and nutritional status associated with chronic diseases [92, 93].

These results suggest that hochuekkito may affect the pathogenesis of the chronic fatigue syndrome or other chronic diseases [84].

2.8 Rikkunshito

Rikkunshito is a traditional herbal medicine used to treat gastrointestinal tract disorders such as functional dyspepsia [94–98] and gastroesophageal reflux [99]. Rikkunshito is prepared by compounding eight herbal medicines listed in the Japanese Pharmacopoeia: atractylodis lanceae rhizoma, ginseng radix, pinelliae tuber, Hoelen, zizyphi fructus, aurantii nobilis pericarpium, glycyrrhizae radix, and zingiberis rhizoma [100]. It has been shown that oral administration of rikkunshito stimulates secretion of the orexigenic peptide, ghrelin, from the stomach [101, 102].

It was shown that rikkunshito promotes improvement of anorexia in a double-blind study in patients with functional dyspepsia (FD) [103]. A combination of rikkunshito plus 5-HT3 receptor antagonist (an antiemetic agent) reduced anorexia and vomiting induced as adverse reactions after chemotherapy in patients with advanced lung cancer, compared with administration of the antiemetic agent alone [104]. Similarly, administration of a selective serotonin reuptake inhibitor (SSRI), fluvoxamine, in combination with Rikkunshito for 8 weeks resulted in a significant reduction in the number of patients who complained of adverse events, especially retching, compared with SSRI administration alone [97]. The gastrointestinal symptom rating score also significantly improved within 2 weeks of starting coadministration of the SSRI with rikkunshito [97]. These findings suggest that rikkunshito suppresses the onset of adverse reactions to frequently prescribed drugs that cannot be treated adequately by adjuvant therapy with current Western medicines [100].

Cisplatin has been shown to cause a significant decrease in plasma ghrelin and food intake in rodents [101], and intravenous injection of exogenous acylated ghrelin inhibited the decrease in food intake after cisplatin administration [100]. Rikkunshito also inhibited the decrease in circulating ghrelin concentration and ameliorated the decrease in food intake caused by cisplatin [100]. Interestingly, coadministration of a ghrelin receptor antagonist, (D-Lys3)-GHRP-6, with rikkunshito abolished this effect [100]. These findings suggest that the mechanism of improvement of anorexia by rikkunshito may involve ghrelin receptor activation via stimulation of ghrelin secretion from the stomach into the plasma [100]. Heptamethoxyflavone, an active ingredient flavonoid in rikkunshito, has been shown to have a pivotal effect on stimulation of ghrelin secretion [100]. In addition, P388-bearing mice showed a tendency for improved survival with rikkunshito treatment, and survival was further improved by treatment with cisplatin in combination with rikkunshito, although the difference was not significant [105]. These results show that administration of rikkunshito has no adverse effect on the anticancer action of cisplatin itself [100].

It has been shown that oral administration of rikkunshito restores disturbed motor activity in the gastrointestinal tract and ameliorates anorexia in rats administered SSRIs [102]. Intraperitoneal administration of fenfluramine or fluvoxamine shifted fasted rats from a fasted-like motor pattern in the antrum and duodenum to fed-like motor activities similar to those seen after feeding [102]. A significant decrease in the plasma concentration of acylated ghrelin, delayed gastric emptying, and decreased food intake was also observed after administration of the SSRI [102]. The SSRIs decrease food intake and fasted motor activities through the 5-HT2c receptor pathway, which requires downstream activation of MC-MC4R signaling for feeding and inhibition of ghrelin-GHS-R signaling for GI motor effects [102]. Concomitant oral administration of rikkunshito with an SSRI suppressed the decrease in plasma acylated ghrelin, changed the fed-like motor activity to fasted activity, suppressed anorexia, and enhanced gastric emptying [100]. These effects were abolished by coadministration of a ghrelin receptor antagonist with rikkunshito [100]. These results indicate a functional divergence of central 5-HT2c receptor pathway [102]. This study has uncovered a novel central 5-HT2c receptor pathway regulating physiologic fasted and fed motor activities, which may represent an integrated mechanism linking feeding behavior and GI motor activities through the gut-brain axis [106, 107]. Cisplatin and SSRIs are widely used in clinical practice [100]. 5-HT is a key factor in adverse reactions to these drugs, since both stimulate production of excess 5-HT and suppress 5-HT metabolism in vivo [100]. The 5-HT2 receptor in appetite control had been shown [108]; specifically, appetite is suppressed when the 5-HT2b receptor in gastric smooth muscle and the 5-HT2c receptor in the central nervous system are activated by receptor agonists [100]. 5-HT produced during treatment with cisplatin or SSRIs binds to various receptor subtypes and is likely to stimulate the 5-HT2b and 2c receptors [100]. A decrease in plasma ghrelin is suppressed by administration of antagonists for these receptors, leading to improvements in food intake and gastrointestinal dysmotility [101, 102]. Isoliquiritigenin, heptamethoxyflavone, and hesperidin are ingredients of rikkunshito that have been shown to antagonize 5-HT2b and 2c receptors [101]; thus, these ingredients are considered to play an important role in the improvement of appetite by rikkunshito [100]. Administration of hesperidin reverses the decrease in plasma ghrelin in cisplatin-treated rats and shifts the fed-like motor pattern induced by SSRI administration to a fasted pattern [100]. Thus, 5-HT2c antagonism by active components in rikkunshito may lead to the improvement of anorexia [100].

More recent report demonstrated that administration of rikkunshito counteracts anorexia of aging via inhibiting a reduced hypothalamic ghrelin receptor reactivity [100]. The data indicated that aging-associated anorexia is caused by an increase in plasma leptin, which results from disturbed reactivity of ghrelin in the hypothalamus and regulation of ghrelin secretion [109]. It has been reported that leptin suppresses the ghrelin-induced activation of NPY neurons [110]. Moreover, leptin activates the PI3K-PDE pathway [111] in NPY neurons. The activation of PI3K-PDE pathway by leptin was recently proposed as a mechanism by which leptin blocks the activity of ghrelin, and it may counteract the adenylate cyclase-cAMP-PKA system implicated in the effect of ghrelin [110]. In this study, oral administration of either the PI3K inhibitor LY-294002 or the PDE3 inhibitor cilostamide ameliorated anorexia in aged mice [109]. Rikkunshito administration also caused a significant reduction in aging-associated anorexia [109]. Similar to cilostamide, the components of rikkunshito may improve appetite by suppressing cAMP downregulation by leptin through PDE3 inhibition in the brain [109].

3 Potentiation of Ghrelin Signaling Attenuates Cancer Anorexia–Cachexia and Prolongs Survival: Modern Translational Approach

Herbal medicines, composed of multiple biologically active compounds, are widely claimed to help a variety of diseases [9]. Our study demonstrated that the integrated mechanism underlying cancer anorexia–cachexia involves lowered ghrelin signaling due to excessive hypothalamic interactions of 5-HT with CRF through the 5-HT2cR and that rikkunshito may be useful in clinical practice for cachectic cancer patients with its potentiation effect of ghrelin signaling [10].

In this study, it was demonstrated that plasma acyl ghrelin concentrations in tumor-bearing rats were higher than those in free-fed normal rats, but lower than those in pair-fed normal rats, and had an inverse relationship with plasma leptin concentrations [10]. These results indicate that changes in ghrelin and leptin secretion in pair-fed animals represent a compensatory mechanism in a persistent catabolic state and that these responses are attenuated in tumor-bearing rats [10]. Peripheral ghrelin administration stimulates food intake in melanoma cell-bearing mice and cancer patients [112] in the short term as well as in lean, healthy men and women [113]. There were similar therapeutic effects of ghrelin on anorexia and GI dysmotility in cachectic animal models, suggesting that high plasma concentrations of ghrelin may overcome resistance to the appetite-stimulating effects of the endogenous peptide in the short term [10]. Rikkunshito, which mimics these ghrelin effects, effectively improved food intake and GI motor activities in this study [10]. Oral administration of rikkunshito increases plasma acyl ghrelin levels in humans, mice [114], rats [101, 102], and dogs [10]. Rikkunshito stimulates ghrelin secretion through 5-HT2b/2c receptor antagonism, and its active flavonoid ingredients such as hesperidin that antagonize 5-HT2b/2c receptor binding have been identified [101].

The central 5-HT system has been implicated in the processes of meal satiation and satiety [10]. 5-HT reuptake inhibitors such as fenfluramine and 5-HT2cR agonists attenuate food intake and weight gain in rodents and humans [115–117], with the involvement of potentiated MC signaling and decreased ghrelin secretion [10]. 5-HT also inhibits NPY/AgRP neurons by activating the 5-HT1bR, leading to decreased orexigenic signaling and an inhibitory drive onto POMC cells [10]. However, the previous study has demonstrated that the 5-HT2cR has a major role in the regulation of physiological fasted and fed motor activities in addition to feeding through changes in endogenous ghrelin [102]. In this study, the decreases in food intake and GI motor activities in tumor-bearing rats were recovered after administration of either a 5-HT2cR antagonist or ghrelin [10]. The 5-HT concentration in the hypothalamus is increased in humans and animals with cancer [118, 119]; in addition, NPY and dopamine concentrations decrease simultaneously, while 5-HT concentration increases in the PVN at the onset of anorexia in tumor-bearing rats [120]. These findings suggest that 5-HT2cR activation in tumor-bearing rats induces anorexia in part via decreased ghrelin secretion [10].

The hypothermia in tumor-bearing rats may be due to a state of negative energy balance or a decrease in the threshold for the activation of thermogenesis, which is involved in starvation-induced hypothermia [121]. IL-1β and leptin [122] decrease the expression of ghrelin mRNA in the stomach, whereas IL-6 produced in various cells, including adipocytes, regulates leptin production [123]. These findings suggest that cytokines have an important role in energy balance through the persistent activation of the leptin system and the inhibition of the ghrelin-NPY/agouti-related peptide orexigenic network in tumor-bearing rats [10]. In addition to NPY and agouti-related peptide, the level of POMC mRNA was also decreased in the hypothalamus of the tumor-bearing rats [10]. Synaptic input organization and mRNA expression of POMC neuron have been shown to be increased in adrenalectomized animals and restored by corticosterone replacement [124]. Thus, activity of hypothalamic POMC neuron may be affected by changes in circulating levels of corticosterone and a state of negative energy balance [10].

Hypothalamic 5-HT and CRF activities are stimulated by proinflammatory cytokines in the circulation and the hypothalamus [125, 126]. A CRF receptor antagonist attenuated cancer anorexia–cachexia, and administration of the 5-HT2cR antagonist or rikkunshito reduced hypothalamic CRF levels and anxiety-related behaviors in tumor-bearing rats [10]. The improvement in anxiety by rikkunshito may lead to a higher quality of life in cancer patients [10]. Some studies suggest that ghrelin induces anxiety, whereas others suggest that the elevated ghrelin helps animals cope with stress by producing anxiolytic-like response [127]. Future studies are needed to sort out the effect of ghrelin on anxiety-like behavior as in the case for NPY [128]. Importantly, a hypothalamic 5-HT-CRF receptor pathway that regulates ghrelin secretion has a major role in cancer anorexia–cachexia [10].

It has been previously shown that a central 5-HT2cR pathway regulates ghrelin secretion without downstream activation of melanocortin 3/4 receptors [102]. The 5-HT2cR is expressed in many brain regions, and its expression is restricted to the central nervous system [10]. Dual-neurohistochemical labeling has revealed that approximately one-half of PVN CRF-containing neurons co-express 5-HT2cR mRNA [129]. In this study, 5-HT activated single CRF neurons isolated from the PVN, and the activities of the CRF neurons were blocked by simultaneous administration of rikkunshito [10]. Moreover, intracerebroventricular administration of CRF decreased plasma acyl ghrelin in fasted rats [10]. These findings suggest that CRF neurons are involved in 5-HT-regulated ghrelin secretion [10].

The GHS-R is reportedly expressed in vagal afferent neurons, and the gastric vagus nerve system is involved in the effect of ghrelin on food intake and GI motor activities [130, 131]. It was demonstrated that ghrelin decreased the afferent activity of the gastric vagus nerve [10]. Gastric ghrelin signaling via vagal afferents stimulated the efferent activities of both the gastric and the celiac branches of the vagus nerve and suppressed the activity of the sympathetic nerve [10]. Peripheral administration of a higher dose of ghrelin increased the discharge rate of the vagal efferent nerve, probably in part through the GHS-R in the ARC of the hypothalamus [10]. It also has been shown that rikkunshito activated the efferent vagus nerve, which may be mediated by both the vagal afferent nerve and the direct central action [10]. In addition, ghrelin-induced cellular signaling in GHS-R-expressing cells was enhanced by pretreatment with rikkunshito and its active components, such as atractylodin, which stimulate ghrelin/GHS-R binding activity [10]. Similar potentiating effects of rikkunshito were observed in rat ARC NPY neurons [10]. These findings suggest that the physiological functions of endogenous ghrelin are enhanced by the dual actions of rikkunshito, which involve the stimulation of ghrelin secretion and the activation of GHS-R activity, possibly due to allosteric changes in the receptor [10]. This potentiation of the ghrelin effect by rikkunshito on NPY neurons could be orexigenic because the activity of ghrelin-responsive NPY neurons is coupled to feeding [110, 132]. As mentioned in the past section, ghrelin strongly stimulates GH secretion in humans

[133–136], which regulates IGF-1 levels, and increases muscle strength [137, 138]. Moreover, ghrelin induces the anti-inflammatory cytokine [139, 140], while suppresses the production of proinflammatory cytokines [139, 141–143], and inhibits the activation of NF-kB which may regulate skeletal muscle proteasome expression and protein degradation [140, 142, 144]. Consequently, potentiation of ghrelin receptor signaling with rikkunshito can be valuable in the treatment of anorexia and muscle wasting which characterize cancer anorexia–cachexia syndrome [10].

The adverse effect of (D-Lys3)-GHRP-6 on survival in tumor-bearing rats has been indicated in this study, suggesting that the potentiation of ghrelin signaling is critical to the attenuation of anorexia–cachexia and the prolongation of survival in subjects with cancer [10]. Rikkunshito and its active component, atractylodin, prolonged survival in these animals, and this effect was enhanced by the concomitant administration of cisplatin [10]. Cancer patients receiving chemotherapy or radiation therapy may experience nausea, vomiting, taste changes, stomatitis, and diarrhea, which could contribute to weight loss and decreased survival [10]. Therefore, cancer anorexia–cachexia syndrome is a major obstacle in cancer chemotherapy [145]. Use of rikkunshito in tumor-bearing rats was effective not only against anorexia–cachexia but also for promoting survival, particularly in combination with chemotherapy [10]. However, daily administration of a 5-HT2c receptor antagonist failed to prolong survival, suggesting that a sensitizing effect on the GHS-R may be essential for ameliorating ghrelin resistance in anorexia–cachexia in the long term [10]. Pancreatic cancer patients generally respond poorly to chemotherapy, resulting in a higher frequency of anorexia–cachexia [10]. The median survival of pancreatic cancer patients treated with gemcitabine was prolonged by the addition of rikkunshito, particularly for those with ascites [10].

In conclusion, these results suggest that rikkunshito may be useful in clinical practice for cachectic cancer patients via its dual action on ghrelin secretion and receptor sensitization [10]. The synergism of activity of the herbs demonstrated in this study highlights the importance of adopting traditional approaches to the utilization of traditional medicines.

4 Concluding Remarks

In recent years, studies on evaluation of the therapeutic and toxic activity of herbal medicinal products became available and popular [146]. The advances in modern biotechnology have led to discovery of many new active constituents [146]. Although the working mechanisms of some of the herbs are unclear and remain to be elucidated, they are worth further studying as newly potential therapy agents [146]. However, it is a constant challenge to establish the pharmacological basis for efficacy and safety of herbal medicinal products [146]. A better understanding of the effects and bioavailability of phytopharmaceuticals can help in discovering suitable and rational therapies [146]. Yet when considering herbal medicines to be used in the treatment (e.g., in the treatment of cancer patients), one must take into account reproducibility of preclinical findings in clinical practice, quality assurance of herbal products, and potential toxicities associated with alternative therapies. All risks and benefits of herbal medicines must be openly discussed and reviewed with the patient [147]. During the process of evaluating traditional herbal remedies, the responsibility of traditional medicine practitioners will be to facilitate the appropriate evaluation of effectiveness, while other medical research techniques provide the capacity and approaches to determine how the therapeutic agents work. This order of activity differs from conventional synthetic or semisynthetic pharmaceutical research for new therapeutic chemical constituents, where the latter has had no marketplace exposure or history of human usage in therapy. However, the multicomponent herbal medicines capable of targeting multiple sites could be useful for future drug discovery. Mechanistic studies and identification of active compounds could lead to new discoveries in biological and biomedical sciences. Prediction of absorption, distribution, metabolism, and excretion (ADME) properties in herbal medicines is now in progress. Herbal medicine seeks disturbances in the human body by analyzing all symptoms and signs in whole-body level, and this makes it possible to treat diseases due to multiple pathogenic factors and some diseases that are not very well understood [1]. Both Western-style modern medicine and Kampo aim to heal patients in a harmonized way and can be developed together into an integrated form of personalized medicine [8]. Modern translational research on Kampo and thus herbal medicines that goes beyond basic science and clinical perspectives should be conducted for further development of complementary and alternative medicine (CAM) and drug discovery for patients with cancer and many other intractable diseases. Further studies, particularly double-blind studies, are needed to verify the efficacy of Kampo and to obtain high-quality evidence to support the use of Kampo.

References

1. Yu F, Takahashi T, Moriya J et al (2006) Traditional Chinese medicine and Kampo: a review from the distant past for the future. J Int Med Res 34:231–239
2. Cheung F (2011) TCM: Made in China. Nature 480:S82–S83. doi:10.1038/480S82a
3. Fuyuno I (2011) Japan: will the sun set on Kampo? Nature 480:S96. doi:10.1038/480S96a
4. Izuo M (2004) Medical history: Seishu hanaoka and his success in breast cancer surgery under general anesthesia two hundred years ago. Breast Cancer 11:319–324. doi:10.1007/BF02968037
5. Ohtake N, Nakai Y, Yamamoto M et al (2004) Separation and isolation methods for analysis of the active principles of Sho-saiko-to (SST) oriental medicine. J Chromatogr B Analyt

Technol Biomed Life Sci 812:135–148. doi:10.1016/j.jchromb.2004.06.051

6. Temel JS, Greer JA, Muzikansky A et al (2010) Early palliative care for patients with metastatic non-small-cell lung cancer. N Engl J Med 363:733–742
7. Qi F, Li A, Inagaki Y et al (2010) Chinese herbal medicines as adjuvant treatment during chemo- or radio-therapy for cancer. Biosci Trends 4:297–307
8. Liu L, Leung EL-H, Tian X (2011) Perspective: the clinical trial barriers. Nature 480: S100. doi:10.1038/480S100a
9. Lam W, Bussom S, Guan F et al (2010) The four-herb Chinese medicine PHY906 reduces chemotherapy-induced gastrointestinal toxicity. Sci Transl Med 2:45ra59. doi:10.1126/scitranslmed.3001270
10. Fujitsuka N, Asakawa A, Uezono Y et al (2011) Potentiation of ghrelin signaling attenuates cancer anorexia-cachexia and prolongs survival. Transl Psychiatry 1:e23. doi:10.1038/tp.2011.25
11. Inui A (2001) Ghrelin: an orexigenic and somatotrophic signal from the stomach. Nat Rev Neurosci 2:551–560. doi:10.1038/35086018
12. Inui A (2003) Neuropeptide gene polymorphisms and human behavioural disorders. Nat Rev Drug Discov 2:986–998. doi:10.1038/nrd1252
13. Olaku O, White JD (2011) Herbal therapy use by cancer patients: a literature review on case reports. Eur J Cancer 47:508–514. doi:10.1016/j.ejca.2010.11.018
14. Mukaida K, Hattori N, Kondo K et al (2011) A pilot study of the multiherb Kampo medicine bakumondoto for cough in patients with chronic obstructive pulmonary disease. Phytomedicine 18:625–629. doi:10.1016/j.phymed.2010.11.006
15. Smith J, Woodcock A (2006) Cough and its importance in COPD. Int J Chron Obstruct Pulmon Dis 1:305–314
16. Kamei J, Yoshikawa Y, Saitoh A (2005) Antitussive effect of Bakumondoto (Mai-men-dong-tang) in guinea-pigs exposed to cigarette smoke. J Tradit Med 22:44–48
17. Aizawa H, Shigyo M, Nakano H et al (1999) Effect of the Chinese herbal medicine, Bakumondo-to, on airway hyperresponsiveness induced by ozone exposure in guinea-pigs. Respirology 4:349–354
18. Aizawa H, Yoshida M, Inoue H, Hara N (2003) Traditional oriental herbal medicine, Bakumondo-to, suppresses vagal neuro-effector transmission in guinea pig trachea. J Asthma 40:497–503
19. Miyata T (2004) Pharmacological characteristics of traditional medicine as curative 'Polypharmacy'. Journal of Traditional Medicines 21:155–165. doi:10.11339/jtm.21.155
20. Miyata T (2007) Pharmacological basis of traditional medicines and health supplements as curatives. J Pharmacol Sci 103:127–131
21. Tsunezuka Y (2010) The efficacy of bakumondoto on prolonged cough after lung cancer surgery. Kampo to Meneki Arerugi (Kampo and Immuno-Allergy) 22:43–55
22. Saiki I (2000) A Kampo medicine "Juzen-taiho-to-" prevention of malignant progression and metastasis of tumor cells and the mechanism of action. Biol Pharm Bull 23:677–688
23. Tsuchiya M, Kono H, Matsuda M et al (2008) Protective effect of Juzen-taiho-to on hepatocarcinogenesis is mediated through the inhibition of Kupffer cell-induced oxidative stress. Int J Cancer 123:2503–2511. doi:10.1002/ijc.23828
24. Saiki I, Yamaura T, Ohnishi Y et al (1999) HPLC analysis of juzen-taiho-to and its variant formulations and their antimetastatic efficacies. Chem Pharm Bull 47:1170–1174
25. Kamiyama H, Takano S, Ishikawa E et al (2005) Anti-angiogenic and immunomodulatory effect of the herbal medicine "Juzen-taiho-to" on malignant glioma. Biol Pharm Bull 28:2111–2116
26. Tatsuta M, Iishi H, Baba M et al (1994) Inhibition by shi-quan-da-bu-tang (TJ-48) of experimental hepatocarcinogenesis induced by N-nitrosomorpholine in Sprague-Dawley rats. Eur J Cancer 30A:74–78
27. Dhuley JN (1999) Anti-oxidant effects of cinnamon (Cinnamomum verum) bark and greater cardamom (Amomum subulatum) seeds in rats fed high fat diet. Indian J Exp Biol 37:238–242
28. Keum YS, Park KK, Lee JM et al (2000) Antioxidant and anti-tumor promoting activities of the methanol extract of heat-processed ginseng. Cancer Lett 150:41–48
29. Chino A, Sakurai H, Choo M-K et al (2005) Juzentaihoto, a Kampo medicine, enhances IL-12 production by modulating Toll-like receptor 4 signaling pathways in murine peritoneal exudate macrophages. Int Immunopharmacol 5:871–882. doi:10.1016/j.intimp.2005.01.004
30. Kawamata H, Ochiai H, Mantani N, Terasawa K (2000) Enhanced expression of inducible nitric oxide synthase by Juzen-taiho-to in LPS-activated RAW264.7 cells, a murine macrophage cell line. Am J Chin Med 28:217–226

31. Inoue H, Seitz HK (2001) Viruses and alcohol in the pathogenesis of primary hepatic carcinoma. Eur J Cancer Prev 10:107–110
32. Kountouras J, Lygidakis NJ (2000) New epidemiological data on liver oncogenesis. Hepatogastroenterology 47:855–861
33. Hussain S, Hofseth L, Harris C (2003) Radical causes of cancer. Nat Rev Cancer 3:276–285
34. Koike K (2006) Oxidative stress and hepatitis C viral infection. Hepatol Res 34:65–73
35. Engstrom PF, Arnoletti JP, Benson AB et al (2009) NCCN Clinical Practice Guidelines in Oncology: colon cancer. J Natl Compr Canc Netw 7:778–831
36. Zuckerman DS, Clark JW (2008) Systemic therapy for metastatic colorectal cancer: current questions. Cancer 112:1879–1891. doi:10.1002/cncr.23409
37. Cassidy J, Misset J-L (2002) Oxaliplatin-related side effects: characteristics and management. Semin Oncol 29:11–20. doi:10.1053/sonc.2002.35524
38. Kono T, Mamiya N, Chisato N et al (2009) Efficacy of goshajinkigan for peripheral neurotoxicity of oxaliplatin in patients with advanced or recurrent colorectal cancer. Evid Based Complement Alternat Med. doi:10.1093/ecam/nep200
39. de Gramont A, Figer A, Seymour M (2000) Leucovorin and fluorouracil with or without oxaliplatin as first-line treatment in advanced colorectal cancer. J Clin Oncol 18 (16):2938–2947
40. Uno T, Ohsawa I, Tokudome M, Sato Y (2005) Effects of goshajinkigan on insulin resistance in patients with type 2 diabetes. Diabetes Res Clin Pract 69:129–135. doi:10.1016/j.diabres.2004.11.017
41. Tawata M, Kurihara A, Nitta K, Iwase E (1994) The effects of goshajinkigan, a herbal medicine, on subjective symptoms and vibratory threshold in patients with diabetic neuropathy. Diabetes Res Clin Pract 26 (2):121–128
42. Usuki Y, Usuki S, Hommura S (1991) Successful treatment of a senile diabetic woman with cataract with goshajinkigan. Am J Chin Med 19:259–263
43. Sato Y, Sakamoto N (1985) Treatment of diabetic neuropathy with Niu-Che-Sen-Qi-Wan. In: Recent Advances in Traditional Medicine in East Asia. Excerpta Medica, Amsterdam, pp 376–383
44. Mamiya N, Kono T, Mamiya K et al (2007) A case of neurotoxicity reduced with goshajinkigan in modified FOLFOX6 chemotherapy for advanced colon cancer. Gan To Kagaku Ryoho 34:1295–1297
45. Shindo Y, Tenma K, Imano H et al (2008) Reduction of oxaliplatin-related neurotoxicity by Gosha-jinki-gan. Gan To Kagaku Ryoho 35:863–865
46. Yamada K, Suzuki E, Nakaki T et al (2005) Aconiti tuber increases plasma nitrite and nitrate levels in humans. J Ethnopharmacol 96:165–169. doi:10.1016/j.jep.2004.09.028
47. Gotoh A, Goto K, Sengoku A et al (2004) Inhibition mechanism of Gosha-jinki-gan on the micturition reflex in rats. J Pharmacol Sci 96:115–123
48. Hu X, Sato J, Oshida Y et al (2003) Effect of Gosha-jinki-gan (Chinese herbal medicine: Niu-Che-Sen-Qi-Wan) on insulin resistance in streptozotocin-induced diabetic rats. Diabetes Res Clin Pract 59(2):103–111
49. Imai A, Horibe S, Fuseya S et al (1995) Possible evidence that the herbal medicine shakuyaku-kanzo-to decreases prostaglandin levels through suppressing arachidonate turnover in endometrium. J Med 26:163–174
50. Yamamoto K, Hoshiai H, Noda K (2001) Effects of shakuyaku-kanzo-to on muscle pain from combination chemotherapy with paclitaxel and carboplatin. Gynecol Oncol 81:333–334. doi:10.1006/gyno.2001.6168
51. Hyodo T, Taira T, Kumakura M et al (2002) The immediate effect of Shakuyaku-kanzo-to, traditional Japanese herbal medicine, for muscular cramps during maintenance hemodialysis. Nephron 90:240
52. Hinoshita F (2003) Effect of orally administered shao-yao-gan-cao-tang (Shakuyaku-kanzo-to) on muscle cramps in maintenance hemodialysis patients: a preliminary study. Am J Chin Med 31:445–453. doi:10.1142/S0192415X03001144
53. Hidaka T, Shima T, Nagira K et al (2009) Herbal medicine Shakuyaku-kanzo-to reduces paclitaxel-induced painful peripheral neuropathy in mice. Eur J Pain 13:22–27. doi:10.1016/j.ejpain.2008.03.003
54. Maeda T, Shinozuka K, Baba K (1983) Effect of shakuyaku-kanzoh-toh, a prescription composed of shakuyaku (Paeoniae Radix) and kanzoh (Glycyrrhizae Radix) on guinea pig ileum. J Pharmacobiodyn 6:153–160
55. Kimura M, Kimura I, Takahashi K et al (1984) Blocking effects of blended paeoniflorin or its related compounds with glycyrrhizin on neuromuscular junctions in frog and mouse. Jpn J Pharmacol 36:275–282

56. Fukuda H, Chen C, Mantyh C et al (2006) The herbal medicine, Dai-Kenchu-to, accelerates delayed gastrointestinal transit after the operation in rats. J Surg Res 131:290–295. doi:10.1016/j.jss.2005.09.018
57. Kehlet H (2001) Review of postoperative ileus. Am J Surg 182:3S
58. Livingston E (1990) Postoperative ileus. Dig Dis Sci 35(121):1990
59. Miedema BW, Johnson JO (2003) Methods for decreasing postoperative gut dysmotility. Lancet Oncol 4:365–372
60. Moriwaki Y, Yamamoto T, Katamura H (1992) Clinical research to the effect of daikenchuto for simple intestinal obstruction. Nihon Touyou Igaku Zassi 43:303, Japanese
61. Furukawa Y, Shiga Y, Hanyu N, Hashimoto Y (1995) Effect of Chinese herbal medicine on gastrointestinal motility and bowel obstruction. Jpn J Gastroenterol Surg 28:956, Japanese
62. Itoh T, Yamakawa J, Mai M (2002) The effect of the herbal medicine dai-kenchu-to on postoperative ileus. J Int Med Res 30:428
63. Shibata C, Sasaki I, Naito H, Ueno T (1999) The herbal medicine Dai-Kenchu-Tou stimulates upper gut motility through cholinergic and 5-hydroxytryptamine 3 receptors in conscious dogs. Surgery 126:918
64. Kurosawa S, Nishikawa S, Kaneko M, Ogiwara S (1998) The herbal medicine Daikenchu-to contracts guinea pig distal colon muscle through acetylcholine release*. Gastroenterology 114:A782
65. Satoh K, Hayakawa T, Kase Y et al (2001) Mechanisms for contractile effect of Daikenchu-to in isolated guinea pig ileum. Dig Dis Sci 46:250–256
66. Andoh T, Ishii K, Suzuki Y et al (1987) Characterization of a mammalian mutant with a camptothecin-resistant DNA topoisomerase I. Proc Natl Acad Sci U S A 84:5565–5569
67. Negoro S, Fukuoka M, Masuda N et al (1991) Phase I study of weekly intravenous infusions of CPT-11, a new derivative of camptothecin, in the treatment of advanced non-small-cell lung cancer. J Natl Cancer Inst 83:1164–1168
68. Fukuoka M, Niitani H, Suzuki A et al (1992) A phase II study of CPT-11, a new derivative of camptothecin, for previously untreated non-small-cell lung cancer. J Clin Oncol 10:16–20
69. Shimada Y, Yoshino M, Wakui A et al (1993) Phase II study of CPT-11, a new camptothecin derivative, in metastatic colorectal cancer. CPT-11 Gastrointestinal Cancer Study Group. J Clin Oncol 11:909–913
70. Masuda N, Fukuoka M, Kudoh S (1994) Phase I study of irinotecan and cisplatin with granulocyte colony-stimulating factor support for advanced non-small-cell lung cancer. J Clin Oncol 12:90–96
71. Kase Y, Hayakawa T, Aburada M et al (1997) Preventive effects of Hange-shashin-to on irinotecan hydrochloride-caused diarrhea and its relevance to the colonic prostaglandin E2 and water absorption in the rat. Jpn J Pharmacol 75:407–413
72. Abigerges D, Armand J (1994) Irinotecan (CPT-11) high-dose escalation using intensive high-dose loperamide to control diarrhea. J Natl Cancer Inst 86:446–449
73. Goncalves E, de Costa L, Abigerges D, Armand JP (1995) A new enkephalinase inhibitor as an alternative to loperamide in the prevention of diarrhea induced by CPT-11. J Clin Oncol 13:2144–2146
74. Kase Y, Hayakawa T, Takeda S et al (1996) Pharmacological studies on antidiarrheal effects of Hange-shashin-to. Biol Pharm Bull 19:1367–1370
75. Rask-Madsen J (1986) Eicosanoids and their role in the pathogenesis of diarrhoeal diseases. Clin Gastroenterol 15:545–566
76. Rask-Madsen J, Bukhave K (1990) Influence on intestinal secretion of eicosanoids. J Intern Med Suppl 732:137–144
77. Rivière PJ, Farmer SC, Burks TF, Porreca F (1991) Prostaglandin E2-induced diarrhea in mice: importance of colonic secretion. J Pharmacol Exp Ther 256:547–552
78. Kono T (2010) Topical application of hangeshashinto (TJ-14) in the treatment of chemotherapy-induced oral mucositis. World J Oncol. doi:10.4021/wjon263w
79. Lalla RV, Pilbeam CC, Walsh SJ et al (2009) Role of the cyclooxygenase pathway in chemotherapy-induced oral mucositis: a pilot study. Support Care Cancer. doi:10.1007/s00520-009-0635-1
80. Scardina GA, Pisano T, Messina P (2010) Oral mucositis. Review of literature. N Y State Dent J 76:34–38
81. Napenas JJ, Shetty KV, Streckfus CF (2007) Oral mucositis: review of pathogenesis, diagnosis, prevention, and management. Gen Dent 55:335–344, quiz 345–6, 376
82. Scully C, Sonis S (2006) Oral mucositis. Oral Dis 14:505–515
83. Sonis ST (2004) The pathobiology of mucositis. Nat Rev Cancer 4:277–284. doi:10.1038/nrc1318

84. Jeong JS, Ryu BH, Kim JS et al (2010) Bojungikki-tang for cancer-related fatigue: a pilot randomized clinical trial. Integr Cancer Ther 9:331–338. doi:10.1177/1534735410383170
85. Sood A, Barton DL, Bauer BA, Loprinzi CL (2007) A critical review of complementary therapies for cancer-related fatigue. Integr Cancer Ther 6:8–13. doi:10.1177/1534735406298143
86. Scheid V, Bensky D, Ellis A (1990) (2009) Chinese herbal medicine: formulas & strategies. Eastland Press, Seattle, WA
87. Kobayashi H, Mizuno N, Teramae H (2004) The effects of Hochu-ekki-to in patients with atopic dermatitis resistant to conventional treatment. Int J Tissue React 26:113–117
88. Kuratsune H (1997) Effect of Kampo Medicine, "Hochu-ekki-to", on chronic fatigue syndrome. Clin Res 74:1837–1845
89. Wang X, Takahashi T, Zhu S (2004) Effect of Hochu-ekki-to(TJ-41), a Japanese herbal medicine, on daily activity in a murine model of chronic fatigue syndrome. Evid Based Complement Alternat Med 1:203–206
90. Satoh N, Sakai S, Kogure T et al (2005) A randomized double blind placebo-controlled clinical trial of Hochuekkito, a traditional herbal medicine, in the treatment of elderly patients with weakness N of one and responder restricted design. Phytomedicine 12:549–554
91. Shin H-Y, Shin C-H, Shin T-Y et al (2003) Effect of bojungikki-tang on lipopolysaccharide-induced cytokine production from peripheral blood mononuclear cells of chronic fatigue syndrome patients. Immunopharmacol Immunotoxicol 25:491–501. doi:10.1081/IPH-120026435
92. Shinozuka N, Tatsumi K, Nakamura A (2007) The traditional herbal medicine Hochuekkito improves systemic inflammation in patients with chronic obstructive pulmonary disease. J Am Geriatr Soc 55:313–314
93. Tatsumi K, Shinozuka N, Nakayama K et al (2009) Hochuekkito improves systemic inflammation and nutritional status in elderly patients with chronic obstructive pulmonary disease. J Am Geriatr Soc 57:169–170. doi:10.1111/j.1532-5415.2009.02034.x
94. Kusunoki H, Haruma K, Hata J et al (2010) Efficacy of Rikkunshito, a traditional Japanese medicine (Kampo), in treating functional dyspepsia. Intern Med 49:2195–2202
95. Takahashi T, Endo S, Nakajima K et al (2009) Effect of rikkunshito, a chinese herbal medicine, on stasis in patients after pylorus-preserving gastrectomy. World J Surg 33:296–302. doi:10.1007/s00268-008-9854-8
96. Oyachi N, Takano K, Hasuda N, Arai H (2008) Effects of Rikkunshi-to on infantile hypertrophic pyloric stenosis, refractory to atropine. Pediatr Int 50:581–583
97. Oka T, Tamagawa Y, Hayashida S et al (2007) Rikkunshi-to attenuates adverse gastrointestinal symptoms induced by fluvoxamine. Biopsychosoc Med 1:21. doi:10.1186/1751-0759-1-21
98. Yagi M, Homma S, Kubota M, Iinuma Y (2004) The herbal medicine Rikkunshi-to stimulates and coordinates the gastric myoelectric activity in post-operative dyspeptic children after gastrointestinal surgery. Pediatr Surg Int 19:760–765
99. Kawahara H, Okuyama H, Nose K et al (2010) Physiological and clinical characteristics of gastroesophageal reflux after congenital diaphragmatic hernia repair. J Pediatr Surg 45:2346–2350. doi:10.1016/j.jpedsurg.2010.08.029
100. Hattori T (2010) Rikkunshito and ghrelin. Int J Pept. doi:10.1155/2010/283549
101. Takeda H, Sadakane C, Hattori T et al (2008) Rikkunshito, an herbal medicine, suppresses cisplatin-induced anorexia in rats via 5-HT2 receptor antagonism. Gastroenterology 134:2004–2013. doi:10.1053/j.gastro.2008.02.078
102. Fujitsuka N, Asakawa A, Hayashi M et al (2009) Selective serotonin reuptake inhibitors modify physiological gastrointestinal motor activities via 5-HT2c receptor and acyl ghrelin. Biol Psychiatry 65:748–759. doi:10.1016/j.biopsych.2008.10.031
103. Harasawa S, Miyoshi A, Miwa T, Masamune O (1998) Double-blind multicenter post-marketing clinical trial of TJ-43 TSUMURA Rikkunshi-to for the treatment of dysmotility-like dyspepsia. J Clin Exp Med 187:207–229, Japanese
104. Tomono H, Ito Y, Watanabe T (2006) Successful antiemetic treatment of TSUMURA Rikkunshi-to Extract Granules for ethical use in addition to other antiemetic agents in neoadjuvant chemotherapy for an advanced breast cancer patient. Gan To Kagaku Ryoho 33:1129–1131
105. Takeda H, Hattori T, Kase Y (2009) Effects of rikkunshito on anorexia induced by anticancer agents. Ulcer Res 36(2):211–215
106. Grundy D, Al-Chaer ED, Aziz Q et al (2006) Fundamentals of neurogastroenterology: basic science. Gastroenterology

130:1391–1411. doi:10.1053/j.gastro.2005.11.060

107. Gershon M (2007) The serotonin signaling system: from basic understanding to drug development for functional GI disorders. Gastroenterology 132:397–414
108. De Vry J, Schreiber R (2000) Effects of selected serotonin 5-HT1 and 5-HT2 receptor agonists on feeding behavior: possible mechanisms of action. Neurosci Biobehav Rev 24:341–353
109. Takeda H, Muto S, Hattori T et al (2010) Rikkunshito ameliorates the aging-associated decrease in ghrelin receptor reactivity via phosphodiesterase III inhibition. Endocrinology 151:244–252. doi:10.1210/en.2009-0633
110. Kohno D, Nakata M, Maekawa F et al (2007) Leptin suppresses ghrelin-induced activation of neuropeptide y neurons in the arcuate nucleus via phosphatidylinositol 3-kinase- and phosphodiesterase 3-mediated pathway. Endocrinology 148:2251–2263. doi:10.1210/en.2006-1240
111. Niswender K, Morton G, Stearns W, Rhodes C (2001) Intracellular signalling: key enzyme in leptin-induced anorexia. Nature 413:794–795. doi:10.1038/35101657
112. Neary NM, Small CJ, Wren AM et al (2004) Ghrelin increases energy intake in cancer patients with impaired appetite: acute, randomized, placebo-controlled trial. J Clin Endocrinol Metab 89:2832–2836. doi:10.1210/jc.2003-031768
113. Laferrère B, Abraham C, Russell CD, Bowers CY (2005) Growth hormone releasing peptide-2 (GHRP-2), like ghrelin, increases food intake in healthy men. J Clin Endocrinol Metab 90:611–614. doi:10.1210/jc.2004-1719
114. Matsumura T, Arai M, Yonemitsu Y et al (2010) The traditional Japanese medicine Rikkunshito increases the plasma level of ghrelin in humans and mice. J Gastroenterol 45:300–307. doi:10.1007/s00535-009-0166-z
115. Halford J, Harrold J, Boyland E, Lawton C (2007) Serotonergic drugs: effects on appetite expression and use for the treatment of obesity. Drugs 67:27–55
116. Vickers SP, Dourish CT, Kennett GA (2001) Evidence that hypophagia induced by d-fenfluramine and d-norfenfluramine in the rat is mediated by 5-HT2C receptors. Neuropharmacology 41:200–209
117. Vickers SP, Easton N, Webster LJ et al (2003) Oral administration of the 5-HT2Creceptor agonist, mCPP, reduces body weight gain in rats over 28 days as a result of maintained hypophagia. Psychopharmacology (Berl) 167:274–280. doi:10.1007/s00213-002-1378-6
118. Wang W, Danielsson A, Svanberg E, Lundholm K (2003) Lack of effects by tricyclic antidepressant and serotonin inhibitors on anorexia in MCG 101 tumor-bearing mice with eicosanoid-related cachexia. Nutrition 19:47–53
119. Makarenko IG, Meguid MM, Gatto L et al (2005) Hypothalamic 5-HT1B-receptor changes in anorectic tumor bearing rats. Neurosci Lett 376:71–75. doi:10.1016/j.neulet.2004.11.026
120. Makarenko IG, Meguid MM, Gatto L et al (2003) Decreased NPY innervation of the hypothalamic nuclei in rats with cancer anorexia. Brain Res 961:100–108
121. Sakurada S, Shido O, Sugimoto N et al (2000) Autonomic and behavioural thermoregulation in starved rats. J Physiol (Lond) 526:417–424, Pt 2
122. Zhao Z, Sakata I, Okubo Y et al (2008) Gastric leptin, but not estrogen and somatostatin, contributes to the elevation of ghrelin mRNA expression level in fasted rats. J Endocrinol 196:529–538. doi:10.1677/JOE-07-0300
123. Turrin N, Ilyin S, Gayle D (2004) Interleukin-1beta system in anorectic catabolic tumor-bearing rats. Curr Opin Clin Metab Care 7:419–426
124. Gyengesi E, Liu Z-W, D'Agostino G et al (2010) Corticosterone regulates synaptic input organization of POMC and NPY/AgRP neurons in adult mice. Endocrinology 151:5395–5402. doi:10.1210/en.2010-0681
125. Chen C-Y, Fujimiya M, Laviano A et al (2010) Modulation of ingestive behavior and gastrointestinal motility by ghrelin in diabetic animals and humans. J Chin Med Assoc 73:225–229. doi:10.1016/S1726-4901(10)70048-4
126. Shintani F, Kanba S, Nakaki T (1993) Interleukin-1 beta augments release of norepinephrine, dopamine, and serotonin in the rat anterior hypothalamus. J Neurosci 13:3574–3581
127. Chuang J (2010) Ghrelin's roles in stress, mood, and anxiety regulation. Int J Pept 2010:1–5
128. Kamiji MM, Inui A (2007) Neuropeptide y receptor selective ligands in the treatment of obesity. Endocr Rev 28:664–684. doi:10.1210/er.2007-0003

129. Heisler LK, Pronchuk N, Nonogaki K et al (2007) Serotonin activates the hypothalamic-pituitary-adrenal axis via serotonin 2C receptor stimulation. J Neurosci 27:6956–6964. doi:10.1523/JNEUROSCI.2584-06.2007
130. Date Y, Murakami N, Toshinai K et al (2002) The role of the gastric afferent vagal nerve in ghrelin-induced feeding and growth hormone secretion in rats. Gastroenterology 123:1120–1128
131. Fujino K, Inui A, Asakawa A et al (2003) Ghrelin induces fasted motor activity of the gastrointestinal tract in conscious fed rats. J Physiol (Lond) 550:227–240. doi:10.1113/jphysiol.2003.040600
132. Muroya S, Yada T, Shioda S, Takigawa M (1999) Glucose-sensitive neurons in the rat arcuate nucleus contain neuropeptide Y. Neurosci Lett 264:113–116
133. Takaya K, Ariyasu H, Kanamoto N et al (2000) Ghrelin strongly stimulates growth hormone release in humans. J Clin Endocrinol Metab 85:4908–4911
134. Arvat E, Maccario M, Di Vito L et al (2001) Endocrine activities of ghrelin, a natural growth hormone secretagogue (GHS), in humans: comparison and interactions with hexarelin, a nonnatural peptidyl GHS, and GH-releasing hormone. J Clin Endocrinol Metab 86:1169–1174
135. Hataya Y, Akamizu T, Takaya K et al (2001) A low dose of ghrelin stimulates growth hormone (GH) release synergistically with GH-releasing hormone in humans. J Clin Endocrinol Metab 86:4552
136. Akamizu T, Takaya K, Irako T et al (2004) Pharmacokinetics, safety, and endocrine and appetite effects of ghrelin administration in young healthy subjects. Eur J Endocrinol 150:447–455
137. Gibney J, Healy ML, Sonksen PH (2007) The growth hormone/insulin-like growth factor-I axis in exercise and sport. Endocr Rev 28:603–624. doi:10.1210/er.2006-0052
138. Velloso CP (2008) Regulation of muscle mass by growth hormone and IGF-I. Br J Pharmacol 154:557–568. doi:10.1038/bjp.2008.153
139. Gonzalez-Rey E, Chorny A, Delgado M (2006) Therapeutic action of ghrelin in a mouse model of colitis. Gastroenterology 130:1707–1720. doi:10.1053/j.gastro.2006.01.041
140. Waseem T, Duxbury M, Ito H et al (2008) Exogenous ghrelin modulates release of pro-inflammatory and anti-inflammatory cytokines in LPS-stimulated macrophages through distinct signaling pathways. Surgery 143:334–342. doi:10.1016/j.surg.2007.09.039
141. Dixit VD, Schaffer EM, Pyle RS et al (2004) Ghrelin inhibits leptin- and activation-induced proinflammatory cytokine expression by human monocytes and T cells. J Clin Invest 114:57–66. doi:10.1172/JCI21134
142. Wu R, Dong W, Zhou M et al (2007) Ghrelin attenuates sepsis-induced acute lung injury and mortality in rats. Am J Respir Crit Care Med 176:805–813. doi:10.1164/rccm.200604-511OC
143. Theil M-M, Miyake S, Mizuno M et al (2009) Suppression of experimental autoimmune encephalomyelitis by ghrelin. J Immunol 183:2859–2866. doi:10.4049/jimmunol.0803362
144. Akamizu T, Kangawa K (2010) Ghrelin for cachexia. J Cachex Sarcopenia Muscle 1:169–176. doi:10.1007/s13539-010-0011-5
145. Inui A (2002) Cancer anorexia-cachexia syndrome: current issues in research and management. CA Cancer J Clin 52:72–91
146. Huang C, Lin S, Liao P, Young S (2008) The immunopharmaceutical effects and mechanisms of herb medicine. Cell Mol Immunol 5:23–31
147. Eng C (2010) Are herbal medicines ripe for the cancer clinic? Sci Transl Med 2:45ps41

Erratum to: Herbal Medicines: New Horizons

Akio Inui

Akio Inui (ed.), *Herbal Medicines: New Horizons*, Methods in Pharmacology and Toxicology,
DOI 10.1007/978-1-4939-4002-8, © Springer Science+Business Media New York 2016

DOI 10.1007/978-1-4939-4002-8_16

The spelling of the editor name Akio Inui was incorrect throughout the book. The correct editor name is given below:

Akio Inui

The online version of the original book can be found under
http://dx.doi.org/10.1007/978-1-4939-4002-8

Akio Inui (ed.), *Herbal Medicines: New Horizons*, Methods in Pharmacology and Toxicology,
DOI 10.1007/978-1-4939-4002-8_16, © Springer Science+Business Media New York 2016

INDEX

Akio Inui (ed.), *Herbal Medicines: New Horizons*, Methods in Pharmacology and Toxicology, DOI 10.1007/978-1-4939-4002-8, © Springer Science+Business Media New York 2016

V

W

Y

Z

Printed by Printforce, the Netherlands